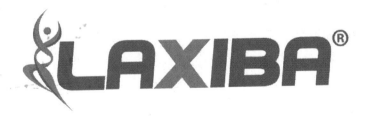

THE IBS NAVIGATOR

The Standard for Irritable Bowel Syndrome

2. Edition, fully revised

The Nutrition Navigator Books Number One

M.SC. J. N. STRATBUCKER

LAXIBA

Houston

ISBN 978-1-941978-28-3
Library of Congress Control Number 2016905916
Cover design by Mahmood Ali
Interior design by Katharina Maas and Mahmood Ali
Layout by Alexandra Krug
E-Mail of the author: John@Laxiba.com

Laxiba GmbH

Rotweinstrasse 12
53506 Rech
Germany

Victoria Botello
2840 Shadowbriar Drive Apt. 314
Houston, Texas, 77077, USA

For companies and institutions:
Are you interested in bulk orders? Visit us at: *https://laxiba.com*

The data set for the algorithmic ordained statements concerning fructose, lactose and sugar-alcohols is from the University of Minnesota Nutrition Coordination Center 2014 Food and Nutrient Database. The reason to acquire the database license for this book were its high quality and scope based on international research. Statements regarding fructans and galactans result from six cited international studies. Nevertheless, the contents of the book bear no guarantee. Neither the author, publisher, any cited scientist nor the University of Minnesota is liable for personal injuries or physical or financial damage. Please note that the quantities of critical ingredients in the mentioned products, which are the foundation for the stated portion sizes, are relative and in part based on derivations. The serving sizes in this book are based on approximations of various details. The precise tolerable portion size of any product varies depending on its processing, country-specific composition, degree of maturity and cultivation.

Manufactured in the United States of America

SECOND EDITION

Acknowledgments

Special thanks to M. Thor and the nutritional research team of the University of Minnesota, J. S. Barrett, J. R. Biesiekierski, P. R. Gibson, K. Liels, J. G. Muir, S. J. Shepherd, R. Rose and O. Rosella as well as the rest of the gastroenterology research team of the Monash University, all other cited scientists for their research, B. Hartmann of the Bundesministerium für Ernährung, Landwirtschaft und Verbraucherschutz, G.-W. von Rymon Lipinski of the Goethe University, and H. Zorn of the Justus Liebig University, for copyediting V. Botello, L. Gomes Domingues, F. Lang, C. R. Mundy, L. Popielinski, and M. Vastolo, for their feedback T. Albert, K. Bayer, U. Blendowske, D. Durchdewald, as well as my friends, especially C. Schlick and I. Kloppenburg, and all other contributors who enabled me to write this book in first place.

To my parents — U. and F. Stratbucker

Contents

Preface

You just lately learned about your irritable bowel or food ingredient sensitivity? Do you not know the trigger of your abdominal discomforts? Alternatively, are you well aware of your disease for many years? In each case, this book will help you, as it makes cooking and eating easy with its portion sizes in standard cooking measures as well as in gram and milliliter: scientifically proven and tested by readers like you. You may have tried out expensive IBS medication or radical regimes like the FODMAP diet. Although the latter really works, it is unnecessarily strict. The aim of this book is to bring you more choice while you avoid your symptoms.

The book's information originates from intensive research and interviews with professors. The food tables in this book show you reliable serving sizes for foods concerning IBS in general and its most likely triggers fructose, fructans and galactans, lactose and sorbitol. Even if you suffer from an intolerance towards several of the mentioned triggers, the design of the tables makes them easy to use. Moreover, they contain several specials. For example, the content of glucose and sorbitol entered the fructose serving size estimations, for results that are more reliable and enable you to eat more of fructose-containing foods by smart combinations. For lactose, you find the additionally tolerated amount per lactase capsule, and you the serving sizes for fructans and galactans, a likely side trigger, on the table right next to it. For sorbitol intolerance, all nine sugar-alcohols entered the portion equations to give you safer results.

You do not have to avoid categorically all foods that contain the trigger. It is enough to avoid eating more of them than you can stomach. By having as much choice as possible while preventing your symptoms, you increase your quality of life. How do you know how much your individual sensitivity allows you to eat? Quite simply, this book will tell you. Curious?

Then read on. In the first Chapter, you will learn about the diagnosis, backgrounds and consequences of the diseases. Then in Chapter 2, you discover how to implement and keep the diet. You will also find a lot of advice there concerning healthy eating in general, recipes, hints of eating-out, strategies to stay motivated to stress management. Afterward, in Chapter 3, you will find the standard portion sizes for more than 1,000 products. Chapter 4 gives you even more advanced techniques to better adapt to your sensitivity and to check alternative triggers. As I deal with an intolerance for a long time, I know about your need for clarity and practical advice.

The focuses of my strategy are quality and suitability for daily use. I wholeheartedly wish you an ongoing success on your way to treat your symptoms and improve your quality of life!

Note:
In case you keep on having symptoms despite following a proper diet, try reducing fructans and galactans, Chapter 2.2.1, and check alternative triggers, see Chapter 4.4.

Despite our aim at the highest quality possible, this book should not be the sole basis for any decision you make. Talk about any diet with your doctor before you begin to limit discomfort. You are responsible for your personal health, including how you choose to interpret data and specialists' advice. I cannot guarantee you a recovery. Several causes for your symptoms are possible—as you will see this book covers most but not all of them.

1

Information

1.1 Why you deserve this book

Congratulations: You take the initiative. By buying this book, you show your will to overcome your discomforts. If you bought this book, you know that a higher well-being is not only good for you but also everyone around you. Turn your back to the symptoms-grumbler. With the proper diet, you will feel healthier and stronger and enjoy more freedom!

Learn all you need to know about your disease, re-evaluate your personal story in that context and learn what you can do to live with it as best as possible. In addition, you find practical advice for a healthier diet in general on page 57 and on page 120 efficient methods to reduce stress, which often worsens your symptoms.

If you bought the book so you could learn to adapt to those in your life suffering from intolerances, you would find out how in Chapter 2.5 and the one following it. Such behavior shows consideration for others that would make anyone glad to be a guest at your table!

That your nutrition affects your happiness is not a secret. It starts with your birth. A full and happy baby makes you happy too. The mother's milk provides the baby with the entire ingredients it needs and tolerates. As an adult, you choose the components of your nutrition yourself. Here it also holds that if you want to be satisfied, you need to eat the food your gut can handle.

Which diagnostic procedure do I have to undergo? Which triggers are possible, which one affects me and how sensitive am I? How much can I eat of foods containing it without hurting myself? Which foods are free of my trigger?

You get the answers for all of the mentioned questions. Explanations of the current scientific results and the most practical food tables for IBS and food intolerances on the market provide you with all you need to take proper action. On top of that, you find the cheat sheets for your wallet that enable you to adapt your diet even when eating out or going to the grocery store. Stop losing valuable energy to abdominal symptoms. Treat them right and start enjoying your life more instead, you deserve it!

1.2 Diagnostic check

Are abdominal pains, bloating, constipation, flatulence or diarrhea your ongoing companion? Without disrespect, we should find a way to get you a better spare time activity. Instead of accepting these discomforts, you should get the appropriate tools to free yourself from them as much as possible in order to spend more of your time enjoying the bright side of life.

The first thing you should do is to find out which of the potential triggers is the one that affects you. Going through all diagnostic procedures can take up half a year but will pay off. You will probably be able to get a handle on your symptoms and by using this book, you will also make sure to avoid unnecessary limitations concerning your diet, as you can stomach small amounts of your relevant trigger(s) without harm.

To determine your profile, you should ask your local doctor to send you to an expert, a so-called gastroenterologist. Just the sound of this word might frighten your troublemakers. The specialist then first checks, whether your symptoms have a different cause than an intolerance. The diagnosis will include a **stool analysis**, an **ultrasonic check** and some camera shots inside your stomach to reject other reasons. These tests will allow the specialist to check whether there is an **abnormal bacterial colonization** of the small intestine. This migration may lead to false positives in uncovering an intolerance towards the **main triggers** covered in this book: **fructose, fructans, galactans, lactose,** and **sorbitol**. The next test looks for **celiac disease**, sensitivity towards gluten, which is an ingredient in grains. In people who have an untreated celiac disease, the tolerance test for the cube sorbitol is often positive, even if they can stomach it if they avoid gluten-containing foods. What you can do in case you suffer from celiac disease, you will learn in Chapter 1.7.1. Following this, you should take a genetic test regarding **hereditary fructose** intolerance. Hereditary fructose intolerance is rare, but it is serious: the fructose test itself can be lethal to those with this disease. If you are affected, you have to abstain from fructose. Use the big smileys in the fructose tables to find fructose free foods.

You ruled out other potential causes, and the brats are probably trembling. Great, as now they are in for: what follows are checks regarding three of the mentioned main triggers. For the so-called breath test, you will take a high dose containing fructose, lactose or sorbitol on different days. If one of these passes through to your large intestine, due to suboptimal absorption by your body, gasses emerge. The doctors measure them to find out if you have an intolerance. When the amount of gas reaches a certain level, the diagnosis is an intolerance toward the respective trigger and have to adapt your diet accordingly. The threshold for a positive diagnosis for a fructose dilution (typically containing 25–50g) is usually 20ppm (parts per million, a concentration measure). This threshold also applies for lactose and sorbitol. The recommended breath test, however, is not available everywhere. In Chapter 2.2.1 you will learn about a substitute test, in case you have no access to the breath test.

Has the breath or substitute test shown that your body has enough capacity to handle even extreme amounts of a trigger? If so, you do not need to take any further attention to that trigger; its consumption will not cause you any harm. Ignore the tables in Chapter three for people that have an intolerance towards a trigger you tolerate. Ignoring triggers you have no intolerance holds for all of them—fructose, fructans and galactans, lactose and sorbitol: there is no point in taking unnecessary diets. If however the test shows that you have for example an intolerance towards lactose, you know which of the triggers you have to render harmless by limiting your consumption of foods in which it is present.

In general, do not accept a diagnosis without a test. If none of the tests comes to a conclusive result, your irritable bowel syndrome is at least—for now—undefined. Irritable bowel just means that your gut reacts sensitively to various types of irritations such as gasses inside it—more on that in Chapter 1.5. The bowel is the final segment of your alimentary canal and the section where your symptoms come to show. Irritable bowel symptoms can be defined—if you have one of the before mentioned intolerances or undefined. If it is undefined, either, you did not take a test or it showed that you do not have an intolerance to one of the mentioned triggers. Note here that no breath-test is available for fructans and galactans as of now, and you will need to test your tolerance yourself, see Chapter 2.2.1. In both cases, the symptoms are similar, because readily fermentable carbohydrates, a group that all triggers belong to, of some sort trigger the symptoms. Incidentally, for up to 90% of patients with an irritable bowel, an intolerance to one or more of the three breath-test-triggers mentioned above causes the symptoms. The remainder of patients will find help as well. One possibility are the fructans and galactans, see Chapter 1.3.3 and 1.3.4, another one alternative triggers mentioned in Chapter 4.4 and a **histamine intolerance**. In the case of the latter, you lack the ability to handle the ingredient histamine. The primary treatment is that of the other triggers as well—by reducing your consumption of histamine-containing foods, you can get a handle on your symptoms. To determine, whether you have a histamine intolerance, proceed according to the third step on page 482 and use the table on *http://www.mastzellaktivierung.info/en/downloads.html#foodlist*. For cooking and purchases, you can also find help in the cheat sheet on page 96.

If you suffer from irritable bowel symptoms, you are not alone: 20% of Americans have an intolerance, i.e., their enzyme worker team is too small for one or more of the three triggers that one tests with a breath test. Worldwide, 10–15% of all people suffer from undefined abdominal discomfort. About 20–30% of Europeans in general, 9% of the Dutch, 22% of the English, 25% of the Japanese and 44% of West Africans are affected. Concerning children, they should only take a diet under medical supervision. By the way, a lactose intolerance can only evolve at an age above five years. All younger children can stomach lactose.

It is also possible that a doctor finds that you are intolerant according to a breath test, but you do not feel symptoms. In such a case you may still want to keep the respective diet if you suffer from depressive moods, see Chapter 1.4.

 ## Summary

If you regularly suffer from abdominal discomfort, visit a specialist, a gastroenterologist. Checks can take up to half a year. Many others share your fate; about 20% of Americans are affected. You are holding in your hands the key to fighting the symptoms!

1.3   Presentation of the triggers

We depict the triggers of an ingredient intolerance as cubes. Why? Just imagine having a big cube in your stomach. Not a good feeling. On the other hand, a cube can have a positive effect, too. Think of a sugar cube that provides a lot of energy. Likewise, the triggers, being sugar related carbohydrates, do provide you with energy, if your stomach makes use for them in that way.

1.3.1   How symptoms emerge

If you have an intolerance against fructose, fructans, galactans, lactose or sorbitol, your body only provides a few enzymes, which you can think of as workers making sure your body uses the cubes for energy, for one or many of the before mentioned triggers. Few workers mean that if you eat too much of foods that contain your trigger cubes, many remain unused by your body and arrive at your large intestine. Now, two processes are responsible for the symptoms: osmosis and fermentation. To understand osmosis, let us imagine two equal fish bowls connected by an underwater tube.

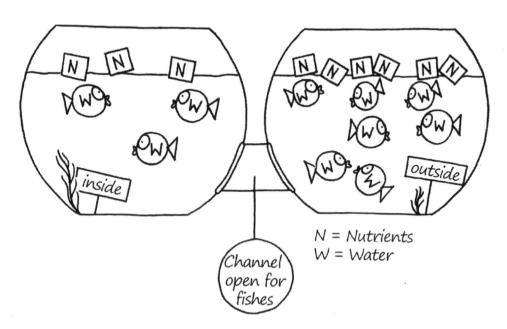

N = Nutrients
W = Water

The glass on the left represents the inside of the bowel and the one on the right for the outside of it. The fishes represent water (W), and their food are either nutrient (N) or trigger cubes that arrive at the inside of the bowel—fructose (F), fructans and galactans (F+G), lactose (L) or sorbitol (S). The channel enables fishes to switch between the bowls. Thus, they always swim to the glass that contains more food. Usually, this would be the outside of the intestine. Thereby, the body detracts the water from the foods—which is a good thing.

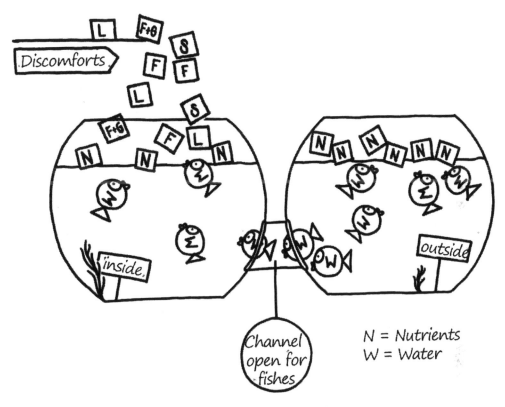

However, if you eat more of foods containing your trigger than your enzyme workers can handle, trigger cubes arrive at the inside of the bowel. Hence, suddenly there is more food in the left fish bowl.

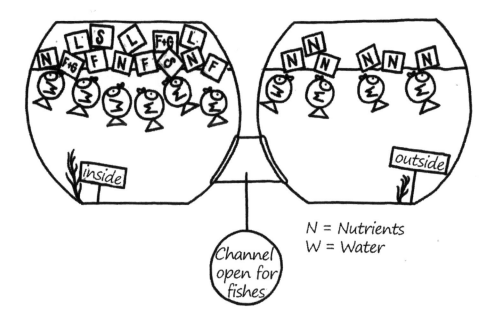

N = Nutrients
W = Water

As the intestinal wall, here represented by the channel, is only partially permeable, the fishes can swim through it, unlike the food. Therefore, some fishes now switch sides and scrimmage on the left. Their movement to the left means that with the cubes, water arrives inside the intestine and you suffer from diarrhea.

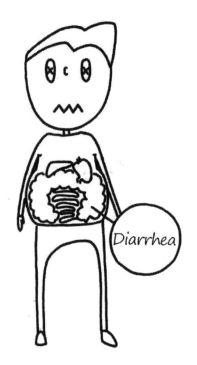

Now you know about osmosis. What causes fermentation?

As you know, you have bacteria inside your bowel, which is normal and that way for any healthy person. The issue is that these bacteria love sweets. Hence, if a trigger cube arrives at the large intestine, they do not falter and immediately consume it to help themselves to some energy.

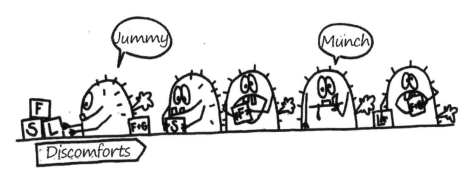

Unfortunately, though, the bacteria are less efficient at consuming the cubes than our body is. When bacteria use the trigger cubes, gas emerges.

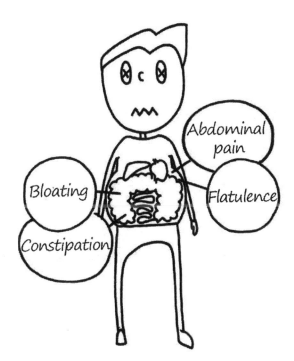

The gas either leaves as bloating or amounts and causes an uncomfortable flatulence. If the pressure increases in some regions of the intestines, this can cause deposits—constipation. If the gas enters the small intestine, it causes, even more, turmoil: it hinders some of the enzymes—the body's cube workers—from doing their job. That is because the enzymes are mainly sitting on the gut wall and the gas reduces the gut wall's contact to the stool.

By the way, linseed can have an alleviating effect on bloating and constipation, see page 57. However, what about the treatment with a diet? In general, it is important for your health to have a diverse diet. The FODMAP approach, which you may have heard of, aims at reducing the fermentation and osmosis by lowering the consumption of all triggers at once. With the IBS standard treatment of this book, you take a more precise aim to give you more freedom concerning your food choice. With it, you only avoid those triggers that are an issue for you, as described in the diagnosis check. First, you should get to know each of your potential triggers.

1.3.2   Lactose or milk sugar

Another name for lactose is milk sugar as it is present primarily in milk and dairy products. Unfortunately, milk sugar is also included in many convenience foods, where you would not expect it to be. Bologna, coating, sauce and even medicine may contain it. Pure milk tends to have the highest share while some dry cheese, like cheddar, is nearly free of it. Luckily, you are still able to stomach a limited amount of lactose despite having a lactose intolerance and there are enzyme capsules to help you increase that amount further. Moreover, nowadays, there are a lot of lactose freed or milk replacement products such as rice milk or soymilk. Be careful though with soymilk. It contains the triggers fructans and galactans and may lead you out of the frying pan into the fire. Rice milk, on the contrary, is also free of that and thus the better alternative.

At the start of your life, lactose is irreplaceable: All small children are dependent on lactose and can tolerate it. At the end of the fifth year, the earliest a lactose intolerance can evolve. About 5 to 17 % of the light-skinned and 50 to 100 % of the rest of the population are affected. Still, not all of them suffer from symptoms at the same level. Most patients tolerate small amounts of lactose and not all of them suffer from a sensitive bowel. Nevertheless, why do some humans react to lactose with symptoms and other do not? How do the symptoms evolve? The following illustrations will show it to you.

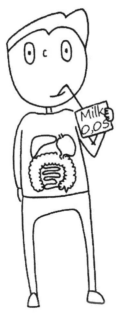

Man <u>with</u> lactose intolerance

Milk contains lactose by nature: 100 mL contain round about 5g of it. In the image, you can see John. Due to his lactose intolerance, he only has a few sips of milk, about 50 mL in total. He knows that he only has a few enzymes to degrade lactose in the small intestine.

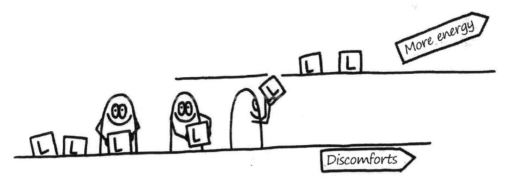

His enzymes, workers, are fine with handling the amount of lactose contained in the 50 mL—in case that is it for this meal. When our body assimilates the lactose (L) by the work of the enzymes, it provides us with energy. The symptoms stay away and everything goes swimmingly.

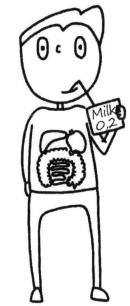

Man with Lactose intolerance

However, now John forgets that his team of lactose enzymes is easy to count. He now drinks a whole pack of milk containing 200 mL and has them work up a sweat.

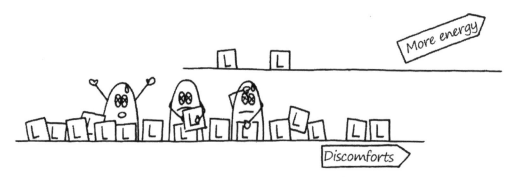

His enzymes cannot handle the load. The sudden flow of lactose is too much for them, and therefore, a lot of it remains on the "conveyor belt". This unprocessed lactose then reaches the large intestine and there it triggers symptoms.

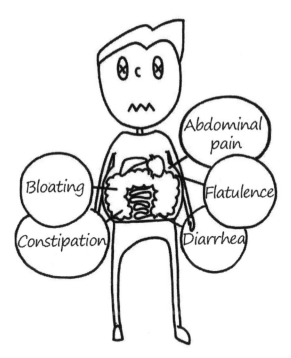

Some hours after the consumption he gets the bill: abdominal pain, bloating, diarrhea and flatulence.

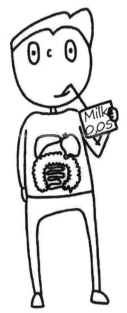

Man <u>without</u> lactose intolerance

Chris, who is also drinking 200 mL, is luckier.

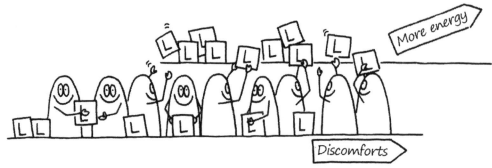

Chris does not have a lactose intolerance and thus has a far bigger team from the start. His many lactose-enzyme labor men work hand in hand are handling the amount quickly and can only smile about their groaning comrades.

The influence of fructans and galactans

In a study, scientists were surprised to find that people suffering from a lactose intolerance were reacting with symptoms to a lactose-free test milk. The reason for this, which I implied is that although the lactose-free milk did not contain lactose, it did still contain other readily fermented (potentially symptom-triggering) carbohydrates, galactans. How much of the latter is contained in milk, depends on the race, month and the lactation period of the animals. The highest average amount is contained in cow milk with 0.137g/100 mL, followed by goat milk with 0.117g/100 mL. Per gram lactose, you can thus add 0.03g to galactans. It thus takes longer to reach the threshold of your sensitivity. However, in combination with other foods like cereals, they can be just the amount that takes it from tolerated to symptoms. That may also be the explanation for the continuing symptoms of some, who consciously avoid lactose, still do not manage to get rid of their discomforts to a satisfying degree.

For some, the intestine reacts even more sensitive to fructans and galactans than towards lactose. Are you one of these unlucky fellows—are you unsatisfied with the symptom reduction by the lactose diet? If so, I recommend you read Chapters 1.3.3 and 1.3.4, where I present both more precisely, as well as take the alternative sensitivity test on page 482.

Your personal sensitivity

If you find that you would rather like to avoid osmosis and fermentation in this context, then batten down the hatches! Make sure that no lactose arrives at your large intestine. Reduce your lactose consumption to the amount that your enzymes can handle. The level that you should not top, in order not to have your enzymes lose the game is usually 10g of lactose per day, which equals about 3.3 gram per meal. With the standard amounts in the nutrition tables at the end of this book, you eat up to 3g of lactose per meal. Here you see how much you can eat of what. By the way, the amount of lactose that medicine contains, which you take in orally, is usually so small that you should be able to tolerate it if you avoid the consumption of other lactose-containing foods during the treatment.

Calcium

If you limit your consumption of milk products, it is important that you take in calcium in alternative ways, as your body needs it. Adults below 50 should take about 1,000mg per day (teenagers even 1,300mg) and women above 50 as well as men above 60, 1,200mg. You can take in calcium via some lactose free milk or milk replacement products, protein powders (1,200mg per 100g), Cheddar cheese, (721mg per 100g), almonds (236mg per 100g), anchovy and salmon (240mg per 100g), spinach in all variants (210mg per 100g) and figs (162g per 100g) or calcium pills. In case you use supplements, try to find some that are lactose-free.

Lactase enzyme capsules

As you can expect to be able to stomach 3g of lactose per meal, it only makes sense to take a capsule if you exceed this amount. For the lactose enzymes you take to have an effect, they have to arrive at the small intestine, where they go to work. There is no use in taking them if the enzymes reach the stomach un-protected. The gastric acid there would only destroy them. Gastric acid resistant capsules are suited best for bringing the enzymes safely to their workplace. By the way, they ought to arrive at the same time that lactose does for an optimal effect. A study showed that the most effective capsule, containing 12,000 FCC[1], was only able to neutralize 2.7g of lactose. Thus, to cover a 237 mL, after sub-tracting the 3g per meal, you still need at least four capsules.

If you are nostalgically thinking of your math class, which you spent freshly in love or crapulous rather below than on you chair and already, have the: "If only I had paid more attention" on your mind: No worries! You do not have to be a master in mental arithmetic to apply this knowledge. You not only find the tolerated amounts but also the additionally tolerated amount per capsules esti-mated for you in the nutrition tables of this book.

---

[1] *Food Chemical Codex, measurement unit for the amount of enzymes.*

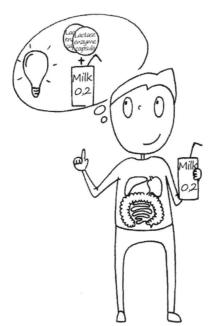

Man <u>with</u> lactose intolerance

John has just gotten smarter. Once more, he wants to drink a whole 200 mL box of milk. As he knows that this amount will cause him an abdominal pain without preparations, he takes four high-dose lactase capsules (12,000 FCC) in advance.

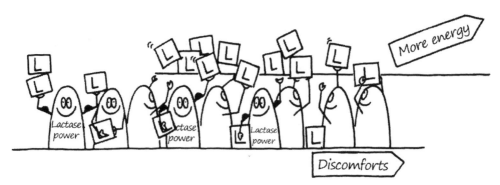

His enzymes thus receive dynamic support and can tackle the incoming amount of lactose. Thereby, John is free from symptoms.

Lactose-free milk (replacement) products

Many lactose freed dairy products as well as milk replacement products, such as soy or rice milk are available in stores. These offer you the opportunity to look at the tables in this book, as you will find many products, such as cheese, of which you can consume quite a lot.

Hint: in case you have a fructans and galactans sensitivity, you should prefer rice to soymilk products, as it is free of it.

1.3.3   Fructans

The name fructans results from the fact that fructose emerges from the degradation of this trigger cube. If bacteria tackle the (short-chained fructans), as you know, gas appears. Although our body absorbs some of them, about 89% just run through our system, giving bacteria a chance to have a free shot. What is more, you stomach other triggers, such as fructose, the worse, the more of fructans you consume. Therefore, if you consume them, your intestine may be more sensitive to other triggers. Some people with a lactose intolerance have even more severe symptoms from fructans than from lactose itself. People without an irritable bowel, on the other hand, have no problem with them.

Thus, in case you have an intolerance and your symptoms stay although you adapt your nutrition accordingly, you should consider fructans as a possible cause. To test this, take the substitute test, see the page 66.

We primarily consume fructans when eating the following (tolerable amounts for the standard sensitivity in parenthesis): garlic (one clove), onions (15g), artichoke (17g), cereals (21–45g) and noodles (147g), as well as pastries like bread, cake, cookies and pizza. There is no relation between fructans and gluten. Even gluten-free bread often contains fructans, albeit about one-third less than ordinary bread. Rice bread is free from fructans as the dough is commonly made without wheat, unlike that for potato or cornbread. In addition, spelt bread is especially well tolerated (250g) compared to rye or wheat bread (one slice each). Some fruits contain fructans as well. Limit yourself, for example, to three-fourths of banana, half a nectarine and two slices of pineapple. The high amount of fructans contained in chicory or Jerusalem and regular artichokes, calls for their avoidance.

Even though the fructans and galactans are often the triggers of ongoing symptoms, we should not demonize them: In amounts you tolerate, fructans have positive effects, so they are added to various foods as inulin. For example, some beverages, brands of butter, candies, cereals, chocolates, ice creams and yogurts contain inulin. The added amounts of inulin are not always certain, aside from the derivations mentioned in the food table of this book. To be on the safe side, you can avoid products that list inulin in their ingredients—ideally, you make a separate test for it according to Chapter 4.4. Another way is to use similar products in the food table of this book as a reference for the consumable amount according to your fructan level. Some people are also allergic to inulin, which has worse effects than a mere sensitivity.

Keeping the limit for fructans only requires little adaptation to your diet. The tables make it easy. Just consider that when you combine fructan-containing foods, the respective single portion sizes decrease. To combine a fructan-containing product with another product that contains fructans or galactans you can, for example, bisect both portion sizes.

Influence on the nutrient supply

A reduction in fructans can require you to plan your intake of proteins, short-chain fatty acids, and fiber as you often lower their consumption with your fructans and galactans diet as well. You can find compensation strategies from Chapter 2.1.4 onward.

1.3.4   Galactans

Our body poorly absorbs short-chain galactans, just as short-chain fructans and they also arrive at the intestine in large chunks. They have another commonality with fructans, and that is their structure. For this reason, both share a tolerance threshold and hence a column in the tables.

Now, you will learn where the saying "every bean has its tone", originates from beans containing much galactans. The absolute safe amount you tolerate in the case of a sensitivity equals one tablespoon of beans. Other foods include them, too. How much you can tolerate of these you find in parenthesis: peas (1 tbsp., 15g), chickpeas (9 tbsp., 135g) and soybeans (3 tbsp., 45g). Vegetarians should pay particular attention to these. Other foods containing considerable amounts are oats (5 tbsp., 75g), lentils (5 tbsp., 75g) and wheat or rye bread (one slice, 42g). Moreover, short-chain galactans are also contained in milk. Agar and carrageenan also contain galactans, but those are more complex and only partially broken down by gut bacteria if at all. At times, people suffering from an irritable bowel are suspicious toward these. Due to a lack of substantial evidence, I ignore them. Still, if you have doubts about them, you can explore their impact yourself by adopting an alternative diet, see Chapter 4.4.

Should you buy prebiotics?

The European Food Safety Authority (*EFSA*) has repeatedly disregarded the claim that prebiotics and probiotics have a positive effect on the gut due to lack of solid proof. It regards them as at best potentially helpful. **Prebiotics** producers assert that artificial galactans contribute to an improved gut flora. A study set up by in collaboration of an employee of a prebiotics producer suggested that 3.5g of a particular kind of artificial galactans improved gut flora and thereby led to an average **improvement** of **37%** regarding symptoms like abdominal pain, bloating, constipation, diarrhea and flatulence. Health claims also concern short-chain fatty acids emerging during the breakdown of galactans by bacteria. Some artificial galactans seem to produce less gas when they bacteria break them down than those that occur naturally. However, as stated before, the EFSA refuses to support prebiotics beyond their statement regarding their potential. Over 80% of participants in a study, who followed this book's **diet** and limited their consumption of fructose and fructans according to the standard sensitivity amounts of our tables experienced **relief** from their symptoms by **about 70%**. Moreover, reducing the number of trigger cubes that arrive at the colon might a have a favorable effect on mood, see page 32. These findings support the recommendation to use the diet to treat the symptoms.

Enzyme capsules

There are special enzyme pills available that may help you to avoid symptoms that by galactans though their effectiveness is in dispute. They contain the enzyme alpha-galactosidase and for their production, the mildew *"aspergillus niger"* is used, though packages may not adequately reflect this information. In addition, they contain the cube mannitol, a sugar alcohol, prevalent in mushrooms, to which some people exhibit allergies. You should be careful with these enzyme capsules if you have a fructose intolerance, as the metabolization of galactans by the enzymes creates fructose. Unless your enzyme workers immediately handle the fructose, it arrives at the intestine. There, gas-producing bacteria rejoice, since you have done some of their work for them. Hence, you gained nothing. These enzyme capsules can only be helpful if you tolerate fructose and sorbitol and do not have an allergy to *aspergillus niger*.

1.3.5 Fructose or fruit sugar

Fruit naturally contains fructose, and that is why another name for it is fruit sugar. Some fruits, like Rhubarb, are free from it, though. Nowadays, fructose is the cause of the sweet taste of many foods. It enters the ingredients as honey, gelling sugars, and corn syrup. In the absence of an intolerance, humans can smoothly break down fructose. Luckily, even in case you do have a fructose intolerance you can consume some of it and to your benefit, foods that contain glucose and enhance your tolerance as shown below.

The way you mainly take in fructose depends on your nutritional habits. In the USA, about two-thirds are taken in as soft drinks, enriched convenience foods, and about one-third as fruit. In Finland, the relations are the other way around. For 39% of those affected by unexplained regular abdominal discomfort, symptoms arise after the consumption of 15g fructose; for 70%, they appear after a dose of 30g. People around the globe consume between 11 and 54g per day, or 4–18g per meal. The following illustrations show you, what happens in the case of a fructose intolerance.

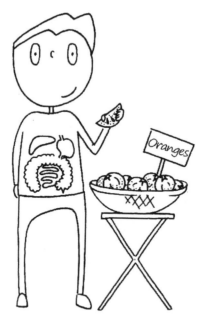

Man __with__ fructose intolerance

Oranges naturally contain fructose: on top of everything, John also has a fructose intolerance and therefore only has a piece of it at breakfast. He knows that he only has a few conveyor belt worker that make sure his body assimilates fructose.

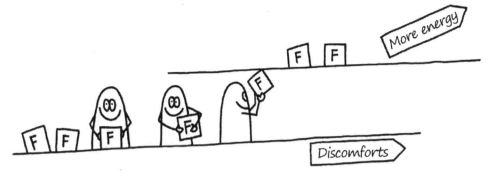

With the amount contained in one piece, his workers can cope—as long as he avoids eating any more products that contain fructose. Thus, his body assimilates the fructose he ate (F), turns it into energy and abdominal discomforts are absent.

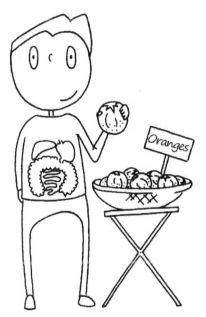

Man with fructose intolerance

However, now John forgets that his team is quite an observable one and eats a whole orange at once. Thus, he makes it sweat a lot.

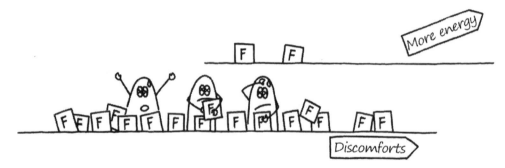

His workers are unable to cope with the sudden fructose load and leave most of it on the belt. This redundant fructose arrives at the large intestine, and there it triggers symptoms.

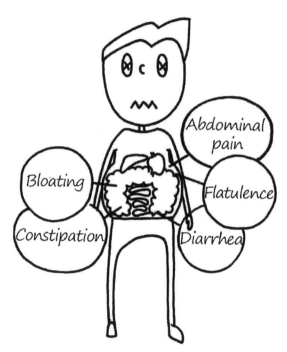

A few hours after the consumptionthe well known ingredient-intolerance symptoms can occur: abdominal pain, bloating, diarrhea and flatulence.

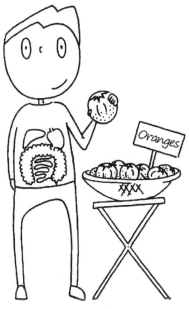

Man _without_ fructose intolerance

When Chris, who also does not have a fructose intolerance, eats a whole orange, it is a different ball game once more.

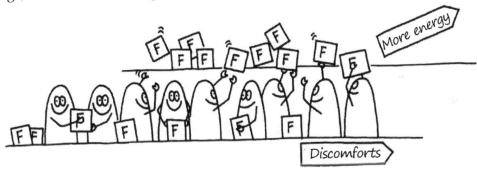

As he has many more fructose employees on the conveyor belt, these handle the load with ease.

Hereditary fructose intolerance

If you suffer from the rare and unfortunately not yet curable hereditary fructose intolerance, consuming fructose can be lethal. Please seek your doctor's advice. You can use the food table in this book to determine foods that are free of fructose. Only eat those with a big smile in the fructose column.

Folic acid deficiency

A folic acid deficiency increases the risk of cardiovascular disease. A fructose intolerance often negatively affects folic acid absorption. Hence, it would be sensible to take suitable supplements. Otherwise, folic acid is contained in Kellogg's® Corn Flakes (323µg/100g), some protein powders (280µg/100g) and short-grain rice (225µg/100g), for example. The recommended daily dose is 300µg for men, 250µg for most women and 400µg for expectant mothers.

Depression

Please see page 32.

Influence of glucose

Glucose does the job for the fructose workers. As soon as glucose meets fructose in effect, they act as if they combined to form table sugar. As you can tolerate much more table sugar than fructose, you can benefit from this effect. To do that, you have to mix food that contains fructose with food containing an equal amount of glucose either in advance or in your mouth.

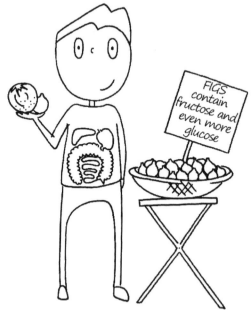

Man with fructose intolerance

As John still loves eating oranges, he now eats it together with a fig, which contains a lot of glucose.

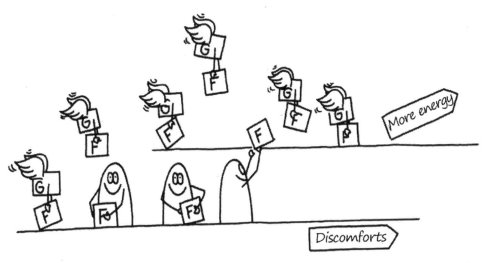

The glucose does it jobs and John's body quickly assimilates the glucose-fructose couple to energy. Despite the fructose load of a whole orange, his team now has a walkover.

Foods that have an abundance of glucose

The following foods are free of other triggers like lactose, sorbitol, and contain a lot of glucose. When consumed with food that is limited by fructose, you can increase the limit by the factors in the following table. If you are interested, just test it out for yourself. You find your multiplier in one of the last four columns of the next table.

Foods	Portion weight	Amount multiplier per portion
Avocado (Florida)	37.5 g	2.25
Fresh figs	50 g	2.0
Maple syrup	30 g	1.5
Mozzarella	28g	1.25
Sweet corn	82g	3.25
Thin slice of pineapple	56.3g	2.25

You can also purchase pure glucose as a powder online though you should avoid a high sugar consumption due to potential health implications (see Chapter 2.1.4).

Influence of sorbitol

Sorbitol and fructose mostly share the same workers. However, if you consume foods that contain sorbitol together with some that contain fructose, the workers always handle sorbitol first. As fewer workers are thus handling the fructose, more remains on the discomforts belt—ends up in the large intestine. For that reason, I accounted for the sorbitol content when estimating the fructose portion sizes you find in the food tables in Chapter 3. The following illustration shows you the interaction of fructose and sorbitol:

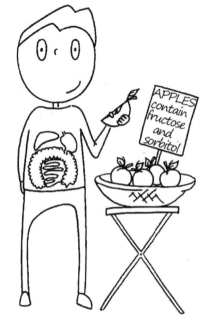

Man <u>with</u> fructose intolerance

Now John eats a piece of apple despite his fructose intolerance…

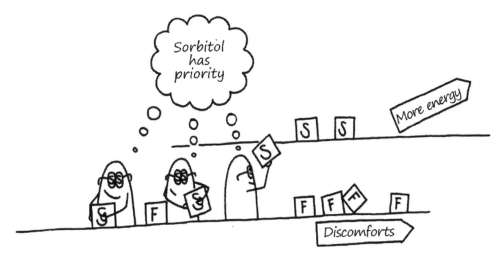

... as an apple contains sorbitol in addition to fructose, and the workers love to handle it most, fructose is left on the belt, and John has symptoms despite eating only a piece.

The impact of sorbitol

Those that do not have a fructose intolerance have enough workers to cope with both fructose and sorbitol. At the utmost, the sorbitol that you consume at a meal can hinder the absorption of the equal amount of fructose by your body. An apple contains 0.56g of sorbitol at most and about 4g of fructose. Thereby the sorbitol contained in an apple can block the handling of 0.56g of fructose at most. Thereby, sorbitol is only an issue for you, as long as you solely suffer from a fructose intolerance, if you consume it together with fructose. If you would add the respective amount of glucose to a glass of apple juice, you could even spare yourself of fructose symptoms entirely as the glucose acts as if it connects to the fructose to form table sugar and sorbitol does not affect this. Therefore, in the case of a sole fructose intolerance, sorbitol is a mere symptoms promoter. In the fructose tables in Chapter 3, the amount of sorbitol that blocks fructose entered the tolerable serving size algorithm according to the example above.

Foods that contain sorbitol

Various fruits and vegetables contain sorbitol. In extreme amounts, you can find it in many products that are sugar-free or for diabetics. Often sorbitol only shows up as the numeric code 420. You should adjust to it in case you are fructose or sorbitol intolerant. Important: If you only have a fructose but not a sorbitol intolerance, it is enough if you eat according to the fructose portions in Chapter 3 as sorbitol has already been accounted for here.

Your personal sensitivity

The amount of fructose that you should limit yourself to per meal is different from person to person. For that reason, you can try whether you can, for example, stomach twice the amount in this book's tables. The standard amount you can tolerate in the case of fructose intolerance is 0.5g of fructose that is unmatched by glucose.

Enzyme capsules

Xylose isomerase is available on the market. The author is aware of only one study that aimed to prove its efficiency, and it showed symptoms improving by about 41%. Whether this justifies the current high sales price, remains for you to decide.

1.3.6   Sorbitol or sugar-alcohols

Sorbitol is one of nine sugar-alcohols that causes symptoms in case of a sorbitol intolerance. As sorbitol is the most popular of the group, though, the label sorbitol intolerance has enforced itself. To make the text more readable, sorbitol refers to all nine sugar-alcohols in this book. Some fruits and vegetables naturally contain sorbitol. Furthermore, sugar-alcohols are sweeteners and carriers for some medicines. Diabetic products like jelly contain up to 12g per portion and chocolate up to 40g per four pieces. Moreover, sorbitol is sometimes included in ice cream, juices, oral hygiene products, sauces, sugar-free chewing gum (up to 2.5 g/piece) and sugar-free mints (up to 2g/piece). As you can see, using diabetic products you can easily top 20g of sorbitol per meal. In one study with 39 healthy participants, 84% of them had symptoms of a sorbitol intolerance after consuming a 20g dose. Consumption of these products thus deserves caution.

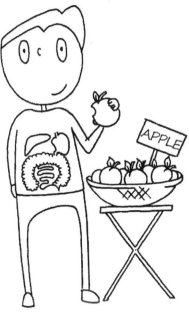

Man <u>with</u> sorbitol intolerance

Apples contain sorbitol by nature. On the picture, you see Tim, who does not know about his sorbitol intolerance. Due to it, he only has a limited amount of workers ensuring that the body makes use of the energy the sugar provides in his small intestine. By eating a whole apple, he puts them under a lot of pressure.

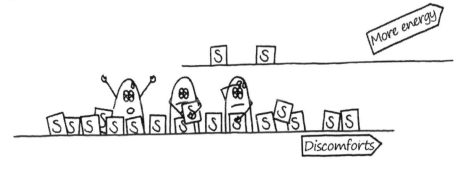

The load overstrains his workers. They are unable to handle the sudden amount of sorbitol and only put a fraction of them on the energy conveyor belt. The remainder arrives at the large intestine and thus causes symptoms.

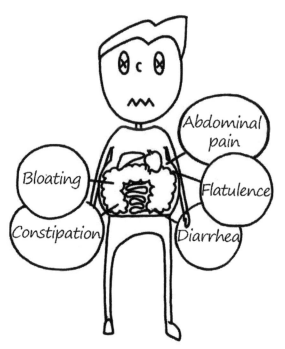

You know the score. A few hours afterward the known assignation occurs— abdominal pain, bloating, diarrhea and flatulence.

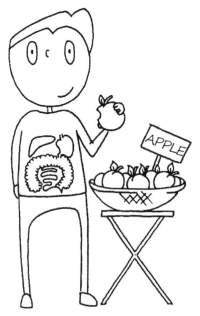

Man _without_ sorbitol intolerance

Lucky Chris is spared from a sorbitol intolerance, too. If he eats an apple…

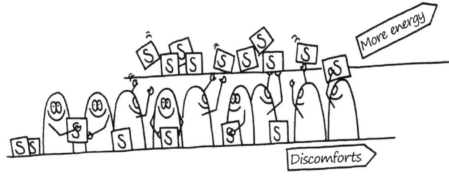

…his workers, can handle the sorbitol load with ease.

Your individual sensitivity

The task is to limit your consumption of sorbitol-containing foods to the amount that your workers can cope with. The standard amount you find in the table is set to avoid sorbitol altogether. If you can tolerate some of it, though, you find the lower sensitivity level one amounts next to it.

Reasons for the standard avoidance of sorbitol in case of an intolerance:

1. The breath test for sorbitol shows an intolerance present at 5g in **58%** of those experiencing abdominal discomfort due to an irritable bowel and **53%** of healthy participants (based on a combination of studies with 564 participants).

2. If you have a fructose intolerance, sorbitol will aggravate your symptoms. Sorbitol hinders the absorption of already-present fructose because fructose and sorbitol share a transportation mechanism where sorbitol is preferred.

3. Sugar-alcohols are causing symptoms to many and can sometimes even lead to a water aggregation in the small intestine, reducing the intestine's ability to metabolize nutrients. On average, 25–40% of consumed sugar-alcohols arrive at the colon. Even small amounts of sorbitol can trigger discomforts.

Hence, it makes sense to test whether you can tolerate more than the standard amounts in the tables in Chapter 3, as you want to be able to consume foods as deliberately as possible.

1.4　Consequences of an intolerance

Physical effects

You are already familiar with the immediate effects of an untreated intolerance: abdominal pain, bloating, diarrhea and flatulence. These alone are certainly enough to have you take action. However, indirectly they can also lead to lower lust, reduced social contacts, lower empathy and less vitality in general. Hence, not handling your intolerance lowers your quality of life. It is not so surprising that this also affects your days off work. A study, done in the USA and the Netherlands, shows that on average people with an untreated intolerance take about twice as many sick leaves from school or work than do their peers. Luckily, you can do something about that. You can recapture your well-being by learning how to adapt your diet to your capacity to absorb your trigger. Ideally, you only limit your nutrition as far as is necessary—a certain amount of fructose, fructans, and galactans, as well as lactose, is usually even tolerable if you are intolerant towards one of these triggers. My aim is to make this as easy as possible for you.

Depression

Note: The main studies underlying the following text included patients suffering from fructose and lactose intolerance only. Whether it also applies to fructans and galactans as well as sorbitol will be the topic of future examinations.

Scientists have found that there is a causal relation between having an untreated intolerance and increased depression scores. The reason for this is a reduced prevalence of a neurotransmitter, serotonin, in case the triggers arrive at the large intestine. Serotonin elevates one's mood. The body produces it from tryptophan, which it derives from food. Presumably, at least, some of the triggers that pass the small intestine—remain on the belt—merge with tryptophan to form a non-absorbable substance. This reaction reduces the amount of available tryptophan and causes the body to produce less serotonin. Hence, the triggers that arrive at the large intestine hinder the body's ability to let positive feelings emerge. In an experiment in which patients lowered their fructose and sorbitol consumption, depression scores normalized for most participants. Keeping the consumption limits that apply to you when choosing your portion sizes can improve your mood (your serotonin metabolism) because fewer triggers arrive at the large intestine. Extra discipline is required to maintain the portion thresholds in cases of depression, however, as a lack of high spirits (tryptophan) can foster the hunger for sweets. Now, candies often contain triggers. If an intolerance is present, the intake sweets containing the respective trigger(s) further lowers one's mood, creating a vicious circle. You can find out how much you can eat for many foods in the lists in Chapter 3. Even if you are not depressed, please remember that in the presence of a dysfunctional metabolism, depression can result from consuming too much of foods that contain problematic ingredients. Affected people should always seek help rather than trying to counter these effects through sheer willpower and bear in mind that they can and should do something about ongoing feelings of sadness, little personal power, and low energy.

Summary

Fructose, fructans, galactans, lactose and sorbitol are carbohydrates that bacteria ferment if they reach the large intestine. In that case, they cause various abdominal symptoms. Many foods contain these potential triggers. The best approach is to determine the ones that are relevant for you—for which one(s) you have too few enzyme workers making sure your body uses them to gain energy before they can reach the large intestine. Once you have determined your trigger(s), you treat your symptoms by adjusting your consumption of these to the capacity of your enzyme workers. To do so, you eat according to the tables showing you the tolerated amount per meal in the third Chapter of this book. This profile-adjusted approach is also the main difference to the FODMAP diet, where one lowers the consumption of all potential triggers. My method is better as a higher quality of life is also associated with more freedom concerning your choice of foods.

1.5   Background of an irritable bowel

Suffering from irritable bowel syndrome symptoms means having a sensitive colon. Like a notorious diva, the intestine shows a lack of robustness and an oversensitivity. It will not allow tampering with, reacts disappointed and offended when ignored by someone that offers her unfitting food. In the case of stress, she pipes up even more vehemently. Many people are carrying such a diva around with them, which repeatedly makes her demands known.

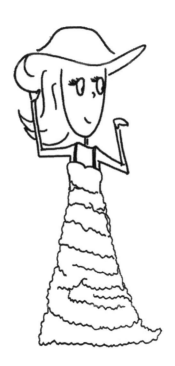

By the way, the exact causes of the diva's show up are unknown. In some cases, infections and emotions play a role. It seems like fortune decided who has an irritable bowel and who does not. In any case, it has nothing to do with the character. Having a diva-tummy not at all means having a diva-like congeniality.

1.6 Abdominal discomfort in kids

In general, abdominal discomforts of your child can have a variety of reasons. A lactose intolerance will not occur before the age of five. Other potential triggers of abdominal pain, bloating and diarrhea in children are fructose and sorbitol: Children ages 14 to 58 months drank 250 mL of apple juice in a study. Afterward, all children who suffered from chronic diarrhea, as well as 65.5% of the healthy children, tested positive for malabsorption-symptoms. Avoiding apple juice led to recovery for **all** of the children. This result corresponds with other research that shows that many children suffer from diarrhea and abdominal pain if they drink too much fruit juice. Liquids that contain high levels of sorbitol are often the trigger. You should give your child a maximum of 10 mL juice per kilogram of body weight. Moreover, you should avoid giving them fruit juices that contain sorbitol or high amounts of free fructose, like apple or peach juice.

1.7 Other possible diseases

The symptoms of the following sicknesses are similar. What concerns the nutrition there are differences, though.

1.7.1 Celiac disease

Celiac disease is an immune reaction of your body towards a protein contained in some types of grain called gluten. If someone with celiac disease consumes it, it causes gastritis. Gastritis leads to a worse digestion in general. The reason for this is a hereditary autoimmune disorder. Thus, your immune system considers gluten as an enemy and shoots instantaneously. If someone that is affected avoids gluten, a complete recovery from the inflammation follows. So, although it is just your immune system playing a trick on you, you have no choice but to avoid strictly gluten-containing foods in case you are affected.

Amount of affected people

In the US, only about 0.8% of the population have celiac disease. About 25 times more suffer from IBS this is like comparing the speed of a bicycle driver with a high-speed train. Important: if you do not suffer from celiac disease, do not start a gluten diet! A gluten free nutrition is not only nutrient-poor but also more expensive.

The symptoms

The early the diagnosis the better. The main symptoms are abdominal pain, diarrhea, flatulence, weight loss and a delay of growth. Affected children already show flatulence and diarrhea at an age between 6 and 18 months of age. The reasons for this is that parents start feeding their kids with gluten-containing foods in this period. What comes along with these symptoms is that the height and weight of the children do not increase at the pace of other children. Another indication is an often loose, pale and bad smelling stool. Additionally, an iron and vitamin deficiency often accompany it. If your child is verifiably affected, you should feed it with gluten free products only and create information material about foods your child can stomach for any host and supervisor of your child. Celiac disease can occur at any age. Now, atypical types of the disease without abdominal symptoms occur. The age of patients at the point of diagnosis is increasing as it is harder to recognize the disease if it is atypical. Symptoms of these uncommon types can be arthritis, herpes-like bubbles in various body regions, chronic hepatitis, thinner enamel, short stature, osteoporosis, a delayed puberty and low fertility or unexplained neurological disorders. The treatment, usually in the form of an appropriate diet, is of utmost importance for the patients' health.

Treatment—avoidance of gluten-containing foods

Should you have celiac disease, you should inform yourself and your family about it in a comprehensive manner. One important aspect if to learn about a proper diet. Due to the indecision of science about a limit as to your tolerance of gluten in the case of celiac disease, you should avoid gluten entirely for now. As you adapt your diet, you should keep an eye on baked goods (mixes, bread, cakes, and waffles), beer, cereals, convenience foods, pasta and breadcrumb coating. These grains contain gluten by nature:

Gluten containing grains (avoid these!)		
Couscous	Groats	Triticale
Spelt/Green kernel	Durum wheat	Whole grain
Einkorn wheat	Khorasan wheat	Wheat in all forms:
Emmer wheat	Malt syrup, -extract	-flakes, -bran, -flour,
Barley	Rye	-protein (hydrolyzate),
Semolina	Wheat gluten (seitan)	-shoots

As you can see on the table, "wheat-free" does not automatically imply that the product is gluten-free as well. Gluten is an ingredient of many other grains as well. All the goods, which contain the ingredient malt should be avoided by you, including barley malt, caramel malt, caramel sweets (caramel color may contain gluten as well), malt beer or coffee and ovaltine, even grannies malt candies. Likewise, maltodextrin and maltose may contain gluten traces. Distilled alcohol, on the other hand, is gluten-free. You should check any lipstick, medicine and food supplements for the term "gluten free" as well before using them. Vegetable gum and modified wheat starch (1404 to 1451) are potential sources of gluten. Potatoes, rice, tapioca or cornstarch, on the other hand, is gluten free. Moreover, you should check convenience foods, especially broth, dressings, ice cream, seasoning mixes (they may include wheat starch), processed meats, yogurt, licorice, milkshakes, chocolate fillings (bars and pralines) sauces (including soy sauce), soup seasoning and frozen potato products, like fries, potato pancakes and hash browns. Critical when eating out are blanched vegetables, burgers, Asian dishes (because of the regular use of gluten-containing sauces), fries (if dusted with flour), meatballs (with breadcrumbs), scrambled eggs (if flour was added) and soups.

Gluten free products		
Amaranth grain	Vegetables	Polenta
Beans	Oatmeal	Quinoa
Buckwheat	Millet	Rice
Chia seeds	Potatoes	Sesam
Eggs	Pumpkin seeds	Sunflower seeds
Pease	Linseeds	Soybeans
Fish	Corn	Sorghum
Meat	Milk	Tapioca
Psyllium	Poppy	Teff
Fruits	Nuts	Wild rice

Although the mentioned foods are gluten-free, contaminate with gluten-containing products may occur during their processing, e.g. by cooking them in the same water or grease laying them into the same shop display as gluten containing foods. Hence, be vigilant and if you are in doubt trust on products that are labeled as "gluten-free" explicitly, especially concerning oatmeal. You should separate gluten-free from gluten-containing foods at home. By the way, the additives glutamate and glutamic acid (INS 620 and 625) are gluten-free as well. However, if "gluten" is a part of the ingredients, you should avoid the product.

To counter the mentioned vitamin deficiency use gluten free supplements. A gluten intolerance can affect your supply with B 6, B-12, calcium, iron, folic acid, copper, and magnesium. However, studies show that even if patients with celiac disease take supplements for vitamin B and folic acid, their levels remain under-average. On the other hand, many overcome their iron deficiency by adhering to a gluten-free diet. Ideally, you have a doctor check your vitamin levels and the prevalence of osteoporosis. Firmly, I advise you to visit a support group to benefit from the experience of other patients. To find a local group in your area, visit this site: *https://www.csaceliacs.org/find.jsp*.

To enhance your quality of life, it is important that you take initiative, see Chapters 2.4.1, 2.4.3 and 2.4.9. You are not alone with their problem. Inform yourself before traveling abroad about the names of local gluten-free products and if necessary tell your airline before your flight. Take it sporty. Professional athletes often change their nutrition and life habits far more than you do as part of your health related diet. Please keep in mind: If you have a celiac disease, following your gluten diet is advisable even if your symptoms disappear. For people that are affected, the diet is a proven way increase your protection from some types of cancer, bone loss, infertility, and vitamin deficiency. Hence, visit your doctor regularly to keep track of your vitamin levels and the effectiveness of your diet.

The challenge of avoiding gluten

To find the best way of keeping your diet when eating out, talk with an experienced patient. Visiting a self-help group would be ideal. The exchange with other patients also facilitates your motivation. On page 95 you will also find the cheat sheet to help assist you.

Another aspect that those with celiac disease should take care of is their fiber supply (see section 2.1.4). Fortunately, you can purchase a variety of gluten-free products, even gluten-free pizza. In Chapter 2.7, you will also find a recipe for it. In case, your symptoms persist despite your avoidance of gluten-containing foods, reconsider if are accidentally eating some that do contain it. Possibly, either, you have an intolerance or IBS on top of your celiac disease. If you are suffering from celiac disease for a long time, up to the tranquillization of your inner intestinal skin (mucosa) by keeping your gluten free diet you do not stomach lactose and sorbitol well.

1.7.2 Colon cancer

 Colon cancer, unfortunately, is the second deadliest cancer. It its precursor are the uncontrolled growth of unwanted cells in the intestine. The illustration shows you the mushroom-like protuberance of primary stage colon cancer called polyp. Its treatment is easy but one often does not have symptoms and can only find it by screening. Possible early stage symptoms are blood in the stool, blood on the toilet paper, an increasing drowsiness and fatigue. If you find blood in your stool, you should seek medical assistance immediately. As the cancer advances, an unexpected weight loss, abdominal cramps, abdominal pain, diarrhea, constipation, a change in bowel movements and the feeling of not having excreted everything after visiting the toilet can occur. Going to the screenings is somewhat like caring for your hair. If you visit your coiffeur regularly, your hair looks great. If you do nothing for your hair and just let it grow, it will probably look terrible after a while. During colonoscopy, the specialist can usually cut off a polyp like a hairdresser your hair. Hence, at first, it requires a screening to find a polyp but the treatment is quite quickly. Afterward, it holds: the more time the cancer had to develop before you find it; the lower is your life expectancy. How often and when do you have to go to a screening? Immidiately, if you have symptoms. Otherwise, it depends on your risk factor. In the case of previous cancer or polyps, ulcerative colitis, Crohn's disease, cancer of other family members, overweight, a high-fat diet, little exercise, smoking and alcohol consumption it is increased. If none of the before mentioned attributes applies to you, start at the age of 50 and let your doctor administer follow-ups (usually every 5 years). If your risk level is increased, ask your specialist to set up an appropriate screening schedule for you right away.

Maybe you imagine the screening as being slightly uncomfortable. In fact, you will not notice anything, as you are asleep during it. Moreover, what is the alternative? Do you want to take a chance and risk having to go through a major surgery and chemotherapy later? Be wise and go to the "hairdresser" to avoid getting "bald". There is **no evidence** that the IBS-diet of this book is of use in case of colon cancer or its prevention. These actions, however, lower your risk:

- Get at least four hours of excercise per week and avoid obesity
- Eat only little processed and red meat, take poultry instead
- Only consume moderate amounts of salt
- Ensure that your calcium and vitamin D levels are adequate
- Eat five servings of fruits and vegetables per day and prefer whole grains
- Be modest with your alcohol consumption

Approximately 5.5% of the population share your fate. The most prevalent cancers affect the breast (13.2%), prostate (17.9%) and lung (6.6%). Remember going to the screening. If you suffer from cancer, rely on a specialist stay brave. There are always people who exceed their forecasts, and you could be such a case. Give your heart to becoming a survivor instead of a victim. Your life depends on it. My uncle died of cancer, yet he was able to exceed his expectation by years and at the end went into the ambulance shaking but standing, inspiring to fight back the nasty enemy. We ourselves or someone in our community could suffer from cancer at any point, and that is a big reason to foster cancer research.

The American Cancer Society® set up a donation account. With your helping hand you support cancer research and treatment: https://donate.cancer.org.

(...)Then out spake brave Horatius,
  The Captain of the gate:
"To every man upon this earth
  Death cometh soon or late.
And how can man die better
  Than facing fearful odds
For the ashes of his fathers
  And the temples of his gods,

"And for the tender mother
  Who dandled him to rest,
And for the wife who nurses
  His baby at her breast,
And for the holy maidens
  Who feed the eternal flame, —
To save them from false Sextus
  That wrought the deed of shame?

"Hew down the bridge, Sir Consul,
  With all the speed ye may;
I, with two more to help me,
  Will hold the foe in play.
In yon strait path a thousand
  May well be stopped by three:
Now who will stand on either hand,
  And keep the bridge with me?"(...)

From "Horatius at the Bridge", Thomas Babington, Lord Macaulay (1800–1859).

1.7.3   Ulcerative colitis

Symptoms: Spasmodic abdominal pain on the left side of the lower abdomen and diarrhea, often bloody, possibly connected to the feeling of not having excreted everything. Furthermore, it results in fatigue, dehydration, weight loss, fever and constipation up to an obstruction of the bowel, in which case surgery is necessary. A specialist diagnoses the disease, which requires continuous treatment. Ulcerative colitis is an inherited autoimmune disease, yet, it comes about less frequent as celiac disease. If you have it, your inner intestinal skin is inflamed over a large area. The colon is the horseshoe inside the bowel of our stick figures, in Chapter 1.3, and you can imagine the mucosa as a bicycle tube therein. With the inflammation your stomach fights an enemy that does not exist, it is shadow boxing. This permanent state of emergency causes discomforts. It is like placing sandbags in front of doors and windows to protect one's house from an expected flood and then leaving them there forever. An untreated ulcerative colitis causes unnecessary obstacles in your everyday life. The inflammation can extend to the joints and the eyes. Should the medication fail or complications occur, it may be necessary to, at least temporarily, use an artificial anus or remove the large intestine. It takes courage to face the disease. Create a strong team for yourself and work confidently with your specialist. Also, be sure to read Chapter 2.4.1.

If you follow the advice of your doctor and correctly adapt your diet, you can regain much of the quality of life you have lost. In the case of intense symptoms, always visit your doctor. Aside from medication, your doctor may also be able to recommend suitable supplements. Especially iron, if you have blood in your stool, as well as calcium and vitamin D to avoid a weakening of your bones, make sense. The following also holds if you are suffering from Crohn's disease: as you are more likely to develop colon cancer, you should have a screening every one or two years.

Often painkillers of the category nonsteroidal inflammatory drugs worsen your symptoms. Therefore, you should only take diclofenac, flufenamic acid, ibuprofen, indomethacin, naproxen and oxicam on the prescription of your doctor. Concerning aspirin, current studies indicate that you can tolerate it, however, to be on the safe side, let your doctor decide about it as well. A safe painkiller is acetaminophen. To treat diarrhea, use loperamide and to fight inflammation antibiotics. Always consider the side effects of any drug with your doctor. Another thing you can do to improve your health is to quit smoking. As the disease progresses, a fructose, lactose and sorbitol intolerance may occur. To treat these, use the individualized diet approach of this book. It helps to reduce the abdominal pressure—flatulence, pain, and diarrhea associated with them. To find out which intolerance you have, proceed according to the outline on page 49 and take the fructans and galactans test. Finally, more tranquility in your life also results in more tranquility in your bowel. In Chapter 2.8 you can find stress management methods that work.

1.7.4 Crohn's disease

Symptoms of Crohn's disease may be an abdominal pain on the right side of the lower abdomen, diarrhea—possibly bloody, vomiting, fever, weight loss, fatigue, and weakness. Furthermore, some patients suffer from fistulas, intestinal blockages, malnutrition and anal fissures. Crohn's disease, like ulcerative colitis, is an autoimmune disease. It usually arises at an age between 20 and 29 years. Instead of pathogens, your security forces are attacking your body. Although they are focusing on the end of the small intestine and the beginning of the colon, they attack all layers of skin there. Rarely, the inflammation can affect your outer skin, joints and eyes as well. The disease occurs in 0.014% of the population. Unfortunately, it often accompanies patients throughout their lives and can worsen over time. On the other hand, there usually are long periods without symptoms.

To treat the disease, proceed as described in the second paragraph of ulcerative colitis. What is more, you have to ensure to supply sufficiently your body with energy and calories. If required, you can take high calorie drinks, like those offered by the company Fresubin®, which your doctor may prescribe to you. To lower your risk of having to undergo surgery, you should quit smoking. To calm your intestine, a liquid diet or nutrition via catheter may be helpful. Meanwhile, the wounds will heal in most cases. A surgical intervention is necessary in 20% of the cases. Reasons for surgery are a dangerous bleeding, intestinal canals or bowel obstruction occur and not achieving the desired effect with medications. During the surgery, doctors remove ulcers, inflamed intestine parts, or at least temporarily set a colostomy.

Although it is difficult, gather your courage and remain upbeat. Exchange with other patients can help you, as well as a reflection on the things you are still able to do. *Nick Vujicic* created inspiring videos on that topic. *Theodore Roosevelt*, the first President of the United States to win the Medal of Honor, would have advised you to "Fight a good fight and keep the faith!". *John Fitzgerald Kennedy* certainly did so and became the president despite of having Crohn's.

1.7.5 Diverticulitis

 This disease is a weakness of the connective tissue of the outer intestinal wall. Here little bags form as shown in the illustration. You can think of it like mini balloons popping out from a garden hose. Constipation is a precursor and companion.

Symptoms usually only develop when the protuberances become infected, e.g. due to food residues inside of them. If that happens, you suffer from sudden severe pain in the left lower abdomen. Bloating, vomiting, fever, diarrhea and constipation and result either. As always, if you can see blood in your stool, in this case usually associated with abdominal cramps, visit your doctor.

The causes of diverticulitis are uncertain. Suspects are a high age, many years of a high fat and low-fiber diet, a lack of exercise, obesity, smoking and the use of those painkillers that mentioned as problematic in the case of ulcerative colitis. The disease usually occurs at an age of 40 years and above. About ten percent of the population have the bags at some point in their life, yet, only about 2% suffer from complaints due to them. Ways to treat an acute diverticulitis are antibiotics, a liquid diet, and a temporary low-fiber diet to reduce the inflammation. In severe cases, e.g. bleeding that does not stop by itself, bowel obstruction, ulcers or fistulas, surgery may be required.

The low fiber diet

Foods that you tolerate well:
- Corn flakes, simple crackers toast, and white bread
- Cooked oatmeal, millet gruel, pearl barley, pasta and white rice
- Cooked and canned fruits without peel, ripe bananas, soft honeydew melon and cantaloupe
- Avocado, tomato sauce and when cooked well: green beans, potatoes without peel, pumpkin without seeds, carrots, mushrooms, spinach and tomato sauce
- Eggs, ice cream, honey, dairy products, fish, meat, pudding and syrup

Foods that you should avoid:
- Seeds, nuts popcorn, seeds, whole grains
- cauliflower, beans, broccoli, cabbage, lentils, corn, horseradish, olives, pickles, sauerkraut, sprouts, tough meat, tofu and onions
- Raw fruits and vegetables and its peel, dried fruits, such as berries, figs, prunes and raisins, jam as well as plum and peach juice

After the inflammation's decay, some scientists suggest you keep a fiber-rich diet. If you want to do that, you should eat much of fructans and galactans rich foods. You can recognize these by small portion statements in the F+G column of the tables in Chapter 3. However, there are no conclusive study results to back up the approach as of now. Thus, you would better note down what you eat in a food diary and determine the foods you tolerate well with a doctor or dietitian. Practitioners also recommend you chew food as well as possible.

2

STRATEGY

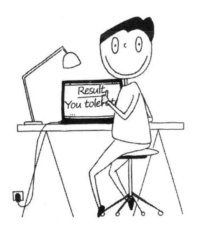

2.1 A gut's change management

No employee likes to stay at a company that always overstrains him. Equally unsatisfactory is to work at a place where one gets the feeling that one does not contribute at all. The typical consequences of both extremes: lack of motivation, an increase in the number of sick leaves up to an incapacity to work at the place anymore. What does that have to do with you? Quite simply: what goes in the professional environment, applies to your bowel as well. Hence, you should strive to work with your enzymes (conveyor-belt workers) in a team instead of over- or under-straining them. Show your leadership qualities and make your staff your motivated allies instead of waiting for them to come to you with their complaints!

How you can get that done, you will find out in this book. Did you ever want to rely on a master plan? If that is so, you will like what follows. According to the following plan, you will first determine the status quo of your symptoms. The next step depends on whether you were able to take a breath test. If you took it, you focus your diet on those triggers you did not tolerate. Otherwise, you follow the full IBS diet—the portion sizes in the IBS tables in Chapter 3. Both holds for three weeks. At the end you determine, whether your symptoms have improved. If so, you can find out whether you can stomach more than the standard amounts—better adapt to the capacity of your workers see Chapter 4.1. If your symptoms did not improve, work on your stress management according to Chapter 2.8 or search for alternative triggers as described in Chapter 4.4.

2.1.1 Signpost

Status-quo-check:	Introduction diet:	Efficiency check:	Adaption:
Note down your symptoms for four days **before** the diet	Keep the IBS diet, or if you did the breath test the diet for your trigger(s) according to the diet plan in Chapter 3.	Note down your symptoms on the last four days of your introductory diet to determine if the diet worked. If not, check alternative causes.	Determination of your trigger(s) with the substitute test and a sensitivity level check.

2.1.2 Roadmap

Step	Action	Target
Duty **1**	**Status-quo-check** Fill out the symptom test sheet Duration: 4 days	Determining your status quo: Which symptoms do you have, and how severe are they?
Optional **2**	**Breath tests at a specialist** Duration: 4 days	Identify the trigger(s) you are intolerant to, which reduces your effort in Step 4.
Duty **3**	**Introductory diet and efficiency check with symptom test sheet** Symptom tracking during the last four days of the diet. Duration of the diet: three weeks	You keep the IBS diet or the diet for (the) trigger(s) you are intolerant to at the breath test with the Chapter 3 tables and fill out the symptom test sheet. Did the diet lower your symptoms satisfactory? **Yes)** Continue with step four, to find out which trigger(s) are relevant for you or, if you did the breath test, step five. **No)** In the case of lactose intolerance retry with half the amounts. Otherwise, act on Chapter 2.8 and if you did the breath test, try the introductory diet for fructans and galactans. Apart from that, check the alternatives see page 482.
Adds to/ replaces step 2 **4**	**Substitute test** Duration: 5 weeks for all most likely triggers	With the substitute test, you check your tolerance for the triggers after the introductory diet without a previous breath test. In case you took the breath test, this step is not required. If your symptoms decreased, do you want to reduce your limitations? Perform the level test (see step 5).
Optional **5**	**Sensitivity-level-test** Duration: 1 trigger ~½ month 2 triggers ~1½ months 3 triggers ~2½ months 4 triggers ~5 months	Enabling you a diet that is as varied as possible while reducing your symptoms is possible by determining your sensitivity level, see Chapter 4.

The goal of the overall strategy is to determine how much you tolerate without causing "the diva" to protest. The first step towards that goal it to determine the status quo, the severity of your symptoms, before changing your diet. The reason for this is that this is the only way to check, whether the diet has an effect. To do so, note down your discomforts in a copy of the following symptom test sheet. **Make sure to keep your symptom test sheets in a folder.** The days at which you note down your symptoms should be average to you. Neither a day on which you sickly vegetated in your bed nor one on which you celebrated the stag party of your best friend or had to master a difficult test count. If you are uncertain about whether it was an average day, cross it out. **Important: This also holds true for all of the subsequent tests. If you are in doubt as to whether the day was "normal," i.e. no circumstances distorted the symptoms, repeat the test to get a more reliable result.** On the days where you track your symptoms, always carry a copy of the symptom test sheet with you. Ideally, you should fill it out right after your main meals, e.g., at 7 am, 1 pm and 7 pm. After the four days of your status quo check, you should also be able to classify the type of stool you usually have. Depending on whether you have constipation, diarrhea or a mix of both, you are an IBS-C, IBS-D or IBS-M type. If you have neither constipation nor diarrhea, your IBS type is unclassified. Take that information with you when you visit the doctor. After tracking your symptoms for four days, you should take the breath test if your gastroenterology specialist offers it. As an alternative, you can take a substitute test after following the introductory diet for IBS and noting down the symptoms at its end to determine the efficiency of that diet (see Chapter 2.2.1). To follow the introductory diet, read on to Chapter 2.3. If you were able to take a breath test, you could disregard those triggers, toward which the breath or substitute test did not indicate a malabsorption. Suppose you only have a fructose intolerance, so you only keep a diet according to the fructose tables in Chapter 3 as part of the introductory diet. In the last week, you then fill out the symptom test sheet to determine the effectiveness. If keeping the diet leads to an improvement of your well-being that you are satisfied with, you should stick to it. You can read how to assess the test sheets more professionally than just laying the one before next to the one after the diet in Chapter 4.3. You can use the efficiency-check-symptom-sheet later as a reference for the sensitivity-level-test, if you decide to take it—it is also included in the advanced techniques-Chapter 4. With the latter, you can adjust your diet to your enzyme worker's capacities. If you still feel no sufficient improvement after keeping the introductory diet, testing your tolerance of fructans and galactans if you took the breath test and otherwise applying our method of identifying alternative triggers are your options, see Chapter 4.4.

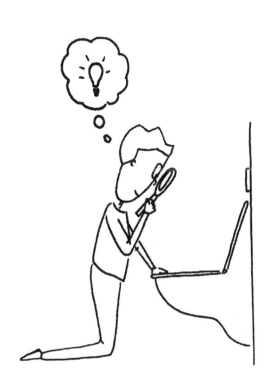

Stool types after Bristol

	Separate hard lumps, like nuts (hard to pass)	**Type A:** Constipation **Value 4**
	Sausage-shaped but lumpy	**Type B:** Constipation Value 2
	Like a sausage but with cracks on the surface	**Type C:** normal **Value 1**
	Like a sausage or snake, smooth and soft	**Type D:** normal **Value 1**
	Soft blobs with clear-cut edges	**Type E:** Diarrhea **Value 2**
	Fluffy pieces with ragged edges, a mushy stool	**Type F:** Diarrhea **Value 4**
	Watery, no solid pieces; **entirely liquid**	**Type G:** Diarrhea **Value 5**

(Based on Lewis & Heaton, 1997; Thompson, 2006)

Types 3 and 4 are the norm. The farther away your type is from these two, the worse your ailments.

2.1.3 Symptom test sheet

Note down your stool type in the morning 🐓, afternoon ☀, and evening ☾ and your stool value from 1 to 5 (see page 52) as well as the number of times you visited the toilet to estimate the stool grade by multiplying the numbers. Also, evaluate bloating and pain from 1 to 5 according to the following scale:

1   No discomfort, like someone without symptoms
2   Hardly any discomfort relative to someone without symptoms
3   Medium discomfort relative to someone without symptoms
4   Severe discomfort relative to someone without symptoms
5   Very severe discomfort relative to someone without symptoms

Test:_____   **End date:**_____

For each test, you need copies of this page!

		Type/ Value	Defecation count	Stool grade	+	Bloating grade	+	Pain grade	= B
Day 1 prior	🐓		x	=					**TEST DAY**
	☀		x	=(+)		+		+	
	☾		x	=(+)		+		+	
			The day's sum A=	=		=			
Day 2 prior	🐓		x	=					**Day 1 after**
	☀		x	=(+)		+		+	
	☾		x	=(+)		+		+	
			The day's sum A=	=		=			
Day 3 prior	🐓		x	=					**Day 2 after**
	☀		x	=(+)		+		+	
	☾		x	=(+)		+		+	
			The day's sum A=	=		=			
Day 4 prior)	🐓		x	=					**Day 3 after**
	☀		x	=(+)		+		+	
	☾		x	=(+)		+		+	
			The day's sum A=	=		=			

Example: The four status quo (1.)/Level (2.) check days

Note down your stool type in the morning 🐓, afternoon ☀, and evening ☾ and your stool value from 1 to 5 (see page 52) as well as the number of times you visited the toilet to estimate the stool grade by multiplying the numbers. Also, evaluate bloating and pain from 1 to 5 according to the following scale:

1 No discomfort, like someone without symptoms
2 Hardly any discomfort relative to someone without symptoms
3 Medium discomfort relative to someone without symptoms
4 Severe discomfort relative to someone without symptoms
5 Very severe discomfort relative to someone without symptoms

Test:_____ **End date:**_____

For each test, you need copies of this page!

	Type/ Value	Defecation count	Stool grade	Bloating grade	Pain grade	
Day 1 prior 🐓	E 2	x 2	= 4	2	2	**TEST DAY**
☀	F 4	x 2	=(+) 8	+ 2	+ 3	
☾	E 2	x 2	=(+) 4	+ 3	+ 2	
		The day's sum	= 16	= 7	= 7	
Day 2 prior 🐓	F 4	x 2	= 8	2	3	**Day 1 after**
☀	E 2	x 1	=(+) 2	+ 3	+ 4	
☾	F 4	x 1	=(+) 4	+ 2	+ 2	
		The day's sum	= 14	= 7	= 9	
Day 3 prior 🐓	E 2	x 1	= 2	2	3	**Day 2 after**
☀	F 4	x 2	=(+) 8	+ 2	+ 4	
☾	E 2	x 1	=(+) 2	+ 3	+ 5	
		The day's sum	= 12	= 7	= 12	
Day 4 prior) 🐓	F 4	x 1	= 4	2	2	**Day 3 after**
☀	E 2	x 1	=(+) 2	+ 2	+ 2	
☾	F 4	x 2	=(+) 8	+ 3	+ 3	
		The day's sum	= 14	= 7	= 7	

Example: The four efficiency check days

Note down your stool type in the morning 🐓, afternoon ☀, and evening ☾ and your stool value from 1 to 5 (see page 52) as well as the number of times you visited the toilet to estimate the stool grade by multiplying the numbers. Also, evaluate bloating and pain from 1 to 5 according to the following scale:

1   No discomfort, like someone without symptoms
2   Hardly any discomfort relative to someone without symptoms
3   Medium discomfort relative to someone without symptoms
4   Severe discomfort relative to someone without symptoms
5   Very severe discomfort relative to someone without symptoms

Test:_____ End date:_____

For each test, you need copies of this page!

		Type/ Value	Defecation count	Stool grade	Bloating grade	Pain grade	
Day 1 prior	🐓	-	x 0	= 0	1	1	TEST DAY
	☀	E 2	x 1	=(+) 2	+ 1	+ 1	
	☾	D 1	x 1	=(+) 1	+ 1	+ 1	
		The day's sum		= 3	= 3	= 3	
Day 2 prior	🐓	D 1	x 1	= 1	1	1	Day 1 after
	☀	-	x 0	=(+) 0	+ 1	+ 1	
	☾	D 1	x 1	=(+) 1	+ 1	+ 1	
		The day's sum		= 2	= 3	= 3	
Day 3 prior	🐓	D 1	x 1	= 1	1	1	Day 2 after
	☀	-	x 0	=(+) 0	+ 2	+ 2	
	☾	E 2	x 1	=(+) 2	+ 1	+ 1	
		The day's sum		= 3	= 4	= 4	
Day 4 prior)	🐓	-	x 0	= 0	1	1	Day 3 after
	☀	D 1	x 1	=(+) 1	+ 1	+ 1	
	☾	D 1	x 1	=(+) 1	+ 1	+ 1	
		The day's sum		= 2	= 3	= 3	

2.1.4 Keeping your balance

Now, you know if the diet provides you benefits and maybe even, how sensitive you are. Still, aside from avoiding the consumption of too much of your trigger, you should also learn some generally advisable nutrition principles.

1	Eat a rich variety of foods, i.e., something different each day and with lots of natural ingredients. Eat with a relaxed posture.	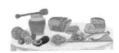
2	Take care of your supply of fiber, e.g., by eating potatoes, flax seeds, lentils, nuts.	
3	Ingest five portions of vegetables (ideally dark green, red or orange) and fruit.	5/day
4	Have some reduced-fat milk products like reduced-fat milk, yogurt or cheese every day.	
5	One or two times a week, eat fish and eggs, as well as 300–600g of low-fat meat, ideally poultry.	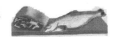
6	Use vegetable oils if possible, like canola oil, and fats.	
7	Reduce your consumption of salt and sugar.	
8	Drink at least 1.5 liters of non-alcoholic drinks per day. Best are unsweetened beverages and water. Drink alcohol moderately or avoid it entirely.	
9	Preferably, cook fresh and at lower temperatures to reduce nutrient leaching.	
+	Stay fit: exercise regularly.	

Compensation needs due to your diet

The consumption of linseeds as described in the following can help you to reduce further your symptoms. Moreover, you will learn that due to short-chained fatty acids you should not entirely dispense milk products even if you are of being intolerant towards lactose.

If you reduce the fructans and galactans in your meals, you might have to compensate for the resulting loss of proteins, short-chain fatty acids and fiber. These three elements belong to a balanced diet. You usually ingest a significant portion through fructans- and galactans-rich wheat products like bread, cereals and noodles and should consider some alternativs, which you will find below. A regular intake of 20 to 38g of fiber, along with moderate exercise, can help to alleviate constipation. As a guideline for your nutrition, find the recommended daily amounts in respective bowls.

Proteins

Proteins
0.66g/kg

One needs 0.66g of protein per kilogram of body weight per day. You can ensure your protein supply by consuming the following products. The rough amount of proteins per portion is shown in parenthesis: 85g meat (28g protein), 85g fish (26g), 150 mL instant coffee with or without caffeine (18g, but standard espresso contains only 0.3g), 200 mL whole milk with added vitamin D (15g), 200 mL whole milk or fat-free milk without additives (6g), 85g corn or wild rice (12g), 90g kidney beans (18g), 140g pasta (15g), 90g soybeans (14g), a medium-sized egg (7.5g), 90g lentils (8g), 110g potatoes (4g), 25g nuts, especially peanuts, peanut butter and almonds (5g), a slice of whole grain bread (5g), 25g cheese (4g), a slice of rice bread (3.5g), 30g cereal (3g), 24g rice bran (3g), 25g dark chocolate (2g) and 50g couscous (1.5g). You may notice that maintaining a supply of protein is rather easy. Vegetarians, however, should plan their protein intake consciously.

Short-chained fatty acids

S.-c. fatty acids
1.2/1.3g/day

Short-chain fatty acids are important energy suppliers. Foods that are particularly rich in short-chain fatty acids include (fatty acids per portion without triglycerides in parenthesis): 10g butter (0.5g), 25g goat's cheese (0.5g), 25g gouda, Swiss cheese, cheddar or Roquefort (0.4g), 50g mozzarella (0.3g), 47g M&M's® (0.3g), 25g blue cheese (0.25g), 20 mL coconut oil (0.2g), 50g coconut meat (0.18g), 150g French fries (0.13g) or 20 mL palm kernel oil (0.08g).

As I said, I recommend the consumption of milk products in tolerable amounts, according to the tables in Chapter 3. Remember that your enzyme-workers should not be undertrained either and that these products are very rich concerning these fatty acids. Experts recommend that short-chain fatty acids amount to 1/60 of the daily amount of consumed fats, which ought to be 70g for women and 80g for men. Thus, the required minimum daily intake is 1.2g per day for females and 1.3g for males. With a lactose intolerance, you can reach this amount easily by eating three slices of cheddar, a cheese that contains hardly any lactose. If you are a vegan, reaching the target is a challenge.

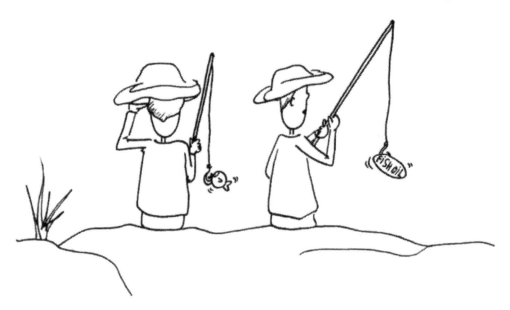

Omega 3 fatty acids

Now talking about fatty acids let me explain another type, which is not impaired by the diet but at times enters the public discussions, omega 3 fatty acids.

Women should take in 6.1g of the omega 3 fatty acid known as alpha-linolenic acid, or ALA while men should take in 7g. Alternatively, maintaining a 2:1 proportion of omega 6 to omega 3 will lead to an intake of up to 9.6g per day for women and 11g for men. ALA fatty acids have a positive effect on your cardiovascular system. The following foods contain high levels (rough ALA amount per portion in parenthesis): 200g fish (4g), 20 mL flaxseed oil (10.5g) for which the consumed amount should be below 100 mL per day (flaxseeds themselves contain 25% oil and thus 24g of flaxseeds, see page 62, at least 3g; however, during pregnancy you should avoid both as it can harm your baby), 20 mL canola oil (1.8g), 20 mL mayonnaise (1g), 20 mL soy oil (0.8g), 100g wheat crackers (0.8g), 70g French fries (0.3g), 16g peanut butter with omega 3 (0.5g), 25g walnuts (0.5g), 10g butter (0.3g) and 10g margarine (0.3g). The data sheds a positive light on the fiber Strategy A as described in the following. You can reach the target amount of 7g for men just by consuming 1 tbsp. flaxseed oil per day. Alternatively, you can arrive at 6g, for example, by eating three portions of salad with 20 mL of canola oil each and a slice of bread with omega 3 peanut butter. Apart from ALA, EPA (eicosapentaenoic acid) and DHA (docosahexaenoic acid) are also essential. Your daily intake of EPA should be 250mg and of DHA, 500mg. If you eat fish at any time during the week, you will usually have covered your need. Krill or fish oil capsules containing these amounts are an alternative.

Fiber

Fiber
20-38g/day

The following products are rich in fiber (fiber per portion in parenthesis): 90g lentils (27.9g), 90g kidney beans (22.5g), 25g almonds (12g), 110g potatoes (8.7g), 30g bran cereals (up to 8.7g for Kellog's® All-Bran®), 24g flaxseeds (6.5g), 100g wild rice (6.2g), 24g rice bran (5g), one 42g slice of rye bread (5g), 30g wheat cereals (3.3g), 25g hazelnuts or pine nuts (2.7g), 25g dark chocolate (2.7g), 25g pecans or pistachios (2.5g), 60g peas (2.4g), 25g walnuts (1.7g), 25g chestnuts or butternuts (1g), 25g peanuts, coconuts or macadamia nuts (0.4g). Fruits and vegetables contain about 1 to 5g per portion, e.g., avocado (1.7g), banana (3g), blackberries (4.4g), cauliflower (1.2g), salad (0.8g), olives (1.2g), orange (2.4g), spinach (7g), tomatoes (1.4g). As fiber may be a challenge, two different compensation strategies follow.

Strategy A: Flaxseeds

Flaxseeds, like chia seeds, contain a high amount of fiber and many omega-3-fatty-acids. They are good at reducing constipation and can help a little against pain and bloating. The downside of this all-around effect is that flaxseeds contain fructans and galactans. If you apply this strategy, the portions you take in for fructans and galactans decrease to 28% of their former quantity. As you take in flaxseeds at three different times of the day, the amount per meal is 24g at most. This way the flaxseeds account for 6.5g of fiber at the highest daily stage. For your body to be acquainted with flaxseeds, start in the first two weeks with one tablespoon combined with at least 75 mL of water at breakfast. In the following weeks, you can then increase the intake amount according to the following table. The numbers printed in normal type relates to the flaxseeds, and the amount in italics to the required minimum amount of water you should drink with it as a dilution:

Week	3–4	5–6	7–8	9–10	11–12	13–14	15–16	17f
Break-fast	1 tsp.	1 tsp.	1 tbsp.	1 tbsp.	1 tbsp.	1 tbsp.	1 tbsp.	1 tbsp.
						1 tsp.	1 tsp.	1 tsp.
	75 mL	*75 mL*	*150 mL*	*150 mL*	*150 mL*	*225 mL*	*225 mL*	*225 mL*
Lunch	1 tsp.	1 tsp.	1 tsp.	1 tbsp.	1 tbsp.	1 tbsp.	1 tbsp.	1 tbsp.
							1 tsp	1 tsp
	75 mL	*75 mL*	*75 mL*	*150 mL*	*150 mL*	*150 mL*	*225 mL*	*225 mL*
Dinner	-	1 tsp.	1 tsp.	1 tsp.	1 tbsp.	1 tbsp.	1 tbsp.	1 tbsp.
								1 tsp.
		75 mL	*75 mL*	*75 mL*	*150 mL*	*150 mL*	*150 mL*	*150 mL*

You can also add flaxseeds to your meals. Whether the flaxseeds are whole or crushed should not make a difference. Make sure that you buy flaxseeds instead of psyllium as study results for suggest that psyllium is less effective. Wheat bran as does not lead to any improvement according to the examinations.

Warning: Do not eat flaxseeds during pregnancy or lactation, as these can disturb your hormonal balance and cause premature birth. Concerning chia-seeds there are no studies yet. To be on the save side avoid these during pregnancy as well, until science rules out any harmful effec. With 24g of flaxseeds, you cover 7g of your fiber demand. One portion of fruits or vegetables contains 2.5g of fiber on average. You can reach your ideal daily fiber intake by eating five of them per day and adding wild rice to one of your meals together with the 17th-week amount of flaxseeds as indicated in the last table.

Strategy B: Brown rice/rice bran

This strategy focuses on rice bran, rather than on flaxseeds as in Strategy A, see page 62. After all, rice bran contains 21g of fiber per 100g and thus accounts for 5g of the daily amount recommended for the plan's optimal stage. The advantage of using rice bran is that your tolerated amounts of fructans and galactans in the food lists remain unchanged. Furthermore, rice bran appears to be unproblematic during pregnancy. If for example: you eat 30g cereal mixed with rice bran for your breakfast, 25g dark chocolate and 20g almonds, as well as two oranges in between; for lunch a portion of tomato salad with avocado and 45g of potatoes; for your dinner eat 45g rice as a side dish, and you will have consumed about 28g of fiber in total. Hence, with a little bit of planning, you can maximize your fiber intake, and minimize your fructans and galactans intake while avoiding fiber supplement capsules.

⊛ Summary

As part of the strategy, you first note down your symptoms before doing anything. Then you start the introductory diet. For it, you reduce the consumption of the four most likely triggers by following the IBS tables or if you took the breath test, those trigger(s) for which you have few enzyme workers. The aim is to check whether the diet lowers your symptoms after all.

So, fill out the symptom-test-sheet before starting the diet. Then follow your diet according to the relevant tables in Chapter 3 for three weeks and fill out the test-sheet once more for the last four days. If you are feeling better now, you should first perform the substitute test—if you did not take the breath test. Afterward, you can also determine your precise sensitivity level; see Chapter 4.

Make sure you keep a balanced diet:

Drink least 1.5 liters of water per day and exercise regularly. Possibly, your diet requires you to compensate with regard to the following ingredients:

Proteins: For example, by eating fish, meat, eggs rice or rice bran.

Short-chain fatty acids: For example, by consuming milk products. If you have a lactose intolerance, take cheese with a moderate amount of it, like cheddar.

Omega 3: For example, by eating flaxseeds or their oil, rapeseed oil or fish.

Dietary fiber: for instance, by having fruit or vegetables five times a day. Furthermore, dark chocolate, a handful of nuts potatoes and rice contribute to it.

Also, ensure to eat a variety of foods, to supply your body with the vitamins that are important for your health. To achieve that, regularly eat fruits and vegetables.

2.2 Your individual strategy

This Chapter describes how to proceed accurately with the introduction of diet and the sensitivity level test. During the introductory diet you keep the portions stated in the tables in Chapter 3. Please note here that the tolerated portions refer to one meal—expecting three meals at intervals of about six hours per day. Follow these steps to find out if the diet has an effect:

First, you take the introductory diet for all triggers by using the IBS column or, if you took a breath test, for those that your breath test showed an intolerance. Four days before starting the diet as well as on the last four days of the third week, you fill out the symptom test sheet on page 53. With it, you can determine the diet's success, see chapter 4.3. The diet is efficient. However, if after three weeks of keeping it, you should not find any improvement; find out whether you unwillingly consumed too much of your trigger(s). One way to do so is to keep a nutrition diary and check it with a specialist or nutrition consultant. If you ruled out an accidental intake of the trigger(s) and are unhappy with the improvement of your well-being, make sure to test fructans and galactans as well by repeating the introductory diet with fructans and galactans and your breath test trigger(s). If you are lactose intolerant, you may be more sensitive than is normal—try half the amounts in the lactose lists to find out. Aside from that, alternative triggers and stress may be the cause. If you are satisfied but did not take the breath test, take the substitute test now, see Chapter 2.2.1.

The test procedure in three levels of escalation

Subsequently, you find an example of the test process for someone with lactose intolerance:

1) Reduce your lactose consumption according to the lactose tables in Chapter 3 for three weeks. Fill out the symptom test sheet for four days before the diet as well as on the last four days. In the third week, if your discomforts improved satisfactory, keep the lactose diet. If you like, you can adjust your sensitivity level further (see Chapter 4). If you remain dissatisfied, act according to step 2).

2) Repeat the introduction with fructans and galactans as well, if you have not already done so. Did your symptoms improve further? If so, keep this diet. In case you are still searching for an improvement, follow step 3).

3) Read the Chapter 2.8 about stress management and the Chapter 4.4 about alternative triggers.

2.2.1 Substitute test

So, you want to figure out, which triggers you can tolerate and which you cannot but your specialist is unable to offer you a breath test? For this situation, I have developed the substitute test. It works this way: You take in the highest conceivable amount of a trigger in a day (under normal circumstances), and then check if you get symptoms from it.

Before taking the substitute test, you have finished the IBS introductory diet and noted an improvement concerning your symptoms. If your symptoms did not improve, the substitute test will not change that and you have to search for other causes as described before. If you symptoms improved, you now keep your introductory diet and perform a provocation test for one of the triggers every four days. You can start the first provocation right after your introductory diet. You will find the trigger load that you consume on the test day on the following page. Warning: If you have symptoms after the first or second of three provocation loads used on some test days, abort the test—you have already found your trigger and it makes no sense to hurt yourself. On the test day and its three subsequent days, you note down your symptoms on the symptom test sheet. After the three observance days, you can continue with the provocation test for the next trigger.

If you are unsure, whether you had symptoms due to a provocation test, you compare your symptoms on the trigger test sheet with the efficiency check sheet you filled out at the end of the introductory diet. If you want to use a mathematical approach to determine the outcome, either download the symptom test tool at *https://laxiba.com*, or follow the level test result calculation table in Chapter 4.3. As soon as you notice symptoms on the test day or the three subsequent days, which you can see mathematically if your Lid grade (**L**) is higher than your K.O.-threshold grade (**K**), you know you have an intolerance. To reduce your abdominal discomfort, drink still mineral water (usually up to three liters per day are salutary) and take a walk. Discuss the tests with your doctor beforehand so that he or she can consider the potential effects to and of your medical treatments and pre-existing conditions. If you have an intolerance towards a trigger, keep the diet for it according to the respective tables in Chapter 3.

For all the tests together, you need a beaker, a 0.5 L bottle, 100g of fructose and 20g of sorbitol, both which you can buy at your local pharmacy, scales and 1 L of reduced-fat cow's milk without additives. If you have an intolerance, you can use the remaining sugars for a sensitivity-level-test later on. On the respective test day, consume the following amounts of the substances.

Lactose test

At breakfast, drink half a liter of the milk, using the 0.5 L bottle. Repeat at lunch unless your symptoms after the breakfast dose are so severe that you can already conclude that you have an intolerance. In addition to the milk, eat in accordance with your IBS diet.

Fructose test

Warning: before doing the test, confirm with your doctor that you do not have a hereditary fructose intolerance! For the check, add 35g of fructose to a clean 0.5 L bottle of water and shake it well. Then drink it completely on the morning of the test. In addition to the fructose, eat according to your IBS diet on the test day and the next three days. You do not need a test for glucose-balanced fructose. If you want to pay attention to it, you can determine the amount you can tolerate by multiplying the tolerated load, for the standard level in this book, it is 0.5g, of fructose by ten. The result applies to g/100g of food, i.e. in the standard case; you tolerate at least 5g of table sugar per 100g of food.

Sorbitol test

Proceed as for the fructose test, but replace the 25g of fructose with 20g of sorbitol.

Fructans and galactans test

Eat a generous portion of wheat cereal in the morning, beans with garlic and onions at lunch, brownies, and crackers in between and a baguette or porridge dish in the evening. Consume them as usual.

2.2.2   It depends on the total load

You feel discomfort as soon as too much of your trigger arrives at your small intestine for your enzyme workers to handle. The more triggers, the worse your symptoms are. In the food tables in the third part of the book, you will find the portion sizes that fit your level. What do you do if you want to combine different foods, e.g., as you prepare to cook a recipe, considering you tolerate a limited amount of some of them? If you used the maximum amount of lactose on the milk for the rice pudding already, do you have to deny yourself the vanilla sauce in the case of a lactose intolerance? Nonessential: reduce the consumption for one or several of the lactose containing foods far enough to not surpass the amount thresholds in sum. Makes sense? Not yet? Here is another example: you want to drink condensed milk in your coffee for breakfast (the tolerable amount is half a portion of 38 ml), and you love mascarpone as a spread (your acceptable portion size for it is 2¼ portions of 30g each). Hence, both foods contain lactose. In order not to surpass your tolerance threshold, restrict yourself to ¼ of a portion of condensed milk (about two teaspoons—10 mL) and one portion of mascarpone. Thus, the total amount of lactose you consume at the meal is below your threshold. If the reduced amounts are too small for you, you may want to look for alternatives. In Chapter 4.4 you can find various cold cut. Your tolerable portion size for Cheddar cheese, for example, is quite high.

2.3   Prevalence of the intolerances

According to an extensive current study in Switzerland, 27% of people with abdominal discomfort suffer from a fructose intolerance, 17% from a lactose intolerance and a further 33% from both. However, the fructose dose of 35g that the study used is high for European conditions, if a Finnish study from 1987 still applies to contemporary diets, and low for American conditions, wherein the average daily amount consumed is 54g. Hence, there is no fixed reference around the world. Another research study using 25g fructose as its base level suggests only a 49% average prevalence of fructose intolerance. An analysis of several studies shows that independent from the investigations mentioned above, 58% of those with irritable bowel symptoms have a sorbitol intolerance. There are no research results concerning the prevalence of a fructans and galactans intolerance known to me at this point.

Are you surprised about the low level of lactose intolerance? Well, you have to account for the fact that it is lowest for Caucasians as they adapted to tolerate milk to cope better with less sunshine in a day. Still, I was amazed that lactose intolerance is not the common type of intolerances according to the studies I read. If you stroll through supermarkets, however, you will hardly find a shelf that holds products for people with sorbitol or fructose intolerance. Instead, the markets have adjusted solely on lactose intolerance—also concerning the labeling. From this perspective, it is better to be lactose intolerant. Those suffering from sorbitol intolerance have to learn the names of nine sugar-alcohols and their assignment numbers instead. Remember sorbitol is also relevant for fructose intolerance due to interaction effects. Go to page 93, to find out more.

2.4 General diet hints

2.4.1 Good reasons for your persistence

Imagine that one of your best friends goes on a two-week vacation leaving his beloved Labrador retriever, *Bailey*, in your care, along with some instructions about the dog's health needs as it has an intolerance towards an ingredient in some dog foods. You run out of dog food after the first week, just as you sat down on the couch to relax—not planning to leave the house again for today. Now you remember that you still have a can of the food you give to the square like dog of your auntie in the basement. If you give *Bailey* some of that, you save an hour drive to the store and back as well as going outside where it started to rain. Annoyingly, the food for your aunt's dog contains the trigger *Bailey* has to avoid. Unlike the happy dog image on the package suggests, giving him this food causes him pain, flatulence, and lethargy; catching a stick will be out of the question for this poor pooch. Maybe, you also imagine your aunt, whose dog feels well, even after consuming what you would never feed him— you remember a cream pie that fell victim to that bitch. "Hogwash!" she would say. "Dogs can eat anything! A dog intolerance? If he only eats enough there will be no farts!"

What is your position at that moment? Back on the couch or driving through the rain to the expert dealer? Now, I am relieved. Therefore, the dog of your friend is worth spending time and money as well as acting considerably. If, at any point it becomes difficult for you to keep your diet, think about the happy *Bailey* and send the square couch potato dog back to your aunt's home!

In the end, I call upon you to take responsibility for your nutrition. Show respect to your body. Acquire the necessary courage and discipline. Your body is a part of you. Just as many vegetarians stand by their dietary choices for the duration of their lives, you should stand by your diet and your body. Be yourself. The key is not starting out perfect, but starting at all and making small improvements every day. That is something you can do! You have the courage and *Bailey* will give you the courage.

Your target should be to change your sustenance day by day, food by food, in such a way as to allow you to lead a mostly symptom-free life. All beginnings are difficult, however, and as you leap the initial hurdles, you will find further motivation and discipline in discovering how much your nutritional changes are paying off for you.

The first step in that direction is to connect that goal with whatever is most important to you in your life. Independent of where your passions lie, you will enjoy them better by gaining more energy and improved wellbeing.

Do you not believe me? Then imagine *Bailey* once more: The retriever sneaks through the house and as he sees a cat pass by through the window, his only reaction is to fart, then, he retreats into his dog hatchet with an abdominal cramp. Curing the food for aunt's dog that got him into the hot water – you do not want to end up likewise. What about this instead: The retriever sneaks through the house, hears steps, stalks to the open window, stops and sees what looks like a burglar nearby the post box (he does not see the letters in his hands). In a flash, *Bailey* is on the road right behind him giving him a good bark! Pure energy!

What triggers your passion? What is your affair of the heart? Gain strength by keeping a diet that is best for you and give it a fresh start. Turn your attention and abilities toward eating in a way that will help you achieve your goals. If you are uncertain whether you can reach, your goals do this: Imagine that you have already done it. How? Cut out the following card and fold it as indicated. Then put it somewhere you can see it every day. Ideally, you can take a picture of yourself after a particularly fruitful milestone and put it on the drawing. Then let it encourage you to continue improving your nutrition each day. *Stephen William Hawking* has never stopped producing outstanding scientific works despite suffering from a myasthenia. Why? Because he is following his heart and because he has a positive attitude about life. Who seeks excuses when they are passionate about something? When it comes to passion, it is all about the how. It is about doing what is possible and thus it is always all about the solution. There are similar examples in sports. *Melissa Stockwell* achieves first class athletic performance despite having lost a leg. Her sport is her passion, and she finds ways to excel in it regardless of the circumstances life gave her.

So what is your passion? Write it down. Then make it clear to yourself that a symptom-reducing diet will positively affect your achievement. Then get on your way to making this nutrition a part of your life. In addition—always remember about your friend, *Bailey,* the dog.

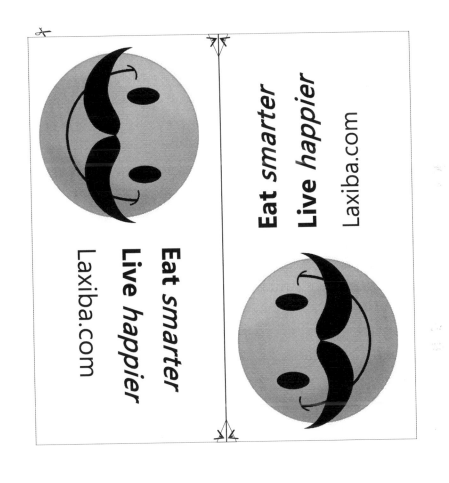

Eat smarter
Live happier
Laxiba.com

Eat smarter
Live happier
Laxiba.com

2.4.2　Mealtimes

Even when and how often you eat can affect your digestion. Who better to ask on that subject than athletes? They, in particular, depend on an optimal nutrient supply. The analysis shows that over 97% of elite Canadian athletes eat at least three times a day; 57% of them also take a snack in the morning, 71% in the afternoon and 58% in the evening. Moreover, regular mealtimes have a positive effect on the cardiovascular system. A study of more than 4,500 children showed that the risk of childhood obesity markedly decreases the more often children eat during the day. How is that? Well, ask the mail carrier of *Bailey's* owner, whether he dares bringing him his letters after eating a gravitationally detrimental meal, his daily ration, in the morning.

2.4.3　Eating out

At home, restricting one's consumption of trigger containing foods is rather easy. Now you want to eat at a restaurant of a friend's house so what do you do? Of course, you understand that a restaurant staff usually does not have the dietician's expertise required to tell you the ingredients of each meal. Luckily, you can help yourself. For example by learning about some foods that you can usually eat without having to think about them. These include eggs, fish or meat without breading or sauce, kiwis, leafy salads dressed with oil, oregano, pepper and salt, oranges, basil pesto, potatoes, rice, and tortillas. Depending on your intolerances, you have to be careful with diabetic products and prepared sauces, as they often contain triggers like sorbitol. What about menus, however? Have you ever spent time at a restaurant considering what the ideal combination of menu items would be for you? The good thing is that you can often ask for a change to menu items without paying extra if you ask the server. You can likewise voice your needs to your hosts when you receive an invitation to a meal. To make it easy, just hand out the safe products list (see Chapter 2.6). You can send it out with the following message, for example:

"Dear [name of the host],

I was glad to receive your invitation to [occasion like your wedding], and I am happy to come. If it is possible for you to cook some of the foods that are included in the attached table separately from the other meals, then I can take part in the meal, as well. Please tell me whether that will be possible so that I can plan accordingly.

Thank you and see you soon!

[Your name]"

The safe products list, see Chapter 2.6, also makes it easier for a restaurant kitchen to find a suitable meal for you. As fast food chains are not as readily equipped to adapt their menus, you will find many fast food chain products and the portion sizes you can stomach in the third part of this book. You can stay on the safe side by always having your book with you. However, it will hardly be always at hand, unlike a foldable list for your purse or wallet. In Chapter 2.5 you will find the fitting cheat sheet for your trigger(s) with the tolerable portion sizes of some common products. This list also includes information on cube names and trigger-free products.

2.4.4   Convenience foods

Unfortunately, fructose, lactose and sorbitol are a part of many convenience foods or are naturally contained in the ingredients. However, you will find exceptions, even when shopping on the cheap, including convenience foods that advertise the use of natural ingredients and those that contain basil pesto. The cheat sheets (see Chapter 2.5) will inform you of which ingredients on a package mean that the food contains your trigger(s).

2.4.5　Medicine and oral hygiene

Anything you take into your mouth can cause symptoms if it contains a cube (trigger) you cannot tolerate. Sorbitol, in particular, is included in many oral hygiene products. An example of a sorbitol-free toothpaste is *JASON® healthy mouth*. Use dental floss without wax, and find a mouthwash such as *TheraBreath® Fresh Breath Oral Rinse*.

For those suffering from sorbitol intolerance it sometimes gets tricky, as sorbitol is not always obvious as n ingredient. If you are in doubt, call the customer service hotline of the respective product and ask them for clarification.

The search for sorbitol-free medicines may be especially hard, so ask your pharmacist for assistance. Many nasal sprays, eye drops, and expectorants contain this additive. However, if you look hard enough, you will usually find alternatives for these as well. Examples of sorbitol-free pharmaceuticals include: *Allegra® 12 Hour Allergy* (allergy), *Allerest® PE Allergy & Sinus Relief—Tablets* [CONTAINS LACTOSE] (frontal sinusitis), *Ayr® Saline Nasal Rinse Kit* (frontal sinusitis), *Florax® DS Diarrhea Relief Vials* (diarrhea), *Hyland's® Earache—Drops* (earache), *Mucinex® 12 Hour Extended Release Expectorant—Tablets* (expectorant), *Mucinex® Sinus-Max Severe Congestion Relief—Tablets* (frontal sinusitis), *SinuCleanse® Neti Pot All Natural Nasal Wash System* (frontal sinusitis) and *Visine-A® Eye Allergy Relief, Antihistamine & Redness Reliever, Drops* (allergy). When considering medicines that contain lactose or fructose, take into account the amount you can stomach at your sensitivity, which is 3g lactose and 0.5g fructose for the standard level. It helps to know that middle-sized capsules contain 0.58g at the most, and the largest, 1.6g per piece while tablets are usually even a little lighter. For mixtures, a teaspoon holds about 5 mL/g and a tablespoon 5–15 mL/g.

Despite your best efforts at researching your intolerance(s), you may find yourself unable to stomach medicine for whatever reason. If you are having symptoms, search for alternatives. If in doubt, use the symptom-test-sheet. Write down your symptoms while using it and compare it with a record of your diet taken when you were not using the medicine, for example, on your efficiency check sheet. You can use any sheet where you recorded your symptoms after refraining from the trigger(s) that causes your symptoms.

2.4.6 Nutritional supplements

If you take vitamin supplements, the following examples are trigger-free:

Nature's Bounty® Vitamin B-12, 1,000mcg, Nature Made® Vitamin B6 100mg Dietary Supplement Tablets, Walgreens® Multivitamin Ultimate Men's Tablets, Walgreens® Multivitamin Ultimate Women's Tablets. A long-term trial did not prove the use of multivitamin supplements. If you take them, make sure not to take too much of certain vitamins. Vitamins that can be unsafe in excess include B3, B6, as well as A, D, E and K, which can cause symptoms of poisoning if you overdose. Thus, you should discuss your intake with your doctor. A viable approach with these vitamins is taking them in three-month cycles. That means taking them for three months and then taking the next three months off.

2.4.7 Protein shakes—nutrition for athletes

There is a partially questionable trend among athletes to take special supplements. If you can cover your protein demand with the products listed in Chapter 2.1.4, you have no need for protein shakes or the like. Some energy bars and electrolyte products contain sorbitol (see Chapter 3.2). You can often find trigger free alternatives in pharmacies.

2.4.8 Fish and meat

Fish and meat by nature are free of triggers. Nevertheless, you have to be careful with breaded and processed fish and meat—these may contain lactose and with sauce, which may contain any of the triggers. To find out about included trigger(s), check the list of ingredients of the product.

2.4.9 These actions lead to lasting change

To achieve lasting success, it is important that you monitor your nutrition. If you find yourself starting to ignore the recommended amounts, you should get back on track and restart your commitment as soon as possible. Write down your goal to adapt your nutrition to the stated food and drink portion sizes to reduce abdominal discomfort and improve your quality of life. Stay conscious of the negative consequences of eating "blindly" covered in the first part of this book. Why is it important to change your habits? Re-read your goal and then write down your five most important reasons for striving toward it. Moreover, answer the following question. Why it is important to act **now**?

Probably, you have made the following experience as well. Filled with motivation and enthusiasm you plunge into something, like a New Year's resolution. One goes right after it and even celebrates first successes. However, this feeling trickles away unless soon afterward even bigger successes surpass the first one. If that does not happen, a slight inertia arises. If you change your diet, this can happen to you as well. It is like there is an angel on your one shoulder to whom you say that you are going to keep at it even if it becomes arduous yet there is an imp sitting on your other shoulder, which is already laughing at his sleeve. In fact, the way gets steeper after the first yards. Many then let things slide, which makes further successes impossible, and the symptoms come back. "Isn't that unfair?" the imp is telling you, "you are putting in your effort for days and how does it pay off? You are having the same symptoms as you had before. Let it be." The angel may have screamed so much that it is croaky by now and shrugs his shoulders exhaustedly. "Sorry, but I tried my best," one excuses oneself trying not to look at the grinning devil.

It is a cognitive bias to believe that it is easier just to accept one's symptoms than to change your diet to avoid them. What about you? Did you catch yourself close to giving up? If so, send the devil on your shoulder to the desert where it belongs.

I can promise you: After you changed your diet to fit your trigger, you will have more energy and a higher quality of life. In addition, after you have mastered staying on the right path for some month, you will find that you are getting used to it, which will make it even easier to stick with it. Getting used to it is something that the imp has deliberately concealed: Once you have taken the first pitch, you get accustomed to quickly assessing foods about their content of the trigger(s) and learns to notice trigger hideouts. Juggling with the amounts becomes so easy that you do not have to think long. At the start, the cheat sheet and this book will serve you well. Later you no longer need both as you know yourself what is right for you. The imp that you sent to the desert now is hot with anger, and you are the one that has a big grin on the face. You have the best arguments to be tenacious!

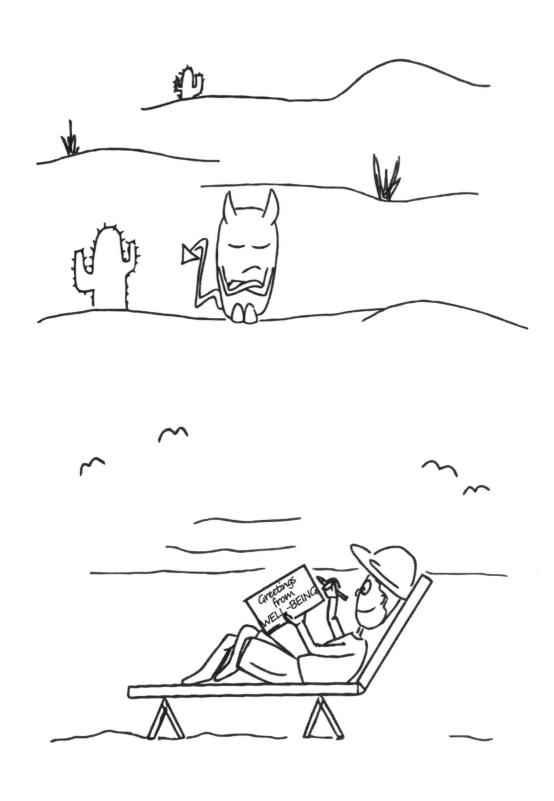

Are you uncertain as to whether you are going to remain motivated? Create an objective agreement with yourself. Note down in writing, why it pays off to you, to endure. Which goal do you want to achieve? For example, like this:

Objective agreement (write it down yourself)

What: comply with the acceptable amounts – Send the devil to the desert.

How to measure it: daily at 7:45 pm (set an alarm on your phone): did I eat dairy products and comply with the portion restrictions?

Consequence: YES, you complied, so give yourself a small reward. NO, you did not so do 10 pushups or mow the lawn (anything you can do, which is good for you but you do not like doing).

Get it done: start within three days and keep on actively managing your diet until you have formed a habit of doing it.

Activities: Put this book into your kitchen and the cheat sheets you need into your wallet; inform those close to you; create reminders in your flat and your car, place your objective agreement somewhere where you can see it at least once a day (e.g. your mirror).

A good way to ensure that you stay committed is to integrate your spouse. Ask them to motivate you and to reflect back to you, which positive changes they notice about you. Another option is to book one of our coaches at *https://laxiba.com/trainer* to help you implement the steps explained in this book. What is more, you will find a way to talk with others and motivate each other at *https://laxiba.com/team*.

The more vivid and multifaceted you can imagine your life after a successful conversion of your diet, the more likely you are to keep moving forward with it and doing what is necessary. Have you been in a rut one day? Forget about it; get the job done better the day after! You can use this book as a compass and correct your course back to being well!

2.4.10 Sweetener's sorbitol content

Pure stevia is sorbitol-free. Aside from that, sorbitol is contained in many sweeteners as well as light and sugar-free products.

2.4.11 Reasons for using the triggers

Why for example is lactose contained in some drugs or sausages? These products have nothing to do with milk! There is a swift explanation. When it comes to processed food, lactose creates certain flavors, makes sausages thicker and saves money. Sorbitol makes products free from table sugar to enable diabetics to consume them as well as keeps chocolates moist. Fructose also can create certain flavours and is often contained in products that contain processed fruits. For drugs, lactose and sorbitol are carriers for active substances because it is simple and works well. There would be alternatives that work well in many cases, which would not cost much more. So far, there is no strong lobby against using triggers in foods or making them easier to avoid, yet. Of course, these triggers also occur naturally, but that is not a valid reason to use them instead of the also naturally occurring Stevia in, for example, chewing gums.

2.4.12 Positive aspects of the diet

Do you want to disagree with me after reading the headline? For many the trigger diet equals abdication. In its original sense, however, diet (from the Greek díaita) means "lifestyle" or "way of life." Are abdication and the feeling of a downer an accurate description of the lifestyle that you want? On the contrary, you perform the diet to lower you symptoms and thus increases your quality of life. As you find out, which foods you can eat concerning your trigger(s) you will automatically start thinking about what you eat in general. The chances are that you will end up eating healthier, and healthy is a much friendlier summary of your lifestyle. Of course, an alternative to the diet would be the use of medicine, like painkillers or drugs to stop diarrhea. Better yet, is to make sure symptoms do not occur in first place. In the case of lactose intolerance, you can use enzymes, which also achieves the latter aim, although as you will learn the food lists for many dairy products, the tolerated amount is larger than you might guess.

2.4.13 Testing yourself

Some of those affected by IBS reportedly struggle to absorb other ingredients like aspartame or maltodextrin. If you have reason to believe that this applies to you, follow the alternative introductory diet outlined in Chapter 4.4.

⊕ Summary

A healthy, balanced diet, fixed mealtimes, and regular exercise are important not only in case of an irritable bowel but for all people. Unfortunately, sometimes triggers are included in products although trigger free alternatives are available. Hence, especially when eating convenience foods or taking drugs, watch out for triggers in the ingredients. Stick to the trigger diet that works. The longer you persist, the easier it gets to maintain it.

2.5   The cheat sheets

Cut out the leaflet(s) that are relevant for your on the following pages. Please fold them along the thick lines. Start with the dotted line. Then fold each leaflet again at the half-dashed line. You can now keep this important information at hand when you are out and about or shopping.

Flyer for lactose, fructans & galactans

Free of lactose despite their name are:

Milk acid	Glucono delta-	Rice and
Milk protein	lactone	almond milk
Lactate	Lactose freed milk products	
Lactase	(INS additive numbers:	
	575, 325-327)	

Products containing lactose:

Lactose	Whey	Yoghurt
Cheese	Kefir, lassi	Milk(-powder)
Curd	Cream	(Concentrated) butter

Asian, Greek, Italian and Spanish meals contain little lactose. Asian rice meals also containing few fructans and galactans. Fish, seafood, meat, black coffee, eggs and oils are also free from lactose. The same holds for fruits and vegetable although some of them contain fructans and galactans.

More lactose sources: LAXIBA®

- Cereals
- Ice cream and sweets like chocolate
- Coffee and milk, condensed milk
- Dairy products, like cream, curd and yoghurt
- Breading, sauces, puréed meat, Tzatziki
- Sweet pastries—biscuits, cakes, tarts, & cream

Primary sources of fructans:

Artichokes, asparagus, banana, blueberries, bread, Brussels sprouts, cabbage, cauliflower, cereals, chicory root, couscous, garlic, leeks, flaxseeds, nectarine, noodles, onions, pastries like biscuits and cake, pineapple, pizza, products that show inulin as an ingredient (like some cereals, chocolates and ice creams) raisins, semolina flour, shallots and sunchoke.

Products that contain much of galactans:

Beans, lentils, flax seeds, oat flakes, peas, soy products, tofu, sprouts, wheat and other grains

Interior left

Lactose, fructans & galactans free:

Apple	Fish and	Oranges
Apricot	Meat	Parmesan
Carrots	Jelly babies	Pear
celery	Ice tea	Peppers
Chocolate sorbet	Ketchup	Potatoes
Coconut	Kiwi	Rice
Drinks without	Lettuce	Spelt flour
milk, yoghurt, etc.	Oil & vinegar	Squash

Low lactose content for average serving sizes

Butter$^{\text{☺; 14g}}$	Margarine$^{\text{21¾P.; 9g}}$	Swiss
Cheddar$^{\text{33¼P.; 30g}}$	Nutella$^{\text{®32¼P.; 37g}}$	cheese
Fondue sauce$^{\text{☺; 53g}}$	Parmesan$^{\text{☺; 5g}}$	☺; 30g

Per active lactase capsule you take in, you can stomach about 75% more of each shown serving size.

These are the portion unit abbreviations:

Exemplar	Cup	Glas	Portion	Slice
E	C	G	P	S

☹=avoid; ☺=nearly free; ☺ =is free of it

Only copy with permission. Copyright © 2016 J. Stratbucker

Interior right

Products with a high amount of lactose

Cacao$^{\text{¼C.; 150g}}$	Kefir$^{\text{¼P.; 220g}}$	Mozzarella$^{\text{9¾P.30g}}$
Casserole$^{\text{½P.; 238g}}$	Mashed-	Pancake$^{\text{½P.; 187g}}$
Cheese-sauce$^{\text{¼P.; 66g}}$	potatoe$^{\text{½P.; 140g}}$	Tart$^{\text{½P.; 87,5g}}$
Condensed milk^{½P}	Milk rice$^{\text{¼P.; 107g}}$	Yoghurt$^{\text{¼P.; 250g}}$
Creme-soup$^{\text{½P.; 245g}}$	Milk$^{\text{¼G.; 200g}}$	

Fructans and galactans rich products

Apple strudel$^{\text{¾ P., 64g}}$	Donut$^{\text{½E., 105g}}$	Plain
Asparagus$^{\text{½P., 85g}}$	French toast$^{\text{¼ P., 131g}}$	dumpling$^{\text{½P., 55g}}$
Baguette$^{\text{1¾S., 42g}}$	Granola bar$^{\text{½P., 27g}}$	Ravioli$^{\text{¼P., 250g}}$
Banana juice$^{\text{½G., 200g}}$	Hamburger$^{\text{½E., 100g}}$	Ryebread$^{\text{¾S., 42g}}$
Cake$^{\text{¼P., 122g}}$	Hot dog$^{\text{¼E., 199g}}$	Sandw.-
Calzone$^{\text{¼P., 168g}}$	Kidney beans$^{\text{¼P., 90g}}$	cookie$^{\text{3E.,14,5g}}$
Cheesecake$^{\text{☹P., 220g}}$	Leeks$^{\text{¼P., 89g}}$	Sandwich$^{\text{☹}}$
Chop Suey$^{\text{¼P., 166g}}$	Lentils$^{\text{¾P., 90g}}$	Shalot$^{\text{¼E., 15g}}$
Cookie$^{\text{½E., 45g}}$	Muesli$^{\text{¼P., 55g}}$	Snowpeas$^{\text{¾P., 85g}}$
Corn Flakes$^{\text{1½P., 30g}}$	Muffin$^{\text{¼E., 113g}}$	Springroll$^{\text{¼P. 140g}}$
Couscous$^{\text{¼P., 140g}}$	Noodles$^{\text{1P., 140g}}$	Tofu$^{\text{½P., 85g}}$
Cracker$^{\text{¼P., 30g}}$	Oat bran$^{\text{1¼P., 55g}}$	Waffles$^{\text{½P., 95g}}$
Crêpe$^{\text{¾E., 55g}}$	Onion Rings$^{\text{¼P., 70g}}$	White whole
Crispbread$^{\text{¼S., 42g}}$	Peas$^{\text{1¼P., 15g}}$	grain wheat
Danish pastry$^{\text{¼E., 125g}}$	Pizza$^{\text{½P., 209g}}$	bread$^{\text{¾S., 42g}}$

Flyer for fructose intolerance

If you mix fructose with sorbitol-containing products, you tolerate less and if you do, so with glucose containing products you can tolerate more fructose. The identifier number for sorbitol is 420. The following table shows you with which factor you can multiply the fructose amounts when you consume or mix the glucose containing foods with them:

Foods	Portion weight	B ×
Avocado (Florida)	37g	2.25
Fresh figs	50g	2.0
Maple syrup	30g	1.5
Mozzarella	28g	1.25
Sweet corn	82g	3.25
Thin slice of pineapple	56g	2.25

Foods that contain fructose:

- Cereals with fructose syrup and HFCS
- Many convenience foods
- Canning sugar, honey and corn syrup
- Some sweeteners
- Most fruits also, when they are dry
- Many soft drinks, fruits, and alcoholic beverages
- Some sauces

Foods that contain sorbitol:

- Fruits, juices and alcoholic beverages
- Products for athletes like protein bars
- Convenience foods and sauces
- chewing gum and mints other than those that only contain stevia and table sugar
- Light und isotonic drinks
- Drugs and oral hygiene products
- Diabetics and dietary products
- Chocolates, cream, and cakes

LAXIBA®

Fructose intolerance serving sizes

Pineapple ¾ P; 140g
Apple ⊗
Apricot ☺ +¾ P/E; 35g
Balsamic vinegar ☺
Banana ☺ +¼ P/E; 118g
Blueberry. muffin. 26 E; 110g
Beer ☺
Big Mac® 5 E; 215g
Bitter lemon ⊗
Pears ½ C; 15g
Lettuces 1¼ P; 85g
Cauliflower ☺

Broccoli 3 P; 85g
Blackberries 1¾ P; 140g
Cranberries ☺
Cinnamon crumble
GoLEAN ☺ ¼ P; 30g
Coca Cola® ½ G; 200ml
Corn flakes ☺ +1½ P/P; 30g
Strawberries ½ P; 140g
Special K® Original ☺
Garden salad 8¼ P; 85g
Ginger Ale ⊗² G; 200ml
Cucumber 4¾ E; 85g
Oatmeal ☺

Portion unit abbreviations:

Exemplar	Cup	Glass	Portion	Tbsp.
E	C	G	P	T

⊗=avoid; ☺=nearly free; ☺=is free of it ☺+=free and contains glucose: B-factor/per unit

Only copy with permission. Copyright © 2016 J. Stratbucker

Raspberries ½, P; 140g
Honey ¼ P 21g
Chicken sweet'n sour 2½T15g
Currants 1 P; 140g
Coffee ☺
Potatoes ☺
Chewing gum ☺
Ketchup ☺ +¼ P/T; 15g
Cherries 1 P; 140g
Kiwi 1 E; 86g
Cabbage ☺ +¾ P/P; 85g
Pumpkin butternut ☺
Long Island Ice tea ¾ G; 200ml
M & M's® ☺
Mango 1 T; 15g
Mate tea ☺
Melon 1¾ T; 15g
Milk ☺
Granola bar ½ E; 30g
Nectarines ¾ E; 142g
Oranges 2¼ E; 140g

Pepper ½ P; 85g
Pepsi® ½ G; 200ml
Peach ☺ +½ P/E; 140g
Plum ☺ +¼ P/E; 15g
Mushrooms ☺
Pizza ☺
Red Bull® ☺+7P/G; 200ml
Rice ☺
Sauerkraut ☺
Chocolate ☺
Champagne ☺
Smacks® ☺ +12 P/P; 30g
Sushi 16 P; 140g
Tomatoes 3 P; 85g
Tonic Water® ⊗² G; 200ml
Grapes ¼ P; 140g
Wine ¾ G; 200ml
Wheat bread ¾ E; 42g
Whopper® 2¾ E; 315g
Lemon ☺
7UP® ⊗² G; 200ml

Front **Flyer sorbitol intolerance**

Tolerated in case of sorbitol intolerance are

Maltodextrin	Sorbic acid	Barley malt syrup
Sodium sorbate	Potassium sorbate	Calcium sorbate
Sorbitan...	Polyoxyethylene(20)-**sorbitan**...	

(INS add. numbers: 200-203, 432-436, 491-495)

These ingredients are sugar alcohols:

Sorbitol	Mannitol	Xylitol
Lactitol	(Ethyl-) Maltol	Hexanhexol
Glucitol	Maltitol/-syrup	Inositol
Isomalt	Palatinit®	Sionon
Erythritol	Pinitol	

(INS add. numbers: 420-21, 636-37, 953, 965-7)

Hence, avoid foods that contain them.

Back **Sugar alcohols like sorbitol are often contained in:**

- Diabetics and dietary products
- Athletes products and energy bars
- Convenience foods and sauces
- Chewing gum and mints except for those that only contain stevia and table sugar
- Some light and isotonic beverages
- Drugs and mouthwashes

- Bars, chocolates, cream, and cream pies
- Moreover, some fruits, their juices, and alcoholic beverages as well as some vegetables

Interior left **Sorbitol intolerance portion sizes**

Pineapple ¾ P-140g
Apple ☺² E; 182g
Apricots ¾ E; 35g
Vinegar balsa. 23 P-15g
Banana 9¼ E; 118g
Blueberry Muffin 88 E; 113g
Beer 10 G-200ml
Big Mac® 6½ E; 215g
Bitter Lemon ☺

Broccoli ☺
Blackberries ☺² P-140g
Cranberries 45¼ P-55g
Froot Loops®☺
Coca Cola®☺
Corn Flakes ☺ P-30g
Strawberries ¼ P-140g
Special K® original ☺
Garden salad 16 P-85g
Ginger Ale ☺

Pear ¼ E; 15g
Lettuces 3 P-85g
Cauliflower 2½ P-85g

Cucumber 1 E; 85g
Oats ☺

If you are sensitive avoid any food but one with ☺

Portion unit abbreviations (gram follows):

Exemplar	Cup	Glas	Portion	Tbsp.
E	C	G	P	T

☹=avoid; ☺=nearly free; ☻=is free of it
Only copy with permission. Copyright © 2016 J. Stratbucker

Interior right

Chicken sweet and sour ☺
Raspberries 1½ P-140g
Honey 1¾ T; 15g
Currants 2½ P-140g
Coffee ☺
Potatoes 45¼ P-110g
Ketchup 3¾ T; 15g
Cherries ¼ T; 15g
Kiwi ☺
Cabbage 58¾ P-85g
Pumpkin butternut ☺
Long Island Icet. 16 G-200ml
M & M's®☺
Mango 4 T; 15g
Mate tea ☺
Mayonnaise ☺
Melon 14¼ P-140g
Milk ☺
Granola bar ☺²
Nectarines 1 T; 15g
Oranges ☺ E; 140g

Peppers ☺ E; 85g
Pepsi®☺ G-200ml
Peach ¼ E; 140g
Plum ¾ T; 15g
Mushroom ¾ T; 15g
Pizza ¾ E; 209g
Red Bull® ☺
Rice ☺
Sauerkraut ¾ T; 15g
Chocolate 48 P-25g
Champaign ¾ G-200ml
Smacks® 83¼ P-30g
Sushi 1½ P-140g
Tomatoes 1 T; 85g
Grapes ½ P-140g
Wine ¾ G-200ml
Wheat bread 26¼ P-42g
Whopper® 1 E; 315g
Lemon ☺
Chewing gum light ☺
7UP® ☺

Front **Cheat sheet celiac disease** &LAXIBA®

Grains to avoid:

Couscous	Pearl barley	Triticale
Spelt/	Durum	Whole wheat
Green spelt	wheat	All kinds of
Small spelt	Khorasan	wheat: -flakes,-
Semolina	Malt, -syrup, -	bran,-flour, -
pudding	-extract	protein (Hy-
		drolysate),
Barley	Rye	
Emmer	Seitan	-shoots

Foods you have to check for gluten:

Asia-food	**Burger**	Seasoning mix
Back mix	Cereals	Yoghurt
Beer	Dressings	Malt drops
Blanched	Ice cream	**Cake**
food	Conve. foods	Licorice
Bread	Meatballs	**Malt beer**
Broth	**Barley malt**	**Caramel drops**

Back **Cheat sheet celiac disease**

Foods you have to check for gluten:

Malt coffee	**Noodles**	Soy sauce
Milkshake	Hash browns	Soups
Potato	Scrambled	Soup
pancake	eggs	seasonings
Ovaltine	Chocolates	Proceeded
Breadcrumb	filled	meat
French fries	Sauces	**Waffles**

Problematic ingredients and products:

1404	to	Maltose	(modified)
1451			wheat starch
Gluten	Maltodextrine	Vegetable Gum	

*gluten free wheat starch, potato-, rice-, tapioca- or cornstarch are harmless. Products in **fat** are gluten rich – avoid these unless they are labelled as gluten-free. Check medicine, tablets and lipstick for gluten, too.

Cheat sheet celiac disease — Gluten free foods (GF)

Amaranth	Vegetables	Polenta
Beans	Oat bran	Quinoa
Buckwheat	Millet	Rice
Chia seed	Potatoes	Sesame
Eggs	Pumpkin seeds	Sunflower seeds
Peas	Linseeds	Soybeans
Fish	Corn	Sorghum
Meat	Milk	Tapioca
Psyllium	Poppy	Teff
Fruits	Nuts	Wild rice
620 to 625 (glutamate and glutamic acid)		

A contamination of gluten free products can happen during their processing, cooking in the same fat or water as well as displaying next to gluten containing foods. Especially, watch out for the gluten free label and icon for oats.

Cheat sheet histamine intolerance — Avoid in case of histamine intolerance

Alcohol	especially	Oranges
Pineapple	smoked/process	Papaya
Aubergine	ed (except for	Plum
Avocado	fresh meat)	Mushrooms
Banana		**Sauerkraut**
Pears	Grapefruits	Hot spices
Beans	Yeast &-extract	**Chocolate**
Protein	Raspberries	**Soy sauce**
Canned veg.	**Cheese (old)**	**Sea fruits**
Strawberry	Kiwis	**Spinach**
Peas	Pumpkin	**Tofu**
Peanuts	Licorice	**Tomatoes**
Vinegar	Lentils	Dry fruits
Con. salad	Mangos	Wheat shoots
Fish/meat	**Nuts**	**Citrus fruits**

Not **fat** means it hinders the histamine absorption. Symptoms? Antihistamine help.

2.5.1   Fructans, galactans, and lactose

Here you can find information on fructan, galactan, and lactose-containing foods. Asian, Greek, Italian and Spanish meals usually contain little lactose. Asian rice meals are also fructans and galactans poor. Fish, other seafood, meat, black coffee, eggs, and oils are also free from lactose. The same holds for fruits and vegetable although some of them contain fructans and galactans.

Despite their name, these ingredients are free from lactose		
Milk acid	Glucono delta-lactone	Rice and almond milk
Milk protein	Lactose freed milk products	
Lactate, lactase	INS additive numbers: 575, 325-327	

These products contain lactose		
Lactose	Yogurt	Whey
Cheese	Kefir, lassi	Milk(-powder)
Curd	(Concentrated) butter	Cream

Attention, lactose is often contained in:

- Cereals
- Ice cream and sweets like chocolate
- Coffee and milk, condensed milk
- Dairy products, like milk, curd, and yogurt
- Breading, sauces, puréed meat, tzatziki
- Sweet pastries like biscuits, cakes, and tarts, cream

High amounts of fructans are present in:

- Artichokes
- Asparagus
- Bananas
- Blueberries
- Brussels sprout
- Cabbage
- Cauliflower
- Cereals
- Chicory root
- Couscous
- Flaxseeds
- Garlic
- Jerusalem artichokes
- Leeks
- Nectarines
- Noodles
- Onions
- Pastries and biscuits, breads and cakes
- Pineapple
- Pizza
- Products that inulin has been added to, such as some cereals, chocolate and ice cream
- Raisins
- Semolina flour
- Shallots

High amounts of galactans are present in:

- Beans
- Flaxseeds
- Lentils
- Oats
- Peas
- Soy products, including tofu
- Sprouts
- Wheat and other grains

2.5.2   Fructose and sugar-alcohols

If you have a fructose intolerance, be mindful of fructose and HFCS while reading the ingredient lists. As you learned before, sorbitol lowers the amount of fructose-containing products you can tolerate. To determine sorbitol-free products, however, you, unfortunately, have to navigate an unbelievable minefield of identifiers, despite the high prevalence of the condition. As I am unaware of studies that tested, if the interaction with fructose is limited to sorbitol, you may want to know the other sugar alcohols in case of fructose intolerance, too:[2]

Caution... these products contain fructose:

- Cereals with high fructose corn syrup (HFCS) or isoglucose, glucose-fructose syrup, fructose-glucose syrup and high fructose maize syrup. Unless they are listed in the food tables of this book you cannot know how much you can tolerate of them
- Many convenience foods
- Preserving sugar
- Honey and corn syrup (fructose quantity is unclear)
- Some sweeteners
- Many fruits, dried fruits, juices, and alcoholic drinks
- Many soft drinks

These foods often contain sugar-alcohols like sorbitol:

- Diabetic and dietary products
- Electrolyte products and energy bars
- Convenience foods and prepared sauces
- Chewing gums and mints, except those sweetened only with Stevia, for example. Sorbitol is either only contained in traces or not contained at all in Wrigley's® Spearmint, Doublemint and Juicy Fruit
- Some "light," i.e., sugar-free, and isotonic beverages
- Medicine and oral hygiene products
- Bars, pralines, sweet pastries, tarts, prepared cream
- Puréed, pickled or breaded sausages, fish, and meat

---

[2] There is an immediate need for simplification here. A proper solution is the declaration "contains sorbitol".

Moreover, some fruits (like apples, apricots, bananas, cantaloupe, carambola, cherries, cranberries, grapes, guava, lowbush cranberries, mango, nectarine, peach, pear, pineapple, plum, pomegranate, raspberries, strawberries and watermelon) and vegetables (artichoke, asparagus, beets, cabbage, carrots, cauliflower, celeriac, celery, chestnuts, chicory, coleslaw, cucumber, eggplant, endive, fennel bulb, garbanzo beans (chickpeas), kale, kohlrabi, leeks, lettuce (Boston), lettuce (green leaf), lettuce (iceberg), lettuce (red leaf), lettuce (romaine), mushrooms, olives, onions, pickled beets, radish, sauerkraut, sour pickles, soybean sprouts, spinach, tempeh, tomatoes and turnip), including juices contain sorbitol. Many alcoholic beverages do, as well, but brandy, gin, rum and whiskey, for example, are often sorbitol-free.

Noncritical ingredients for sorbitol intolerance[3]

Maltodextrin	Sorbic acid	Barley malt syrup
Sodium sorbate	Potassium sorbate	Calcium sorbate
Sorbitan...	Polyoxyethylene (20) –sorbitan-...	

Critical ingredients for sorbitol intolerance[4]

Sorbitol	Mannitol	Xylitol
Lactitol	(Ethyl-) Maltol	Hexanhexol
Glucitol	Maltitol/-syrup	Inositol
Isomalt	Palatinit®	Sionon
Erythritol	Pinitol	

---

[3] INS additive numbers: 200–203, 432–436, 491–495.
[4] INS additive numbers: 420–21, 636–37, 953, 965–67.

2.5.3 Celiac disease

Grains to avoid:

Couscous	Pearl barley	Triticale
Spelt/green spelt	Durum wheat	Whole wheat
Small spelt	Khorasan	All kinds of wheat:
Semolina pudding	Malt, -syrup, -extract	-flakes,-bran,-flour,
Barley	Rye	-protein (Hydrolysate),
Emmer	Seitan	-shoots

Foods you have to check for gluten:

Asia-food	Chocolates filled	**Noodles**
Backmix	Conve. foods	**Ovaltine**
Barley malt	Dressings	Potato pancake
Beer	French fries	Proceeded meat
Blanched food	Hash browns	Sauces
Bread	Ice cream	Scrambled eggs
Breadcrumb	Licorice	Seasoning mix
Broth	**Malt beer**	Soup seasonings
Burger	**Malt coffee**	Soups
Cake	Malt drops	Soy sauce
Caramel drops	Meatballs	**Waffles**
Cereals	Milk shake	Yogurt

Problematic ingredients and products:

INS: 1404 to 1451	Maltose	(modified) wheat starch*
Gluten	Maltodextrine	Vegetable Gum

*gluten free wheat starch, potato-, rice-, tapioca- or corn-starch are harmless. Products in **fat** are gluten rich and have to be avoided unless marked as gluten free. Check medicine, tablets and lipstick for gluten, too.

Foods you have to check for gluten:

Amaranth	Milk	Quinoa
Beans	Millet	Rice
Buckwheat	Nuts	Sesame
Chia seed	Oat bran	Sorghum
Corn	Peas	Soy beans
Eggs	Polenta	Sunflower seeds
Fish	Poppy	Tapioca
Fruits	Potatoes	Teff
Linseeds	Psyllium	Vegetables
Meat	Pumpkin seeds	Wild rice
620 to 625 (glutamate and glutamic acid)		

Otherwise a contamination of gluten free products can occur during their processing, cooking in the same fat or water as well as display next to gluten containing foods. Especially, watch out for the gluten free label and icon of oats.

2.5.4 Histamine intolerance

Not **fat** means it only hinders the histamine absorbtion. Fat means it contains histamine. Symptoms? Antihistamine help.

Avoid in case of histamine intolerance

Alcohol	Grapefruits	Plum
Aubergine	Hot spices	Protein
Avocado	Kiwis	Pumpkin
Banana	Lentils	Raspberries
Beans	Licorice	**Sauerkraut**
Canned vegetables	Mangos	**Sea fruits**
Cheese (old)	Mushrooms	Soy sauce
Chocolate	**Nuts**	Spinach
Citrus fruits	Oranges	**Strawberry**
Con. salad	Papaya	**Tofu**
Dry fruits	Peanuts	**Tomatoes**
Fish and meat especially if it is smoked and processed. If you cook your meat from fresh, it is usually tolerable.	Pears	**Vinegar**
	Peas	Wheat shoots
	Pineapple	Yeast & -extract
	Grapefruits	Plum

2.6 The safe products list

Likely, if you yourself do not have it, someone in your circle of acquaintances has the irritable bowel syndrome or an intolerance towards some ingredient. As a good host, you may have already been in a situation to consider those to make sure that none of your guests encounters an uneasy feeling after an invitation.

If you ask your guests to tell you about any problematic ingredient you should accustom to, you are prepared professionally: Such a question will always leave a positive impression as it shows that your guest's well-being is important to you. You are well accustomed to any guest, if you make sure that some foods that are usually tolerable for anyone are on the menu. How can you achieve that? It is quite simple: make sure to offer the sauces separately from the side dishes. Hence, provide a bowl of potatoes, another bowl with butter, a third one with salad and lastly one with dressings. By the way, with some exceptions like garlic and onions anyone can tolerate most herbs and spices. The table on the following page shows you some usually safe foods.

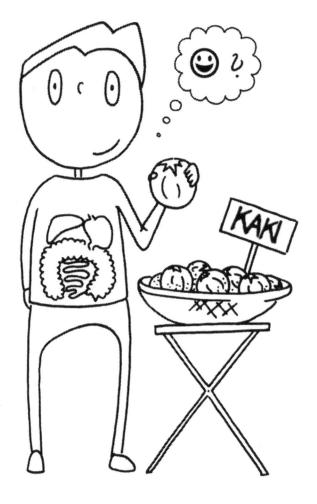

Check it with the Laxiba App!

1. Get it on the App Store or on Google Play and subscribe

2. Choose "Yes" or your tolerance level for your sensitivities

3. Find the answer with the text or category search option

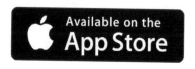
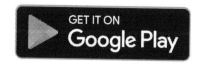

Fruit	Vegetables	Warm dishes
Blackberries	Avocado, green	Brandy vinegar
Currants	Basil	Caviar
Dates, fresh	Chard	Chinese oyster sauce
Figs, fresh	Chives	Fish, meat, shrimp and
Goji berries	Coriander	shellfish*
Lemon zest	Green peppers	Kraft® Italian Dressing
Loganberry	Horseradish	
Papaya	Kelp	Kraft® Mayonnaise
Passion fruit	Oregano	Oils
Rhubarb	Parsnips	Kraft® Thousand Island
	Peppermint, fresh	Dressing®
	Rice	Pepper and salt
	Rosemary	Rice bread
	Rutabaga	Rice noodles
	Squash: Butternut, cala-bash, giant and spaghetti	Soy oil
	Thyme	Spelt flour
	Yam	Tabasco® sauce

*Non pureed and without breading and sauce.

Beverages	Other	
Black coffee	Baking powder	Pecan nuts
Brandy	Brazil nuts	Pine nuts
Gin	Brown sugar	Pistachios
Jasmine tea	Cashews	Pumpkin seeds
Maté tea	Coconut	Rice bread
Peppermint tea	Gelatin	Spelt
Rum	Ginkgo	Walnuts
Tequila	Licorice	White sugar
Tonic Water	Macadamia nuts	
Vodka	Maple syrup	
Water	Peanut butter	
Whiskey	Peanuts	

2.7 Recipes

2.7.1 Apricot cuts

Fructose	☺
Fructans + galactans	1 and ½ pieces
Lactose	☺
Sorbitol	☹

What you need:

4 tbsp. of apricot jam
4/5 cup of dried, fine sliced apricots
One cup of butter
One cup of flour (in case of celiac disease, use gluten free flour)
3/5 cup of rice flour
One tsp. of vanilla-extract
2/5 cup of sugar, as well as some to dust over

Preparation:

Preheat the oven at 390 °F top and bottom heat or 360 °F convection heat. Then, lay out an eight in deep backing tray with baking paper. Now add the apricots and jam in a small pan with 4 tbsp. water. Simmer over medium heat until they are thick. Then squash the apricots a little with a fork and let them cool down. Add the butter, vanilla extract and sugar in a bowl and mix with the blender. Afterward, add the rice flour and the flour and whip with a spoon or your hands to form a dough. Then, divide the dough into two equal pieces. Spread one-half of the dough on the baking sheet. Knead the remaining dough into an eight in² square piece and place it on top. Press alongside the edge of the dough and stab some small holes into it with a fork. Bake for 25-30 minutes until the corners turn golden. Leave it in the baking mold for the cool down and sprinkle powdered sugar over it. Slice three cuts to the top and the sides and that is it.

2.7.2   Banana cake

Fructose	15 pieces
Fructans + galactans	½ piece
Lactose	☺
Sorbitol	☹

What you need:

Two ripe bananas
A handful of banana chips
One packet of baking powder (celiac disease? Use gluten-free baking powder)
3/5 cup of butter and something for the baking mold
Two large eggs
1/5 cup of icing
3/5 cup of flour (use gluten free flour if gluten intolerant)
3/5 cup of sugar

Preparation:

Preheat the oven to 390 °F top and bottom heat or 360 °F circulating air. Meanwhile spread some butter into a marble cake mold. Gently mix the butter and sugar together. Then slowly add the eggs and some flour. Afterward, stir the rest of the flour, baking powder and bananas into the mix. Place the dough in a baking mold and bake the cake for about 30 minutes until it well rises. Now let it cool down in the mold for about 10 minutes. Following, prepare the frosting with two teaspoons of water, douse the cake with it and decorate with the banana chips.

2.7.3   Creamy rice pudding

Fructose   ☺
Fructans + galactans ☺
Lactose   ☺
Sorbitol   ☹

What you need (for four servings):

One tbsp. butter

2/5 cup of cranberries

One egg

3/5 cup of rice

2 cups of rice milk

One pinch of salt

½ tsp. of vanilla extract

¼ cup of sugar

Preparation:

Cook the rice in water. Then add 350g of cooked rice with ¾ of the milk, the sugar and a pinch of salt in a new pan, stir from time to time and let the mix cook for another 3 minutes. Meanwhile, beat the egg in a small bowl with a wire whisk. At the end of the cooking time, add to the mix with the rest of the milk and the cranberries and let it simmer it yet another 3 minutes. It is important that you always stir it. Now remove the pan from the plate and mix with the butter and the vanilla extract – Bon appetite.

2.7.4 Spring chicken bowl

Fructose   ☺

Fructans + galactans   ¼ serving

Lactose   ☺

Sorbitol   ☹

What you need (five servings):

1 and ½ cups of broccoli, finely chopped
3/5 cup of green beans
Two cups of chicken fillet
Two cloves of garlic
1 and ½ cups chard
One tbsp. olive oil
Two tbsp. of green pesto
1 and 4/5 cup of Brussels sprout
One-bunch of chives
One and ¼ cups of sweet potato

Preparation:

Heat the oil in a large heavy saucepan. Fry the chicken on each side slightly until golden brown. Cook, it with the potatoes in a large pot afterwards. Add a crushed garlic clove and pepper to the cooking water. After 15 minutes, add the Brussels sprouts and the beans. After another 15 minutes add the broccoli and chard. Heat for 5 minutes more. Before serving, mix the pesto - finished.

2.7.5 Kiwi sauce (e.g. with ice)

Fructose	1 and ½ servings
Fructans + galactans	☺
Lactose	☺
Sorbitol	☺

What you need (one serving):

Three tsp. of maple syrup
Two ripe green kiwi fruits
Two tsp. of lime or lemon juice

Preparation:

Peel the kiwis, dice them and blend them afterwards together with the lime or lemon juice. If you love pure green, sieve out the remaining black seeds later on.

2.7.6   Fruit salad

Fructose   ☺

Fructans + galactans   two servings

Lactose   ☺

Sorbitol   ☹

What you need (four servings):

4/5 cup of pineapple
One banana, ½ cup
One cup of strawberry
One orange, 3/5 cup
One cup of cranberries
One tbsp. of lemon juice

Preparation:

Peel the pineapple, remove the stem and cut into finger-thick pieces. Now peel the orange, remove the seeds and chop up, also cut the strawberries. Place the pieces in a bowl and pour the lemon juice over them. Stir well now and you did it. If you suffer from a fructose intolerance, it is better if you blend the salad and make sorbet, because your tolerance depends on the glucose content of the cranberries.

2.7.7 Fruit salad with curd

Fructose	☺
Fructans + galactans	4 and ½ servings
Lactose	3 and ¼ servings
Sorbitol	☹

What you need (eight servings):

Maple syrup
Two cups of canned pineapple (if fresh the curd turns bitter)
One and ¼ cup of cranberries
One and ¼ cup of canned mandarins
Two cups of sour cream or cottage cheese with a little milk

Preparation:

Cut the pineapple into finger-thick pieces. Now place the fruit and sour cream in a bowl. After stirred well, season well with the maple syrup. To consume enough glucose-containing cranberries, puree the fruits with a blender.

2.7.8 Lemon bar

Fructose	~ 30 piece
Fructans + galactans	2-4 piece
Lactose	10 piece
Sorbitol	☺

What you need:
For the dough:

3/5 cup of butter
¾ cup of flour (celiac disease? Use gluten free flour)
One tbsp. milk
1/5 cup of rice flour
4/5 cup of brown sugar

For the topping:

Three eggs
2 tbsp. of flour (celiac disease? Use gluten free flour)
Icing sugar
The zest of three lemons
4/5 cup of mL lemon juice
4/5 cup of sugar

Preparation:

Preheat the oven at 430 °F top and bottom heat or 390 °F air circulation. Cover a 9 in. baking tray with baking paper. Mix the butter, the flour, rice flour and sugar in a bowl, until only small lumps form. Then add the milk and spread the dough on the baking tray. Let it bake for 17 minutes until golden brown. Then remove the tray and reduce the oven temperature to 390 °F top and bottom heat or 360 °F air circulation. Whisk the lemon juice and the eggs, the sugar, the flour and the lemon zest in a bowl. Pour this concentrate over the dough and bake the lemon bars for another 15 minutes until the surface almost firm. Let it cool down on the tray. Finally, cut and powder - ready to enjoy.

2.7.9 Orange-peppermint-salad

Fructose	2 and ¼ servings
Fructans + galactans	☺
Lactose	☺
Sorbitol	☺

What you need (for four servings):

12-pitted dates cut lengthwise

Four oranges

A small bunch of mint: some leaves finely cut and a few left a whole

One tbsp. of water

Preparation:

Peel the orange and place it together with the liberated juice in a bowl. Afterward, add the date pieces and the chopped peppermint leaves to the water and mix gently. Finally, top it with whole mint leaves.

2.7.10 Pancakes

Fructose	☺
Fructans + galactans	1-2 pieces
Lactose	☺
Sorbitol	☺

What you need:

One egg
Half a cup of flour (celiac disease? Use gluten free flour)
1 and ¼ cup of rice milk
Sunflower oil

Preparation:

Put the flour into a bowl and make a hole in the middle, in which you put the egg together with the rice milk. Now whisk everything well with a mixer. Add a quarter of the rice milk and continue to add the rest once the batter is lump free. Now let the dough rest and after 20 minutes whisk it again. Preheat a small non-stick frying pan and pour the oil into it. Cover the whole bottom of the pan with a thin layer of dough. Fry the pancakes on each side, until golden brown. Place some baking paper between the pancakes when you pile them, so they remain crispy. Serve with any filling.

2.7.11 Pizza dough

Fructose	☺
Fructans + galactans	1 piece of pizza
Lactose	☺
Sorbitol	☺

What you need:

7g (one filled tsp) yeast (celiac disease? Use dry gluten-free yeast. First, let it rise with a tsp. of sugar in a cup that is half-full of water. After that, mix it with the rest of the water and flour. Often, it takes some time until the dough has risen.) One and ½ cups of flour (celiac disease? Use gluten-free flour, here you may have to experiment a bit)
One 1/5 cups of water

Preparation:

Put the flour with a tsp. salt, yeast and 275 mL lukewarm water in a bowl and mix everything for about 5 minutes to form a dough. Now, take out the dough and let it rise it in a lightly oiled bowl until it rises about twice the size. Knead the dough afterwards for a bit, then cut it in half and roll out each of both parts on a thin layer of flour as thin as possible. Now garnish the pizza as desired and bake in the oven at 430 °F air circulation.

2.7.12 Rhubarb, roasted

Fructose   ☺

Fructans + galactans   ☺

Lactose   ☺

Sorbitol   ☺

What you need (five servings):

1 and 1/3 cup of Rhubarb

1/3 cup of brown sugar

Preparation:

Preheat the oven at 390 °F top and bottom heat or 360 °F air circulation. Wash the Rhubarb then shake off the water. Cut the end and the middle of the sticks into small finger-sized pieces. Cover a closed baking tray with a baking sheet and spread the Rhubarb on it. Sprinkle some sugar over it and cover the Rhubarb with it. Bake the Rhubarb for about 15 minutes with baking paper on top. Then remove the baking paper and shake the plate slightly. Then continue baking for about five minutes. When the Rhubarb is ready, it is soft, but not mushy.

2.7.13 Rhubarb cake

Fructose	☺
Fructans + galactans	1 and ½ pieces
Lactose	☺
Sorbitol	☺

What you need:

One packet of baking powder (celiac disease? Use gluten-free baking powder)
Four large eggs
One cup of flour (celiac disease? Use gluten free flour)
Icing sugar
Pre-roasted Rhubarb, as described before.
One cup of sweet cream butter and even something for the baking tray
One tsp. vanilla extract
3/5 cup of custard
One cup of brown sugar

Preparation:

First, prepare the roasted Rhubarb and drain the juice. Preheat now the oven at 390 °F top and bottom heat or 180 degrees air circulation. Wipe a nine in cake springform pan with butter. Put 3 tbsp. of the vanilla pudding in a separate bowl. The rest you whisk up creamy with butter, the flour, baking powder, eggs and sugar in a bowl. Pour one-third of the mix in the cake form and place about half of the Rhubarb over it. Put one more third of dough over this layer and flatten it as smooth as possible. Cover the top with the rest of the Rhubarb and pour the remaining mixture over it, this time, the surface remains rough. Then use the remaining 3 tbsp. of the vanilla pudding to place on top. Bake the cake for 40 minutes, until it rises and becomes golden. Cover it with baking paper and leave it baking for another 15 minutes. The cake is ready when you stab it with a toothpick, and it comes out clean. Sprinkle some icing sugar over the cake after it cooled down.

2.7.14 Rhubarb-smoothie

Fructose	☺
Fructans + galactans	One serving
Lactose	☺
Sorbitol	☹

What you need (for two servings):

One small banana
One cup of cranberry juice
2/5 cup of frozen Rhubarb
Five tbsp. (1/2 cups) of vanilla yogurt or lactose-free vanilla yogurt (1/2 cup)

Preparation:

Cut the banana into small pieces and puree everything together in a blender.

2.7.15 Rucola salad

Fructose	☺
Fructans + galactans	3 servings
Lactose	½ to ¾ serving
Sorbitol	☺

What you need (for 2-3 servings):

Four tsp. vinegar from vinegar essence-water mixture
Two cups of grill cheese (e.g., halumi)
Three tbsp. of olive oil
Three medium, skinned oranges
One small bunch of chopped peppermint
3/5 cup of Rocket salad
1/5 cup (3 tbsp.) of roasted walnuts

Preparation:

Heat up a pan in which you fry the 1/3 in. sized grill cheese slices for about 1 to 2 minutes until they begin to melt. Mix the oranges with the juice from the peeling; the mint leaves and the vinegar gently in a bowl. Now add the walnuts and the rocket salad and mix well. Place the cheese slices on top. Finally, season the salad with black pepper - good appetite.

2.7.16 Spaghetti al salmone

Fructose   ☺
Fructans + galactans   ¼ serving
Lactose   ☺
Sorbitol   ☺

What you need (for 2-3 portions):

Two small finely ground chillies
Four tbsp. capers without the water from the glass
Two cloves of garlic
½ cup of mL extra virgin olive oil
4/5 cup of rocket salad
Two cups of spaghetti (celiac disease? Use gluten-free pasta)
200g salmon pieces
Two tbsp. of small cubes of white bread (celiac disease? Use gluten-free bread or go without croutons)
Lemon zest, meaning the yellow skin of a well-washed lemon

Preparation:

Heat up two tbsp. of olive oil in the pan and toast in the bread cubes over medium heat for three to four minutes, until golden brown. Place in a small bowl afterwards. Cook the spaghetti in salted water until al dente. Meanwhile, squeeze out the garlic cloves and heat the garlic with the chili powder and the remaining oil in the pan. Please make sure not to fry the garlic. Let the pasta drain and place them in a preheated bowl. Next, put the grated lemon zest and capers into the oil. Pour it over the pasta and spread it well. At last, you mix everything with the salmon and the rocket salad. Sprinkle the croutons over it before serving—et voila.

2.7.17 Sweet potato- or salami & pesto-pizza

Fructose   ☺
Fructans + galactans   ½ Pizza
Lactose   ¼ Pizza
Sorbitol   ☺

What you need (for two servings):

3/5 cup of ciabatta bread-dough mixture
½ cup of mozzarella balls
Two tsp. Olive oil, one for pizza and one for the baking tray
Two tbsp. green pesto
A handful of rocket salad
4/g cup of sweet potatoes (or salami)

Preparation:

Peel the potatoes, cut them into slices and boil them for 15 minutes in salted water. Then drain and let cool down briefly. Meanwhile, preheat the oven to 430 °F. Form the dough into a pizza shape and place it on a pre-oiled baking sheet. Now wait for 15 minutes. Spread the pesto on the pizza base. Sprinkle half of the mozzarella over it. The next layer is the potatoes (or salami) and on top of it is the rest of the mozzarella. Let the pizza bake for 15 to 18 minutes until the crust is golden brown and the cheese bubbles. Finally, put the rocket salad on the pizza and season with black pepper.

2.7.18 Tuna pizza

Fructose	☺
Fructans + galactans	One piece of pizza
Lactose	One piece of pizza
Sorbitol	☺

What you need (for eight servings):

A pack of cream cheese (225g)
2/3 cup of finely sliced mozzarella
Pepper
One and 2/3 cups (400g) pizza dough (celiac disease? Use gluten-free dough)
Small bunch chives
A can of tuna

Preparation:

Preheat the oven to 430 °F. Bake the dough briefly. Spread the cream cheese over it. Now cover the pizza base with tuna and mozzarella, season the pizza with pepper and finish baking. Meanwhile, wash the chives and cut it finely to spread it on the pizza, when it is ready.

2.7.19 Tropical fruit salad

Fructose	½ Portion
Fructans + galactans	☺
Lactose	☺
Sorbitol	☺

What you need (six servings):

One and 2/3 cups of pieced cantaloupe
Two peeled kiwis
One and 2/3 cups of lychees
Three peeled oranges
Two stalks of lemongrass
1/3 cup of brown sugar

Preparation:

Cut the lemon grass into pieces and crush it with a rolling pin. Peel the lychees and remove the seeds, catch the juice. Mix the juice with the sugar and the lemongrass and heat it up for about a minute in a pan until the sugar has melted. Then let the broth cool down and sprinkle it over the fruits.

2.8   Stress management

tress can affect your stomach and worsen irritable bowel symptoms. Hence, it is important to reduce it. To find out its effect on you, fill out your symptom-test-sheet on a day when you have a lot of stress. Developing a solution-oriented way to manage your worries can help you do so. How does that help? The more you stress over something, the more brain areas that you need for a reasonable decision are being set off. The body does so, because, in a certain way, our bodies are prepared for an earlier historical era. Dangerous situations like an attack by a wolf pack left us with three options: fight, flight or playing dead. If we spent too much time thinking in such a situation, it was game over! Hence, we are poled to stop thinking as soon as we feel we are in danger—which is not always helpful in our modern time.

If nowadays your boss storms into your office with some tricky and pressing demands of a huge client, neither a spontaneous attack nor jumping out of the window or acting as dead will be recommendable. Seriously, nowadays usually much different factors trigger stress than it was a few thousand years ago. Aside from noise, extreme temperatures, and air pollution, it is especially the feeling of losing control in a situation, which feels threatening to us. Fear can grab you, when a project is particularly delicate and important, something fundamental has to change, and you are under time pressure.

At the advent of fear, the release of hormones supports fight and flight reactions that enable us to make quick, even if ill-conceived, decisions. Everything inside of you screams "Do something immidiately, no matter what!" Large parts of our brain are set aside for that purpose. You feel stress and tend to make impulsive rather than rational decisions. The hormones lead to a shut down of vast areas of your brain at that moment; you feel stress. The third option your mind conceives in a dangerous situation, playing dead, somewhat corresponds to the extreme modern-day phenomena that is widely known as burnout.

So you have the impulses of a Stone Age hunter but the tasks of a top manager: how can you make that fit together? The only option you have to resist your impulse is to take command of your body and mind. To react appropriately, you are required not to have your hormones to turn off your resources for rational decision-making.

Once your body feels in danger, it is a challenge to halt the rolling wheel of your body's emergency reactions abruptly. Hence, the best thing you can do is to prevent these stress reactions from evolving in the first place. Yoga and progressive muscle relaxation before work are useful stress preventers. Using such techniques before going to work is sensible, as it is seldom possible to take an hour off during the workday. Breaks and disruptions during your working hours are also **counterproductive** if you are dealing with complex tasks; they often lead to poor decisions, more stress, and a short temper. Thus, try to avoid disruption when dealing with sophisticated tasks. You will agree if you imagine working on a complex calculation while your phone is ringing and your colleague enters to chat with you and a technician wanting to maintain your printer is waiting in front of the door. Therefore, try to avoid distractions when you are dealing with challenging tasks.

However, interruptions of simple mental or physical labor lasting a few minutes, rather than seconds, result in slight positive effects. Taking breaks from hard physical labor, meanwhile, show even stronger benefits, lowering the risk of injuries and enhancing endurance. You do not want to be following a printer printing during your break. To make the best use of it, close your eyes and focus on your breathing. Whenever thoughts come up, focus your whole attention bad on your breath without evaluating the thoughts. What makes this better is counting the times that you breathe out and feeling your breath leave your mouth.

Still, relaxation alone might not be the solution. Often, you can identify general worries that effect your mood. So how do you deal with such concerns? Many try to evade them by trying to ignore them, distract themselves or even take alcohol or other supposed comforters. Instead of bringing you closer to your goal, such a reaction, makes matters worse in most cases. The only thing that will help you resolve your troublesome thoughts is actively dealing with them. Only if you can name them, you can find solutions. Also, consider this; ignorance may well be one of the leading causes of failure.

Of course, for most worries no one hands you the solution on a silver platter. You have to take action. An open examination of your concerns and the right strategy can lead you towards a feasible solution. There is an immediate positive effect of this, independent from what solution you find: you avoid panic actions that one tends to in charged situations. If you regularly call a spade a spade and rationally seek solutions to situations you worry about you reduce the number of poor decisions.

By doing so, you can even use your fears—through the process of conquering them—to help you become more successful in your everyday life. What I recommend you do is sit down at a quiet desk at the beginning or end of the day. Next, think about what you are worried about right now and which steps you need to take to prevent the feared outcomes.

It is helpful to create an Excel spreadsheet for doing so or to purchase the standardized and printer-optimized edition at *www.Laxiba.com*. If you want to create the table by yourself, call the first sheet "Worries" and the second one "Task List." Next, write down the following task headings in the first spreadsheet: "Current Worries," "Preventive Measure A," "Preventive Measure B" and "Preventive Measure C." Then enter the following column titles in the second spreadsheet: "Task," "Priority," "Deadline," "Who does it?" and "Done."

You should write down your concerns in the first column of the first sheet. Then, think about what you will need to do to prevent these worries from becoming a reality. Think of three alternatives for each outcome. Enter these into the "Preventive Measure A–C" fields next to each worry, A being the action you want to take first. Then, transfer "Preventive Measure A" to the "Task List" sheet. Next, prioritize the tasks by employing an adapted version of the "Eisenhower method," an organization technique that takes importance and urgency into account, from A to E:

Task is important	**A** *ction now*	**B** *etter do it soon*
Task is unimportant	**C** *hance to do the task if you completed all A and B duties.*	**D** *ull moment task*
E *fface, don't do task*	**Task is urgent**	**Postponable task**

In the order from A to D, you then execute your duties on a daily basis. The category E is for tasks that are ineffective and therefore, you leave it. Hence, you prevent worrying and free yourself from doubting whether you are currently doing the right thing. After assessing the tasks from A to D, you fill out the column "Deadline," into which you enter the date at which you want to accomplish the task. Furthermore, you either note "I" or the name of the person that you want to delegate the work to in the column "Who does it?" Finally, you tick off the cell in the column „Done", when you have finished the task.

Another important aspect is keeping your life balanced. A fulfilled family life and friendships also help to improve your stress resistance. To name an example: taking a healthy exercise is beneficial for all areas of your life. Brought to an extreme, though, let's say if you spend ten hours per day at a fitness center, this will take too much of your time away from your other areas—unless you are a personal trainer. The four quadrants of your life are like the four legs of a stool you sit on. Let us call it your life-stool. If each leg is just as long as the others and all are adequately thick, you will sit well and safe. In however you chop off some from one or more legs repeatedly and strengthen another leg, you will start to waggle—until at some point, there is a crack, and you land on your patoot. You have to avoid this "breakdown". Of course, I know that this is exactly the dilemma that burdens many people nowadays. You feel that you have to perform continuously in all areas. Fathers do not only have to work. They also have to spend time with their family. They ought to bring their children to the violin tuition. Then in the evening, they should foster their social contacts and engage in the summer festival of their city. Having a well-trained body is necessary for many. On top of that, you ideally are relaxed and well groomed. For woman and mothers, the expectations are just as high. They feel like they have to perform like men at work and still manage their family, organize the spare time and stay fit. Expectations appear to rise everywhere.

So do not get me wrong: keeping your life in a healthy balance means finding the **right** balance between those things that are important to you personally. It is not about which expectations others have concerning your life's quadrants! It is not about what the society expects from you. What is important is that you consider the key aspects of your individual life. In the table below these are work, relaxation, family and spare time. For you, the quadrants may be different. You set the priorities yourself. Free yourself as much as possible from the influence of the acknowledgment by others, follow the saying "great horses jump tight" and develop a healthy self-confidence and composure.

Instead of delivering an over-the-top performance in one area but lousy results in all others, you want to do at least a satisfying job in all sectors, to remain capable in the end. Which of the family, spare time, relaxation and work quadrants are important is up to you, along with the results you are aiming for with them, such as spending time with those closest to you, taking daily walks, pursuing your hobbies and getting your work done properly. Furthermore, it is important to resist basing your success on external measures. You should nourish a healthy self-confidence and serenity in yourself. Thus, you need to know when finished the task you are doing well enough. Some people get into time trouble because they over deliver on some tasks and then have little time left to take care of other important tasks, which then causes stress. Often it takes 80% of the time to improve on the last 20% of a job, so it pays off if you know if the last 20% are worth it.

Family:	**Relaxation:**
Spend time with those closest to you	*Go out for a walk on a daily basis*
Spare time:	**Work:**
Pursue your hobbies regularly	*Get your work done properly*

You can measure your progress about the four quadrants on a monthly basis on a scale of 1 (very good) to 7 (very poor). Always assign 7 points to the area that you are happiest with and other numbers to the remaining quadrants in relation to that one. Afterward, consider whether you want to make any changes to how you are approaching these areas of your life and how you can make those changes. You can also use the spreadsheet you created to manage your worries.

One final point on the topic of stress, even if it may seem trivial: be mindful of your mood, and try to stay upbeat! What you need to do that depends on you. Your mood only partially depends on circumstances. Sometimes simply deciding to be in a good mood can do more than most people realize. Everyone has a load of problems to carry, and it is easier to take it if you commit yourself to a positive outlook.

Do things that excite you as often as possible. Perform activities that contribute to what is most important to you. Is it your family? Then plan an excursion with your family! Is it a sport? Then ask someone to go jogging with you, for example. Consciously take the time to do those things that are close to your heart. Maybe you now object that you do not have time for that and that such self-serving activities would only lead to more stress. Try it out! I bet this qualitatively precious time will not incur losses but help you to mount every day with more tranquility. Plan your activities around what is most important to you in your life. What that means is obviously personal to you! It is your treasure, per se, so you have to dig it out yourself. *Abraham Lincoln* had this to say, to send you on your way: "That some achieve great success is proof to all that others can achieve it as well."

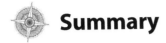

Summary

Stress can foster irritable bowel syndrome and intolerance symptoms. Increase your resistance to stress by training to use relaxation techniques, naming fears and worries, developing and noting down solution strategies and adding priorities to them. Make sure you keep your life in the right balance by trading-off between the areas that are important to you. Keep your eye on your goal.

2.9   General summary

1. What you are dealing with

Do you have an irritable bowel syndrome or an intolerance and symptoms? Then certain probably certain food ingredients irritate your gut. The symptoms occur because of your body's limited capacity to absorb the respective trigger substance before it reaches the large intestine, where it causes the discomforts. IBS and food intolerances are often a chronic but do not cause cancer. In most cases, following a fitting diet reduces the symptoms to an acceptable level.

2. Are you a unique case?

According to the *World Gastroenterology Organisation (WGO)*, up to one billion people have a dietary intolerance or IBS around the globe. In a way, you are lucky, as you can use this book to help you to reduce your symptoms.

3. Good reasons to follow this diet

An intolerance accompanies you for a long time, maybe for the rest of your life. If the diet works, it is far cheaper than medical treatment and sometimes even more efficient. Many medicines also have side effects. By examining different triggers one by one, you can find the one(s) that your body cannot tolerate. You learn, as well, how to balance your diet despite reducing the consumption of certain foods. If the diet works for you, it will also lead to a general improvement in your wellbeing. You should find that you are ill less often, better able to concentrate, better at fulfilling social obligations, stronger at sports—your new diet can even enhance your love life!

4. Why you want to take the level test

Sensitivities differ in their severity. The fewer dietary restrictions you face, the more you save yourself the effort and can enjoy a more varied selection of food.

5. What you should pay attention to for the diet

Two things: First, adhere to your portion sizes, which you find in the tables for your trigger. Thus, only eat as much of the trigger containing foods as your enzyme workers can handle. If you have a fructose or lactose intolerance, you should keep eating foods containing the trigger(s) in tolerable amounts, as fruits contain healthy vitamins and cheese vital fatty acids. Second, eat in a balanced way by consuming oats, fiber, and proteins each day, see Chapter 2.1.4.

6. Dealing with setbacks

You have decided to change your diet and have made the first steps in that direction. Now, you have to stick to it. Moreover, that means to assess properly short-term setbacks. Rebounds are a part of any change process. What is important is that you get back up! The experience of meeting success after facing a blow will strengthen you immensely and ensure that you will be able to get back up even faster next time around. At some point, your experiences and successes will make it a habit for you to persevere and stick to your diet.

It may help you to set a time each Sunday to fill out the symptom test sheet—independent of the other tests. Doing this will remind you of your goal and let you break down the necessary steps toward it on a weekly basis. What is also important is that you become aware of the hurdles you will face. It will be hard to restrict yourself concerning the consumption of some foods that you have come to love. Particularly at the beginning, it will be unnerving to ask for dietary considerations as a dinner guest. Your nutrition plan will be new to others; you may feel criticized for your insistence on maintaining your new eating habits. Explain that you need to do it for the sake of your health. At the same time, express your appreciation for others' support. Moreover, try not giving dietary advice unless someone asks you for it — respecting the eating habits of others. They are more likely to accept yours in turn.

The adversary left for you to face is not standing next to you at the buffet and believes to know better what you can consume. The best captains are always standing ashore. The adversary is in your head and regularly cries "do it as you did it before. Before it was easier!" The influence of our old habits is often greater than we think. After a few days of tenacity, this caller has his big appearance. As soon, as our vigilance is lower he whispers in our ear "This is how you have always done it, and it has always been good, everything else is too exhaustive for you. Simply, show your adversary your weekly symptom test sheet--it works like garlic against vampires. It is the best mean to get rid of old habits, and form new ones! If you always readjust your heading—your diet to your goal, you will come close to it in the end. If you proceed like that, you have a good chance to win against the trigger and old habit imp.

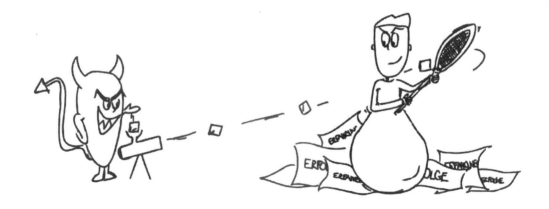

7. FAQs

What do you recommend concerning the diet? Drink at least 1.5 L of water every day. Eat a variety of foods. Even if you are lactose intolerant, you can try to eat dry cheese (for example) to cover your need for short-chain fatty acids. If you are fructose intolerant, try to eat as many fruits as you can to ensure a natural supply of vitamins. If you are a vegan, you should plan your protein intake, and consider your fiber consumption, if you are restricting your fructans and galactans intake. In addition to following your portion sizes and taking in flaxseeds or rice bran and a handful of nuts, you might also like to eat beans, lentils, peas and so forth. It is ok to eat foods that contain your trigger(s); they can even be good for you as long as you keep within your restrictions. The latter does not apply to people with celiac disease and hereditary fructose intolerance, may not apply to people with sorbitol intolerance and concerning the other conditions covered in other chapters you should discuss this with your doctor. To do even more for your health, work out regularly.

What can you do if a drink contains too much of your trigger(s) to drink a regular glass full? By diluting it with water, you can multiply your tolerable portion. Another option in case of fructose or lactose intolerance is to take fitting enzyme capsules.

How can you save on cooking time? Cook larger portion sizes. Usually, it only takes a little longer than preparing small ones, and warming the food up is quick. You can keep rice and potatoes in the fridge for days, for instance. Purchase lockable glass containers to store your food keeping it fresh longer.

I have acute symptoms, what can I do? Take a walk and drink up to three liters of drinking water per day.

8. The LAXIBA® quickie

Fructans galactans sensitivity: Eat fewer beans, lentils, peas and grain products, such as pastries and noodles.

Fructose intolerance: Avoid apple and peach juices and drink orange juice instead, for example. Be careful with sweet non-alcoholic beverages.

Lactose intolerance: Reduce your consumption of milk or use replacement products such as rice milk. Dry cheese like cheddar contains only a little lactose.

Sorbitol intolerance: Be wary of diabetic, diet and light products, as well as dried fruit.

Do not start any diet, especially one for celiac disease, without a proper diagnosis in advance. The gluten free products contain fewer healthy nutrients but are free from the symptom trigger for people with celiac disease. If you want to do something for your health, in general, stick to the advice see the Chapters starting on pages 69 and 120.

FEEDBACK

Congratulations, you have mastered the background and strategy chapter. I hope that you have found the trigger(s) of your symptoms. Around the globe, the brand *LAXIBA* represents an improved quality of life in connection with abdominal diseases and stress. Our goal is to offer you scientific solutions that you can implement swiftly to improve your life. To find out about our latest innovations, visit us at *https://laxiba.com* and register for our useletter.

Many improvements make this second edition the gold standard. Each contribution can help to make the book even better in the future. Thus, I am glad to learn about your experiences and your wishes! There are still grey areas, and regularly new foods enter the market that fit our tables well. To deal with the disease, it is important that you adapt your diet to the capacity of your enzyme workers. Therefore, we are interested in any food you are missing.

Would you like to take part in a coaching concerning the implementation of the diet or a workshop on stress management? We will have an offer that suits you. Visit us at *https://laxiba.com*. We look forward to getting to know you. Finally, I wish you prosperity, happiness and an improvement in your quality of life.

Your author,

Jan Stratbucker – *John@Laxiba.com*

3

FOOD TABLES

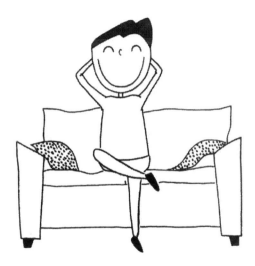

3.1 Introduction to the tables

In the following section, you will learn about the tolerable portion sizes for IBS as well as an intolerance towards fructose, fructans, galactans, lactose and sorbitol (the sum of nine sugar-alcohols). If you cannot take the breath test, stick to the IBS diet for three weeks before continuing with the substitute test. The statements all relate to **one meal**, assuming **three meals** per day and that only eat one food containing your trigger. The stated amounts expect you to consume three meals per day, one at roughly 7 am, 1 pm and 7 pm, i.e., each with about **six hours** in between. However, the times are mainly just a reference point just make sure to keep the gaps! If you read the book carefully, you have also learned that eating in between the big meals can have a positive effect on your health. For each food, you can find out how much you can tolerate both in a suitable unit as well as in gram. These statements make cooking as well as eating out easy.

The lists are ordered by category. Apple juice is listed under beverages-juices, for example. The idea behind this is that you can easily find alternatives should your tolerated amount be small. At the end of the tables, you also find a food index, though, see page 501, which you can use if you are solely interested in finding out how much orange juice you can stomach. The tables are set up in a manner that is easy to understand. For each trigger, you find one page. Next to lactose stands the sum of fructans and galactans, as sometimes a fructans and galactans sensitivity accompanies a lactose intolerance. Following is fructose and next to it is sorbitol. Each page contains about 14 foods. In the tables, you find the category title in the first cell of each table. Below it, you can see the food names and next to them the tolerated amount explained by a proper unit or a smiley. Afterward, you find an explanation as well as the amount in gram. This procedure also concerns the B-factors for fructose—they indicate that the food is free of fructose and contains glucose. Due to this fact, you enhance your ability to eat foods containing fructose if you eat glucose containing foods with it. For the first time, the tables account for the interactions of fructose with glucose sorbitol as well as all nine sugar-alcohols to determine the sorbitol portion sizes to allow for a more reliable diet. For lactose, you also find the additionally consumable amount per lactase capsule with 12,000 FCC regarding the selected unit as well as in gram in the last column. In the following the symbols and units will be explained further.

It is important to us that the data quality is excellent. Except for fructans and galactans, all figures originate from an analysis conducted by the *University of Minnesota*. Note: If you only suffer from fructose but not sorbitol intolerance, it is sufficient if you eat according to the fructose table only as the amount of sorbitol has already been accounted for there.

Note if you have a sorbitol intolerance: Even if you stick to the standard portion sizes in the following tables, look at the low sensitivity amount as well. If the amount there is high, you can probably tolerate the food, because the standard portion sizes mean that you completely avoid sorbitol.

3.1.1   Explanation of the symbols

Here you will find an explanation of the symbols, assuming you find them in the fructose lists. The symbols show you at a glance how many units you can tolerate of the respective food. If you can see a smiley in the list, you will not find an amount. If the smiley looks sad, you should avoid the product if you have a fructose intolerance. If it smiles, you can enjoy it to your heart's content—if there is a big smile this also hold if you have a hereditary fructose intolerance.

Symbol	Meaning
	An average sized potion
	Slice(s)
	Piece(s)
	Hand(s) full
	Tablespoon(s)
	Bar
	Pinch
	Cup, 150 mL
	Glass, 200 mL
	Avoid the consumption. You can tolerate less than ¼ of the lowest amount due to the high fructose load of the food.
	Nearly free of fructose, hence, you can tolerate it unless you suffer from a hereditary fructose intolerance. Note: For fructans, galactans, lactose and sorbitol this food is safe, as the hereditary issue is unique to fructose (unless your doctor tells you otherwise).

Free consumption as the food is free of fructose.

Glucose

The food is free of fructose. Moreover, it contains more glucose than fructose. Thus, the simultaneous intake of a portion measurement unit of the respective food can enable you to eat up to B-[number] times the amount of other fructose-containing foods. To be on the safe side, divide the [number] by two, as you partially absorb glucose by the mouth and sometimes the food you do not chew thoroughly. Hence, to profit from the glucose of another food, you should either mix both in advance or chew them together.

For example, for an ice cream you find "B ×3". For grapes, the tolerated amount is ¼. Hence, if you eat the grapes together with the ice cream, you can now consume ¼ plus ¼ ×3 and thus 1 unit. If you want to be on the safe side, divide the B-number by two, and you can consume about half a unit of grapes. Hint: If you can tolerate more than the standard amount, be aware that the B-multiplier works for the norm level only, i.e. calculate the additionally consumable amount by using the standard amount in the table.

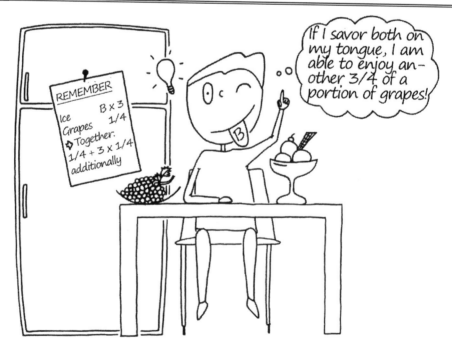

3.1.2 Explanation of the statements

Label	Meaning
Standard amount	In this column, you find the name of the unit or the meaning of the smiley. Behind it, in brackets, is stated how much gram one unit has followed by the tolerated amount per meal in total. For products that contain more glucose than fructose, you will also find the B-factor definition.
¼, ½, ¾, 1, 1¼, 1½, 1¾, 2, etc.	The tolerated amount of the respective unit, e.g., "cookie ½ piece" means you tolerate half a cookie of the type per meal, and "soup 1¾ portion" means one and three-fourths of a portion of the soup.
Avoid consumption.	Avoid the consumption of the food; it contains much of the respective trigger.
Avoid consumption!	Avoid the consumption of the food; it contains very much of the respective trigger.
Avoid consumption!!	Avoid the consumption of the food; it contains an extreme load of the respective trigger.
Lactase capsules	In the last column, you can find the additionally consumable amount per strong, 12,000 FCC, lactase capsule. Important: The additionally consumable amount is independent of your sensitivity level. For example, you can find + ¼ for an ice cream. The tolerable amount (stated in the column in front of it) is a ¼ portion, 28g. Now, per lactase capsule you take, you can tolerate ¼ of a portion in addition to the amount your enzyme workers can cover themselves. Doing the math, we get ¼ + ¼, which makes ½ a portion (56g). You can purchase fitting lactase capsules on our homepage, https://laxiba.com.
F+G amount	Here you find the portion sizes if you take the fructans and galactans diet. The sources for these values are: Biesiekierski et al., 2011; Muir et al., 2009; Muir et al., 2007; Shepherd and Gibson, 2006; van Loo et al., 1995; Muir et al., 2007; Van Loo et al., 1995 as well as Monash University, 2014.

Note: Please always look at the ingredients as stated on the food packages as well. Especially, if the list does not mention a producer, the composition may vary. In addition, you should consider the weight of one unit in gram. The average portion sizes underlying the statements may be larger or smaller than you expect. For example, 30g of cornflakes can fill an entire bowl while you can eat 30g of dark whole grain bread in three bites. If you suffer from a fructose intolerance only, it is sufficient to base your consumption decisions on the fructose portions only, as the sorbitol has been accounted for here already. For sorbitol, the low sensitivity amount column in the tables refers to sensitivity level 1 and the standard amount to level 0.

3.1.3   Your personal sensitivity levels

Level multiplier and tolerable amount per meal by level

Trigger	Level	g	Table amount multiplier	Your level
Fructose g/meal	Standard	0.5	base	
	1	1	×2	
	2	2	×4	
	3	3	×6	
Lactose g/meal	0	1.5	÷2	
	Standard	3	base	
	2	6	×2	
	3	9	×3	
Sorbitol and other sugar alcohols g/meal	Standard	0	×0	
	1	0.1	base	
	2	0.4	×4	
	3	0.7	×7	
Fructans and galactans g/meal	Standard	0.5	base	
	1	1	×2	
	2	2	×4	
	3	3	×6	

CATEGORY LIST-INDEX

3.2 Athletes

Athletes	LACTOSE		Standard amount	
Clif Bar®, Chocolate Chip	9		Piece (68g); 612g in total.	+7½
Clif Bar®, Crunchy Peanut Butter		🙂	Free of lactose.	
Clif Bar®, Oatmeal Raisin Walnut		🙂	Free of lactose.	
Electrolyte replacement drink		🙂	Free of lactose.	
Gatorade®, all flavors	6¼		Glass (240g); 1,500 mL in total.	+5
Gatorade®, from dry mix, all flavors		🙂	Free of lactose.	
Glaceau® Vitaminwater 10		🙂	Free of lactose.	
Glaceau® Vitaminwater Energy		🙂	Free of lactose.	
Glaceau® Vitaminwater Essential		🙂	Free of lactose.	
Glaceau® Vitaminwater Focus		🙂	Free of lactose.	
Glaceau® Vitaminwater Power-C		🙂	Free of lactose.	
Glaceau® Vitaminwater Revive		🙂	Free of lactose.	
High-protein Bar, generic	39¼		Piece (65g); 2,551g in total.	+32¾
Power Bar® 20g Protein Plus, Chocolate Crisp	3		Piece (61g); 183g in total.	+2½
Power Bar® 20g Protein Plus, Chocolate Peanut Butter	3		Piece (61g); 183g in total.	+2½

Athletes	IBS	Standard amount	F+G	amount
Clif Bar®, Chocolate Chip	¾ 🍰	Piece (68g); 51g in total.	¾ 🍰	
Clif Bar®, Crunchy Peanut Butter	2½ 🍰	Piece (68g); 170g in total.	🙂	
Clif Bar®, Oatmeal Raisin Walnut	1¾ 🍰	Piece (68g); 119g in total.	1¾ 🍰	
Electrolyte replacement drink	🙂	Free of triggers.	🙂	
Gatorade®, all flavors	7½ 🥛	Glass (200g); 1,500 mL in total.	41½ 🥛	
Gatorade®, from dry mix, all flavors	🙂	Free of triggers.	🙂	
Glaceau® Vitaminwater 10	🙁	Avoid consumption!	🙂	
Glaceau® Vitaminwater Energy	🙁	Avoid consumption!	🙂	
Glaceau® Vitaminwater Essential	🙁	Avoid consumption!	🙂	
Glaceau® Vitaminwater Focus	🙁	Avoid consumption!	🙂	
Glaceau® Vitaminwater Power-C	🙁	Avoid consumption!	🙂	
Glaceau® Vitaminwater Revive	🙁	Avoid consumption!	🙂	
High-protein Bar, generic	¾ 🍰	Piece (65g); 49g in total.	🙂	
Power Bar® 20g Protein Plus, Chocolate Crisp	🙁	Avoid consumption!!	4 🍰	
Power Bar® 20g Protein Plus, Chocolate Peanut Butter	🙁	Avoid consumption!!	17 🍰	

Athletes	FRUCTOSE		Standard amount
Clif Bar®, Chocolate Chip	B ×10	😊+	Free of fructose. Per Piece (68g) you eat with it, add B-no × F-limit.
Clif Bar®, Crunchy Peanut Butter	B ×10	😊+	Free of fructose. Per Piece (68g) you eat with it, add B-no × F-limit.
Clif Bar®, Oatmeal Raisin Walnut	B ×10	😊+	Free of fructose. Per Piece (68g) you eat with it, add B-no × F-limit.
Electrolyte replacement drink	B ×9¾	😊+	Free of fructose. Per Glass (200 mL) you drink with it, add B-no × F-limit.
Gatorade®, all flavors	B ×1¼	😊+	Free of fructose. Per Glass (200 mL) you drink with it, add B-no × F-limit.
Gatorade®, from dry mix, all flavors	B ×10	😊+	Free of fructose. Per Glass (200 mL) you drink with it, add B-no × F-limit.
Glaceau® Vitaminwater 10		☹	Avoid consumption.
Glaceau® Vitaminwater Energy		☹	Avoid consumption!
Glaceau® Vitaminwater Essential		☹	Avoid consumption!
Glaceau® Vitaminwater Focus		☹	Avoid consumption!
Glaceau® Vitaminwater Power-C		☹	Avoid consumption!
Glaceau® Vitaminwater Revive		☹	Avoid consumption!
High-protein Bar, generic	¾	🍰	Piece (65g); 49g in total.
Power Bar® 20g Protein Plus, Chocolate Crisp		☹	Avoid consumption!
Power Bar® 20g Protein Plus, Chocolate Peanut Butter		☹	Avoid consumption!!

Athletes	Sorbitol standard		SORBITOL Low sensitivity amount	
Clif Bar®, Chocolate Chip	☹	Avoid	2¼ 🍰	Piece (68g); 153g in total.
Clif Bar®, Crunchy Peanut Butter	☹	Avoid	2½ 🍰	Piece (68g); 170g in total.
Clif Bar®, Oatmeal Raisin Walnut	☹	Avoid	1¾ 🍰	Piece (68g); 119g in total.
Electrolyte replacement drink	☺	Free	☺	Free of sorbitol.
Gatorade®, all flavors	☺	Free	☺	Free of sorbitol.
Gatorade®, from dry mix, all flavors	☺	Free	☺	Free of sorbitol.
Glaceau® Vitaminwater 10	☹	Avoid	☹	Avoid consumption!!
Glaceau® Vitaminwater Energy	☺	Free	☺	Free of sorbitol.
Glaceau® Vitaminwater Essential	☺	Free	☺	Free of sorbitol.
Glaceau® Vitaminwater Focus	☺	Free	☺	Free of sorbitol.
Glaceau® Vitaminwater Power-C	☺	Free	☺	Free of sorbitol.
Glaceau® Vitaminwater Revive	☺	Free	☺	Free of sorbitol.
High-protein Bar, generic	☹	Avoid	76¾ 🍰	Piece (65g); 4,989g in total.
Power Bar® 20g Protein Plus, Chocolate Crisp	☹	Avoid	☹	Avoid consumption!!
Power Bar® 20g Protein Plus, Chocolate Peanut Butter	☹	Avoid	☹	Avoid consumption!!

Athletes	LACTOSE	Standard amount	
Power Bar® 30g Protein Plus, Chocolate Brownie	2	Piece (70g); 140g in total.	+1½
Power Bar® Harvest Energy®, Double Chocolate Crisp	2¾	Piece (65g); 179g in total.	+2¼
Power Bar® Performance Energy®, Banana		Free of lactose.	
Power Bar® Performance Energy®, Chocolate		Free of lactose.	
Power Bar® Performance Energy®, Cookie Dough		Free of lactose.	
Power Bar® Performance Energy®, Mixed Berry Blast		Free of lactose.	
Power Bar® Performance Energy®, Vanilla Crisp		Free of lactose.	
Powerade®, all flavors	6¼	Glass (240g); 1,500 mL in total.	+5

Athletes	IBS Standard amount		F+G amount	
Power Bar® 30g Protein Plus, Chocolate Brownie	2	Piece (70g); 140g in total.	3¼	
Power Bar® Harvest Energy®, Double Chocolate Crisp	¼	Piece (65g); 16g in total.	¼	
Power Bar® Performance Energy®, Banana	¼	Piece (65g); 16g in total.	10½	
Power Bar® Performance Energy®, Chocolate	¼	Piece (65g); 16g in total.	3¼	
Power Bar® Performance Energy®, Cookie Dough	¼	Piece (65g); 16g in total.	10½	
Power Bar® Performance Energy®, Mixed Berry Blast	¼	Piece (65g); 16g in total.	10½	
Power Bar® Performance Energy®, Vanilla Crisp	¼	Piece (65g); 16g in total.	10½	
Powerade®, all flavors	7½	Glass (200g); 1,500 mL in total.	41½	

Athletes	FRUCTOSE		Standard amount
Power Bar® 30g Protein Plus, Chocolate Brownie	B ×1½	☺+	Free of fructose. Per Piece (70g) you eat with it, add B-no × F-limit.
Power Bar® Harvest Energy®, Double Chocolate Crisp	B ×5¾	☺+	Free of fructose. Per Piece (65g) you eat with it, add B-no × F-limit.
Power Bar® Performance Energy®, Banana	¼		Piece (65g); 16g in total.
Power Bar® Performance Energy®, Chocolate	¼		Piece (65g); 16g in total.
Power Bar® Performance Energy®, Cookie Dough	¼		Piece (65g); 16g in total.
Power Bar® Performance Energy®, Mixed Berry Blast	¼		Piece (65g); 16g in total.
Power Bar® Performance Energy®, Vanilla Crisp	¼		Piece (65g); 16g in total.
Powerade®, all flavors	B ×1¼	☺+	Free of fructose. Per Glass (200 mL) you drink with it, add B-no × F-limit.

Athletes	SORBITOL Stand.		SORBITOL Low sensitivity amount	
Power Bar® 30g Protein Plus, Chocolate Brownie	☺	Nearly free	☺	Nearly free of sorbitol
Power Bar® Harvest Energy®, Double Chocolate Crisp	☹	Avoid	10¾	Piece (65g); 699g in total.
Power Bar® Performance Energy®, Banana	☺	Nearly free	☺	Nearly free of sorbitol
Power Bar® Performance Energy®, Chocolate	☹	Avoid	76¾	Piece (65g); 4,989g in total.
Power Bar® Performance Energy®, Cookie Dough	☺	Nearly free	☺	Nearly free of sorbitol
Power Bar® Performance Energy®, Mixed Berry Blast	☹	Avoid	19	Piece (65g); 1,235g in total.
Power Bar® Performance Energy®, Vanilla Crisp	☺	Nearly free	☺	Nearly free of sorbitol
Powerade®, all flavors	☺	Free	☺	Free of sorbitol.

3.3 Beverages

3.3.1 Alcoholic

Alcoholic	LACTOSE	Standard amount	⊕
Ale	🙂	Free of lactose.	
Amaretto	🙂	Free of lactose.	
Apple juice or cider, made from frozen	🙂	Free of lactose.	
Apple juice or cider, unsweetened	🙂	Free of lactose.	
Applejack liquor	🙂	Free of lactose.	
Aquavit	🙂	Free of lactose.	
Beer	🙂	Free of lactose.	
Beer, low alcohol	🙂	Free of lactose.	
Beer, low carb	🙂	Free of lactose.	
Beer, non alcoholic	🙂	Free of lactose.	
Black Russian	🙂	Free of lactose.	
Bloody Mary	🙂	Free of lactose.	
Bourbon	🙂	Free of lactose.	
Brandy	🙂	Free of lactose.	

Alcoholic	IBS Standard amount		F+G amount
Ale	10	Glass (200g); 2,000 mL in total.	☺
Amaretto	¼	Glass (200g); 50 mL in total.	☺
Apple juice or cider, made from frozen	☹	Avoid consumption!	☺
Apple juice or cider, un-sweetened	☹	Avoid consumption!	☺
Applejack liquor	☺	Free of triggers.	☺
Aquavit	☺	Free of triggers.	☺
Beer	10	Glass (200g); 2,000 mL in total.	☺
Beer, low alcohol	☺	Free of triggers.	☺
Beer, low carb	10	Glass (200g); 2,000 mL in total.	☺
Beer, non alcoholic	☺	Free of triggers.	☺
Black Russian	8¼	Glass (200g); 1,650 mL in total.	☺
Bloody Mary	½	Glass (200g); 100 mL in total.	☺
Bourbon	☺	Free of triggers.	☺
Brandy	☺	Free of triggers.	☺
Brandy, flavored	¼	Glass (200g); 50 mL in total.	☺

Alcoholic	FRUCTOSE	Standard amount
Ale	☺	Free of fructose.
Amaretto	B ×5 ☺	Free of fructose. Per Glass (200 mL) you drink with it, add B-no × F-limit.
Apple juice or cider, made from frozen	☹	Avoid consumption!
Apple juice or cider, un-sweetened	☹	Avoid consumption!
Applejack liquor	☺	Free of fructose.
Aquavit	☺	Free of fructose.
Beer	☺	Free of fructose.
Beer, low alcohol	B ×2¼ ☺	Free of fructose. Per Glass (200 mL) you drink with it, add B-no × F-limit.
Beer, low carb	☺	Free of fructose.
Beer, non alcoholic	☺	Free of fructose.
Black Russian	☺	Nearly free of fructose, avoid at hereditary fructose intolerance.
Bloody Mary	1 🥛	Glass (200g); 200 mL in total.
Bourbon	☺	Free of fructose.
Brandy	☺	Free of fructose.
Brandy, flavored	B ×5 ☺	Free of fructose. Per Glass (200 mL) you drink with it, add B-no × F-limit.

Alcoholic	SORBITOL Stand.		SORBITOL Low sensitivity amount
Ale	☹ Avoid	10	Glass (200g); 2,000 mL in total.
Amaretto	☹ Avoid	¼	Glass (200g); 50 mL in total.
Apple juice or cider, made from frozen	☹ Avoid	☹	Avoid consumption!
Apple juice or cider, unsweetened	☹ Avoid	☹	Avoid consumption!
Applejack liquor	☺ Free	☺	Free of sorbitol.
Aquavit	☺ Free	☺	Free of sorbitol.
Beer	☹ Avoid	10	Glass (200g); 2,000 mL in total.
Beer, low alcohol	☺ Free	☺	Free of sorbitol.
Beer, low carb	☹ Avoid	10	Glass (200g); 2,000 mL in total.
Beer, non alcoholic	☺ Free	☺	Free of sorbitol.
Black Russian	☹ Avoid	8¼	Glass (200g); 1,650 mL in total.
Bloody Mary	☹ Avoid	½	Glass (200g); 100 mL in total.
Bourbon	☺ Free	☺	Free of sorbitol.
Brandy	☺ Free	☺	Free of sorbitol.
Brandy, flavored	☹ Avoid	¼	Glass (200g); 50 mL in total.

Alcoholic	LACTOSE	Standard amount	
Burgundy wine, red	🙂	Free of lactose.	
Burgundy wine, white	🙂	Free of lactose.	
Campari®	🙂	Free of lactose.	
Cape Cod	🙂	Free of lactose.	
Champagne punch	🙂	Free of lactose.	
Champagne, white	🙂	Free of lactose.	
Chardonnay	🙂	Free of lactose.	
Club soda	🙂	Free of lactose.	
Cognac	🙂	Free of lactose.	
Cointreau®	🙂	Free of lactose.	
Creme de Cocoa	🙂	Free of lactose.	
Creme de menthe	🙂	Free of lactose.	
Curacao	🙂	Free of lactose.	
Daiquiri	🙂	Free of lactose.	
Eggnog, regular	🥛	Glass (240g); Avoid consumption!!	0.2
Fruit punch, alcoholic	🙂	Free of lactose.	

Alcoholic	IBS	Standard amount	F+G amount
Burgundy wine, red	½	Glass (200g); 100 mL in total.	☺
Burgundy wine, white	¾	Glass (200g); 150 mL in total.	☺
Campari®	¼	Glass (200g); 50 mL in total.	☺
Cape Cod	25	Glass (200g); 5,000 mL in total.	☺
Champagne punch	½	Glass (200g); 100 mL in total.	☺
Champagne, white	¾	Glass (200g); 150 mL in total.	☺
Chardonnay	¾	Glass (200g); 150 mL in total.	☺
Club soda	☺	Free of triggers.	☺
Cognac	☺	Free of triggers.	☺
Cointreau®	¼	Glass (200g); 50 mL in total.	☺
Creme de Cocoa	2½	Glass (200g); 500 mL in total.	☺
Creme de menthe	¼	Glass (200g); 50 mL in total.	☺
Curacao	¼	Glass (200g); 50 mL in total.	☺
Daiquiri	☺	Free of triggers.	☺
Eggnog, regular	¼	Glass (200g); 50 mL in total.	1½
Fruit punch, alcoholic	½	Glass (200g); 100 mL in total.	☺

Alcoholic	FRUCTOSE		Standard amount
Burgundy wine, red		☺	Free of fructose.
Burgundy wine, white		☺	Free of fructose.
Campari®	B ×5	☺+	Free of fructose. Per Glass (200 mL) you drink with it, add B-no × F-limit.
Cape Cod	B ×5	☺+	Free of fructose. Per Glass (200 mL) you drink with it, add B-no × F-limit.
Champagne punch	½	🥛	Glass (200g); 100 mL in total.
Champagne, white		☺	Free of fructose.
Chardonnay		☺	Free of fructose.
Club soda		☺	Free of fructose.
Cognac		☺	Free of fructose.
Cointreau®	B ×5	☺+	Free of fructose. Per Glass (200 mL) you drink with it, add B-no × F-limit.
Creme de Cocoa		☺	Nearly free of fructose, avoid at hereditary fructose intolerance.
Creme de menthe	B ×5	☺+	Free of fructose. Per Glass (200 mL) you drink with it, add B-no × F-limit.
Curacao	B ×5	☺+	Free of fructose. Per Glass (200 mL) you drink with it, add B-no × F-limit.
Daiquiri		☺	Free of fructose.
Eggnog, regular	B ×4¾	☺+	Free of fructose. Per Glass (200 mL) you drink with it, add B-no × F-limit.
Fruit punch, alcoholic	½	🥛	Glass (200g); 100 mL in total.

Alcoholic	SORBITOL Stand.	SORBITOL Low sensitivity amount	
Burgundy wine, red	☹ Avoid	½	Glass (200g); 100 mL in total.
Burgundy wine, white	☹ Avoid	¾	Glass (200g); 150 mL in total.
Campari®	☹ Avoid	¼	Glass (200g); 50 mL in total.
Cape Cod	☹ Avoid	25	Glass (200g); 5,000 mL in total.
Champagne punch	☹ Avoid	1	Glass (200g); 200 mL in total.
Champagne, white	☹ Avoid	¾	Glass (200g); 150 mL in total.
Chardonnay	☹ Avoid	¾	Glass (200g); 150 mL in total.
Club soda	☺ Free		Free of sorbitol.
Cognac	☺ Free		Free of sorbitol.
Cointreau®	☹ Avoid	¼	Glass (200g); 50 mL in total.
Creme de Cocoa	☹ Avoid	2½	Glass (200g); 500 mL in total.
Creme de menthe	☹ Avoid	¼	Glass (200g); 50 mL in total.
Curaçao	☹ Avoid	¼	Glass (200g); 50 mL in total.
Daiquiri	☺ Free		Free of sorbitol.
Eggnog, regular	☺ Free		Free of sorbitol.
Fruit punch, alcoholic	☹ Avoid	1	Glass (200g); 200 mL in total.

Alcoholic	LACTOSE	Standard amount	🔒
Gibson	🙂	Free of lactose.	
Gin	🙂	Free of lactose.	
Grand Marnier®	🙂	Free of lactose.	
Grasshopper	1 🥛	Glass (240g); 240 mL in total.	+¾
Harvey Wallbanger	🙂	Free of lactose.	
Kamikaze	🙂	Free of lactose.	
Kirsch	🙂	Free of lactose.	
Light beer	🙂	Free of lactose.	
Liqueur, coffee flavored	🙂	Free of lactose.	
Long Island iced tea	🙂	Free of lactose.	
Mai Tai	🙂	Free of lactose.	
Malt liquor	🙂	Free of lactose.	
Manhattan	🙂	Free of lactose.	
Margarita, frozen	🙂	Free of lactose.	
Martini®	🙂	Free of lactose.	
Merlot, red	🙂	Free of lactose.	

Alcoholic	IBS Standard amount		F+G amount
Gibson	3¼	Glass (200g); 650 mL in total.	🙂
Gin	🙂	Free of triggers.	🙂
Grand Marnier®	¼	Glass (200g); 50 mL in total.	🙂
Grasshopper	¾	Glass (200g); 150 mL in total.	7
Harvey Wallbanger	¼	Glass (200g); 50 mL in total.	🙂
Kamikaze	1	Glass (200g); 200 mL in total.	🙂
Kirsch	¼	Glass (200g); 50 mL in total.	🙂
Light beer	12½	Glass (200g); 2,500 mL in total.	🙂
Liqueur, coffee flavored	2½	Glass (200g); 500 mL in total.	🙂
Long Island iced tea	¾	Glass (200g); 150 mL in total.	🙂
Mai Tai	1¾	Glass (200g); 350 mL in total.	🙂
Malt liquor	10	Glass (200g); 2,000 mL in total.	🙂
Manhattan	½	Glass (200g); 100 mL in total.	🙂
Margarita, frozen	7	Glass (200g); 1,400 mL in total.	🙂
Martini®	3¼	Glass (200g); 650 mL in total.	🙂
Merlot, red	½	Glass (200g); 100 mL in total.	🙂

Alcoholic	FRUCTOSE		Standard amount
Gibson		🙂	Free of fructose.
Gin		🙂	Free of fructose.
Grand Marnier®	B ×5	🙂+	Free of fructose. Per Glass (200 mL) you drink with it, add B-no × F-limit.
Grasshopper	B ×1½	🙂+	Free of fructose. Per Glass (200 mL) you drink with it, add B-no × F-limit.
Harvey Wallbanger	62½	🥛	Glass (200g); 12,500 mL in total.
Kamikaze	B ×1¾	🙂+	Free of fructose. Per Glass (200 mL) you drink with it, add B-no × F-limit.
Kirsch	B ×5	🙂+	Free of fructose. Per Glass (200 mL) you drink with it, add B-no × F-limit.
Light beer	B ×¼	🙂+	Free of fructose. Per Glass (200 mL) you drink with it, add B-no × F-limit.
Liqueur, coffee flavored		🙂	Nearly free of fructose, avoid at hereditary fructose intolerance.
Long Island iced tea	¾	🥛	Glass (200g); 150 mL in total.
Mai Tai	B ×½	🙂+	Free of fructose. Per Glass (200 mL) you drink with it, add B-no × F-limit.
Malt liquor		🙂	Free of fructose.
Manhattan	½	🥛	Glass (200g); 100 mL in total.
Margarita, frozen	B ×¼	🙂+	Free of fructose. Per Glass (200 mL) you drink with it, add B-no × F-limit.
Martini®		🙂	Free of fructose.
Merlot, red		🙂	Free of fructose.

Alcoholic	SORBITOL Stand.		SORBITOL Low sensitivity amount
Gibson	😞 Avoid	3¼	Glass (200g); 650 mL in total.
Gin	😊 Free	😊	Free of sorbitol.
Grand Marnier®	😞 Avoid	¼	Glass (200g); 50 mL in total.
Grasshopper	😞 Avoid	¾	Glass (200g); 150 mL in total.
Harvey Wallbanger	😞 Avoid	¼	Glass (200g); 50 mL in total.
Kamikaze	😞 Avoid	1	Glass (200g); 200 mL in total.
Kirsch	😞 Avoid	¼	Glass (200g); 50 mL in total.
Light beer	😞 Avoid	12½	Glass (200g); 2,500 mL in total.
Liqueur, coffee flavored	😞 Avoid	2½	Glass (200g); 500 mL in total.
Long Island iced tea	😞 Avoid	16½	Glass (200g); 3,300 mL in total.
Mai Tai	😞 Avoid	1¾	Glass (200g); 350 mL in total.
Malt liquor	😞 Avoid	10	Glass (200g); 2,000 mL in total.
Manhattan	😞 Avoid	2	Glass (200g); 400 mL in total.
Margarita, frozen	😞 Avoid	7	Glass (200g); 1,400 mL in total.
Martini®	😞 Avoid	3¼	Glass (200g); 650 mL in total.
Merlot, red	😞 Avoid	½	Glass (200g); 100 mL in total.

Alcoholic	LACTOSE	Standard amount	
Merlot, white	☺	Free of lactose.	
Mint Julep	☺	Free of lactose.	
Mojito	☺	Free of lactose.	
Muscatel	☺	Free of lactose.	
Non-alcoholic wine	☺	Free of lactose.	
Ouzo	☺	Free of lactose.	
Pina colada	☺	Free of lactose.	
Port wine	☺	Free of lactose.	
Riesling	☺	Free of lactose.	
Rob Roy	☺	Free of lactose.	
Rompope (eggnog with alcohol)	¼ 🥛	Glass (240g); 60 mL in total.	+¼
Root beer	☺	Free of lactose.	
Rose wine, other types	☺	Free of lactose.	
Rum	☺	Free of lactose.	
Rum and cola	☺	Free of lactose.	
Rusty nail	☺	Free of lactose.	

Alcoholic	IBS	Standard amount	F+G amount
Merlot, white	¾	Glass (200g); 150 mL in total.	☺
Mint Julep	☺	Free of triggers.	☺
Mojito	☺	Free of triggers.	☺
Muscatel	☹	Avoid consumption!	☺
Non-alcoholic wine	2¼	Glass (200g); 450 mL in total.	☺
Ouzo	¼	Glass (200g); 50 mL in total.	☺
Pina colada	4	Glass (200g); 800 mL in total.	☺
Port wine	☹	Avoid consumption!	☺
Riesling	¾	Glass (200g); 150 mL in total.	☺
Rob Roy	¼	Glass (200g); 50 mL in total.	☺
Rompope (eggnog with alcohol)	¼	Glass (200g); 50 mL in total.	2¾
Root beer	½	Glass (200g); 100 mL in total.	☺
Rose wine, other types	¾	Glass (200g); 150 mL in total.	☺
Rum	☺	Free of triggers.	☺
Rum and cola	1	Glass (200g); 200 mL in total.	☺
Rusty nail	¾	Glass (200g); 150 mL in total.	☺

Alcoholic	FRUCTOSE		Standard amount
Merlot, white	¾		Glass (200g); 150 mL in total.
Mint Julep		☺	Free of fructose.
Mojito		☺	Free of fructose.
Muscatel		☹	Avoid consumption!
Non-alcoholic wine	2¼		Glass (200g); 450 mL in total.
Ouzo	B ×5	☺+	Free of fructose. Per Glass (200 mL) you drink with it, add B-no × F-limit.
Pina colada	B ×1¼	☺+	Free of fructose. Per Glass (200 mL) you drink with it, add B-no × F-limit.
Port wine		☹	Avoid consumption!
Riesling		☺	Free of fructose.
Rob Roy	¼		Glass (200g); 50 mL in total.
Rompope (eggnog with alcohol)		☺	Free of fructose.
Root beer	½		Glass (200g); 100 mL in total.
Rose wine, other types	¾		Glass (200g); 150 mL in total.
Rum		☺	Free of fructose.
Rum and cola	1		Glass (200g); 200 mL in total.
Rusty nail	B ×2	☺+	Free of fructose. Per Glass (200 mL) you drink with it, add B-no × F-limit.

Alcoholic	SORBITOL Stand.	SORBITOL Low sensitivity amount
Merlot, white	🙂 Free	🙂 Free of sorbitol.
Mint Julep	🙂 Free	🙂 Free of sorbitol.
Mojito	🙂 Free	🙂 Free of sorbitol.
Muscatel	☹ Avoid	½ 🥃 Glass (200g); 100 mL in total.
Non-alcoholic wine	☹ Avoid	50 🥃 Glass (200g); 10,000 mL in total.
Ouzo	☹ Avoid	¼ 🥃 Glass (200g); 50 mL in total.
Pina colada	☹ Avoid	4 🥃 Glass (200g); 800 mL in total.
Port wine	☹ Avoid	½ 🥃 Glass (200g); 100 mL in total.
Riesling	☹ Avoid	¾ 🥃 Glass (200g); 150 mL in total.
Rob Roy	☹ Avoid	2½ 🥃 Glass (200g); 500 mL in total.
Rompope (eggnog with alcohol)	🙂 Free	🙂 Free of sorbitol.
Root beer	🙂 Free	🙂 Free of sorbitol.
Rose wine, other types	🙂 Free	🙂 Free of sorbitol.
Rum	🙂 Free	🙂 Free of sorbitol.
Rum and cola	🙂 Free	🙂 Free of sorbitol.
Rusty nail	☹ Avoid	¾ 🥃 Glass (200g); 150 mL in total.

Alcoholic	LACTOSE	Standard amount
Sake	🙂	Free of lactose.
Sambuca	🙂	Free of lactose.
Sangria	🙂	Free of lactose.
Schnapps, all flavors	🙂	Free of lactose.
Scotch and soda	🙂	Free of lactose.
Screwdriver	🙂	Free of lactose.
Seabreeze	🙂	Free of lactose.
Singapore sling	🙂	Free of lactose.
Sloe gin	🙂	Free of lactose.
Sloe gin fizz	🙂	Free of lactose.
Southern Comfort®	🙂	Free of lactose.
Sylvaner	🙂	Free of lactose.
Tequila	🙂	Free of lactose.
Tequila sunrise	🙂	Free of lactose.
Tokaji Wine	🙂	Free of lactose.

Alcoholic	IBS Standard amount		F+G amount
Sake	☹	Avoid consumption!	☺
Sambuca	¼ 🥃	Glass (200g); 50 mL in total.	☺
Sangria	¾ 🥃	Glass (200g); 150 mL in total.	☺
Schnapps, all flavors	½ 🥃	Glass (200g); 100 mL in total.	☺
Scotch and soda	☺	Free of triggers.	☺
Screwdriver	¼ 🥃	Glass (200g); 50 mL in total.	☺
Seabreeze	2½ 🥃	Glass (200g); 500 mL in total.	☺
Singapore sling	4½ 🥃	Glass (200g); 900 mL in total.	☺
Sloe gin	¼ 🥃	Glass (200g); 50 mL in total.	☺
Sloe gin fizz	1½ 🥃	Glass (200g); 300 mL in total.	☺
Southern Comfort®	☺	Free of triggers.	☺
Sylvaner	¾ 🥃	Glass (200g); 150 mL in total.	☺
Tequila	☺	Free of triggers.	☺
Tequila sunrise	3¼ 🥃	Glass (200g); 650 mL in total.	☺
Tokaji Wine	☹	Avoid consumption!	☺
Tom Collins	16½ 🥃	Glass (200g); 3,300 mL in total.	☺

Alcoholic	FRUCTOSE	Standard amount
Sake	☹	Avoid consumption!
Sambuca	B ×5 ☺+	Free of fructose. Per Glass (200 mL) you drink with it, add B-no × F-limit.
Sangria	5½ 🥛	Glass (200g); 1,100 mL in total.
Schnapps, all flavors	B ×2½ ☺+	Free of fructose. Per Glass (200 mL) you drink with it, add B-no × F-limit.
Scotch and soda	☺	Free of fructose.
Screwdriver	1 🥛	Glass (200g); 200 mL in total.
Seabreeze	B ×5¼ ☺+	Free of fructose. Per Glass (200 mL) you drink with it, add B-no × F-limit.
Singapore sling	B ×¼ ☺+	Free of fructose. Per Glass (200 mL) you drink with it, add B-no × F-limit.
Sloe gin	B ×5 ☺+	Free of fructose. Per Glass (200 mL) you drink with it, add B-no × F-limit.
Sloe gin fizz	B ×¾ ☺+	Free of fructose. Per Glass (200 mL) you drink with it, add B-no × F-limit.
Southern Comfort®	☺	Free of fructose.
Sylvaner	☺	Free of fructose.
Tequila	☺	Free of fructose.
Tequila sunrise	B ×¼ ☺+	Free of fructose. Per Glass (200 mL) you drink with it, add B-no × F-limit.
Tokaji Wine	☹	Avoid consumption!
Tom Collins	22½ 🥛	Glass (200g); 4,500 mL in total.

Alcoholic	SORBITOL Stand.		SORBITOL Low sensitivity amount
Sake	😞 Avoid	½	Glass (200g); 100 mL in total.
Sambuca	😞 Avoid	¼	Glass (200g); 50 mL in total.
Sangria	😞 Avoid	¾	Glass (200g); 150 mL in total.
Schnapps, all flavors	😞 Avoid	½	Glass (200g); 100 mL in total.
Scotch and soda	😊 Free		Free of sorbitol.
Screwdriver	😞 Avoid	¼	Glass (200g); 50 mL in total.
Seabreeze	😞 Avoid	2½	Glass (200g); 500 mL in total.
Singapore sling	😞 Avoid	4½	Glass (200g); 900 mL in total.
Sloe gin	😞 Avoid	¼	Glass (200g); 50 mL in total.
Sloe gin fizz	😞 Avoid	1½	Glass (200g); 300 mL in total.
Southern Comfort®	😊 Free		Free of sorbitol.
Sylvaner	😞 Avoid	¾	Glass (200g); 150 mL in total.
Tequila	😊 Free		Free of sorbitol.
Tequila sunrise	😞 Avoid	3¼	Glass (200g); 650 mL in total.
Tokaji Wine	😞 Avoid	½	Glass (200g); 100 mL in total.
Tom Collins	😞 Avoid	16½	Glass (200g); 3,300 mL in total.

Alcoholic	LACTOSE		Standard amount	
Triple Sec		🙂	Free of lactose.	
Vodka		🙂	Free of lactose.	
Whiskey		🙂	Free of lactose.	
Whiskey sour		🙂	Free of lactose.	
White Russian	1¼	🥃	Glass (240g); 300 mL in total.	+1
Wine spritzer		🙂	Free of lactose.	

Alcoholic	IBS		Standard amount	F+G	amount
Triple Sec	¼	🥃	Glass (200g); 50 mL in total.		🙂
Vodka		🙂	Free of triggers.		🙂
Whiskey		🙂	Free of triggers.		🙂
Whiskey sour	6¼	🥃	Glass (200g); 1,250 mL in total.		🙂
White Russian	1½	🥃	Glass (200g); 1,650 mL in total.	9	🥃
Wine spritzer	1	🥃	Glass (200g); 200 mL in total.		🙂

Alcoholic	FRUCTOSE		Standard amount
Triple Sec	B ×5	😊+	Free of fructose. Per Glass (200 mL) you drink with it, add B-no × F-limit.
Vodka		😊	Free of fructose.
Whiskey		😊	Free of fructose.
Whiskey sour	7¼	🥛	Glass (200g); 1,450 mL in total.
White Russian		😊	Free of fructose.
Wine spritzer		😊	Free of fructose.

Alcoholic	SORBITOL Stand.		SORBITOL Low sensitivity amount	
Triple Sec	☹️ Avoid	¼	🥛	Glass (200g); 50 mL in total.
Vodka	😊 Free		😊	Free of sorbitol.
Whiskey	😊 Free		😊	Free of sorbitol.
Whiskey sour	☹️ Avoid	6¼	🥛	Glass (200g); 1,250 mL in total.
White Russian	☹️ Avoid	8¼	🥛	Glass (200g); 1,650 mL in total.
Wine spritzer	☹️ Avoid	1	🥛	Glass (200g); 200 mL in total.

3.3.2 Hot beverages

Hot beverages	LACTOSE		Standard amount	➕
Americano, decaf, without flavored syrup		☺	Free of lactose.	
Americano, with flavored syrup		☺	Free of lactose.	
Americano, without flavored syrup		☺	Free of lactose.	
Brown sugar		☺	Free of lactose.	
Cafe au lait, without flavored syrup	½	☕	Cup (150g); 75 mL in total.	+¼
Cafe latte, with flavored syrup	½	☕	Cup (150g); 75 mL in total.	+¼
Cafe latte, without flavored syrup	½	☕	Cup (150g); 75 mL in total.	+¼
Camomile tea		☺	Free of lactose.	
Cappuccino, bottled or canned	½	☕	Cup (150g); 75 mL in total.	+½
Cappuccino, decaf, with flavored syrup	½	☕	Cup (150g); 75 mL in total.	+¼
Cappuccino, decaf, without flavored syrup	½	☕	Cup (150g); 75 mL in total.	+¼
Chai tea		☺	Free of lactose.	
Chicory coffee		☺	Free of lactose.	
Coffee substitute, prepared		☺	Free of lactose.	
Coffee, prepared from flavored mix, sugar free		☺	Nearly free of lactose	

Hot beverages	IBS Standard amount		F+G amount
Americano, decaf, without flavored syrup	☺	Free of triggers.	☺
Americano, with flavored syrup	☺	Free of triggers.	☺
Americano, without flavored syrup	☺	Free of triggers.	☺
Brown sugar	☺	Free of triggers.	☺
Cafe au lait, without flavored syrup	½ 🍵	Cup (150g); 75 mL in total.	6½ 🍵
Cafe latte, with flavored syrup	½ 🍵	Cup (150g); 75 mL in total.	3 🍵
Cafe latte, without flavored syrup	½ 🍵	Cup (150g); 75 mL in total.	2¾ 🍵
Camomile tea	¾ 🥛	Glass (200g); 100 mL in total.	¾ 🥛
Cappuccino, bottled or canned	½ 🍵	Cup (150g); 75 mL in total.	4 🍵
Cappuccino, decaf, with flavored syrup	½ 🍵	Cup (150g); 75 mL in total.	3 🍵
Cappuccino, decaf, without flavored syrup	½ 🍵	Cup (150g); 75 mL in total.	2¾ 🍵
Chai tea	☺	Free of triggers.	☺
Chicory coffee	☹	Avoid consumption!!	☹
Coffee substitute, prepared	☺	Free of triggers.	☺
Coffee, prepared from flavored mix, sugar free	☺	Nearly free of F+G.	☺

Hot beverages	FRUCTOSE	Standard amount
Americano, decaf, without flavored syrup	😊	Free of fructose.
Americano, with flavored syrup	😊	Free of fructose.
Americano, without flavored syrup	😊	Free of fructose.
Brown sugar	😊	Free of fructose.
Cafe au lait, without flavored syrup	😊	Free of fructose.
Cafe latte, with flavored syrup	😊	Free of fructose.
Cafe latte, without flavored syrup	😊	Free of fructose.
Camomile tea	😊	Free of fructose.
Cappuccino, bottled or canned	😊	Free of fructose.
Cappuccino, decaf, with flavored syrup	😊	Free of fructose.
Cappuccino, decaf, without flavored syrup	😊	Free of fructose.
Chai tea	😊	Free of fructose.
Chicory coffee	🙂	Nearly free of fructose, avoid at hereditary fructose intolerance.
Coffee substitute, prepared	😊	Free of fructose.
Coffee, prepared from flavored mix, sugar free	😊	Free of fructose.

Hot beverages	SORBITOL Stand.	SORBITOL Low sensitivity amount
Americano, decaf, without flavored syrup	😊 Free	😊 Free of sorbitol.
Americano, with flavored syrup	😊 Free	😊 Free of sorbitol.
Americano, without flavored syrup	😊 Free	😊 Free of sorbitol.
Brown sugar	😊 Free	😊 Free of sorbitol.
Cafe au lait, without flavored syrup	😊 Free	😊 Free of sorbitol.
Cafe latte, with flavored syrup	😊 Free	😊 Free of sorbitol.
Cafe latte, without flavored syrup	😊 Free	😊 Free of sorbitol.
Camomile tea	😊 Free	😊 Free of sorbitol.
Cappuccino, bottled or canned	😊 Free	😊 Free of sorbitol.
Cappuccino, decaf, with flavored syrup	😊 Free	😊 Free of sorbitol.
Cappuccino, decaf, without flavored syrup	😊 Free	😊 Free of sorbitol.
Chai tea	😊 Free	😊 Free of sorbitol.
Chicory coffee	☹ Avoid	11 ☕ Cup (150g); 1,650 mL in total.
Coffee substitute, prepared	😊 Free	😊 Free of sorbitol.
Coffee, prepared from flavored mix, sugar free	☹ Avoid	66½ ☕ Cup (150g); 9,975 mL in total.

Hot beverages	LACTOSE	Standard amount	⊕
Dandelion tea	😊	Free of lactose.	
Demitasse	😊	Free of lactose.	
Dove® Promises, Milk Chocolate	¼	Cup (150g); 38 mL in total.	0.22
Earl Grey, strong	😊	Free of lactose.	
Espresso, without flavored syrup	😊	Free of lactose.	
Evaporated milk, diluted, skim (fat free)	¼	Cup (150g); 38 mL in total.	+¼
Fennel tea	😊	Free of lactose.	
Frappuccino®	½	Cup (150g); 75 mL in total.	+½
Frappuccino®, bottled or canned	½	Cup (150g); 75 mL in total.	+½
Frappuccino®, bottled or canned, light	½	Cup (150g); 75 mL in total.	+½
Green tea, strong	😊	Free of lactose.	
Herbal tea	😊	Free of lactose.	
Hershey's® Bliss Hot Drink White Chocolate, prepared	¼	Cup (150g); 38 mL in total.	+¼
Hot chocolate, homemade	¼	Cup (150g); 38 mL in total.	+¼
Instant coffee mix, unprepared	😊	Free of lactose.	
Irish coffee with alcohol and whipped cream	3¾	Cup (150g); 563 mL in total.	+3

Hot beverages	IBS Standard amount		F+G amount
Dandelion tea	¾	Glass (200g); 150g in total.	¾
Demitasse	☺	Free of triggers.	☺
Dove® Promises, Milk Chocolate	¼	Cup (150g); 35 mL in total.	1¼
Earl Grey, strong	¾	Glass (200g); 100 mL in total.	1¾
Espresso, without flavored syrup	☺	Free of triggers.	☺
Evaporated milk, diluted, skim (fat free)	¼	Cup (150g); 35 mL in total.	1¾
Fennel tea	¾	Glass (200g); 100 mL in total.	¾
Frappuccino®	½	Cup (150g); 75 mL in total.	3¾
Frappuccino®, bottled or canned	½	Cup (150g); 75 mL in total.	3½
Frappuccino®, bottled or canned, light	½	Cup (150g); 75 mL in total.	4
Green tea, strong	☺	Free of triggers.	☺
Herbal tea	¾	Glass (200g); 150g in total.	¾
Hershey's® Bliss Hot Drink White Chocolate, prepared	¼	Cup (150g); 35 mL in total.	2
Hot chocolate, homemade	¼	Cup (150g); 35 mL in total.	2
Instant coffee mix, unprepared	☹	Avoid consumption!	☺
Irish coffee with alcohol and whipped cream	3¾	Cup (150g); 550 mL in total.	21

Hot beverages	FRUCTOSE	Standard amount
Dandelion tea	☺	Free of fructose.
Demitasse	☺	Free of fructose.
Dove® Promises, Milk Chocolate	☺	Free of fructose.
Earl Grey, strong	¾ 🥛	Glass (200g); 150 mL in total.
Espresso, without flavored syrup	☺	Free of fructose.
Evaporated milk, diluted, skim (fat free)	☺	Free of fructose.
Fennel tea	☺	Free of fructose.
Frappuccino®	☺	Free of fructose.
Frappuccino®, bottled or canned	☺	Free of fructose.
Frappuccino®, bottled or canned, light	☺	Free of fructose.
Green tea, strong	☺	Free of fructose.
Herbal tea	☺	Free of fructose.
Hershey's® Bliss Hot Drink White Chocolate, prepared	B ×½ ☺	Free of fructose. Per Cup (150 mL) you drink with it, add B-no × F-limit.
Hot chocolate, homemade	25½ ☕	Cup (150g); 3,825 mL in total.
Instant coffee mix, unprepared	4 ☕	Cup (150g); 600 mL in total.
Irish coffee with alcohol and whipped cream	☺	Free of fructose.

Hot beverages	SORBITOL Stand.	SORBITOL Low sensitivity amount
Dandelion tea	🙂 Free	🙂 Free of sorbitol.
Demitasse	🙂 Free	🙂 Free of sorbitol.
Dove® Promises, Milk Chocolate	🙂 Free	🙂 Free of sorbitol.
Earl Grey, strong	🙂 Free	🙂 Free of sorbitol.
Espresso, without flavored syrup	🙂 Free	🙂 Free of sorbitol.
Evaporated milk, diluted, skim (fat free)	🙂 Free	🙂 Free of sorbitol.
Fennel tea	🙂 Free	🙂 Free of sorbitol.
Frappuccino®	🙂 Free	🙂 Free of sorbitol.
Frappuccino®, bottled or canned	🙂 Free	🙂 Free of sorbitol.
Frappuccino®, bottled or canned, light	🙂 Free	🙂 Free of sorbitol.
Green tea, strong	🙂 Free	🙂 Free of sorbitol.
Herbal tea	🙂 Free	🙂 Free of sorbitol.
Hershey's® Bliss Hot Drink White Chocolate, prepared	🙂 Free	🙂 Free of sorbitol.
Hot chocolate, homemade	☹ Avoid	66½ ☕ Cup (150g); 9,975 mL in total.
Instant coffee mix, unprepared	☹ Avoid	☹ Avoid consumption!
Irish coffee with alcohol and whipped cream	🙂 Free	🙂 Free of sorbitol.

Hot beverages	LACTOSE		Standard amount	
Jasmine tea		☺	Free of lactose.	
Light cream	5¼	🥣	Portion (15g); 79g in total.	+4½
Milk, lactose reduced Lactaid®, skim (fat free)		☺	Free of lactose.	
Milk, lactose reduced Lactaid®, whole		☺	Free of lactose.	
Milk, unprepared dry powder, nonfat, instant	¼	🥣	Portion (22.64g); 6g in total.	0.22
Mocha, without flavored syrup	½	☕	Cup (150g); 75 mL in total.	+¼
Nestle® Hot Cocoa Dark Chocolate, prepared	¼	☕	Cup (150g); 38 mL in total.	+¼
Nestle® Hot Cocoa Rich Milk Chocolate, prepared	¼	☕	Cup (150g); 38 mL in total.	+¼
Oolong tea		☺	Free of lactose.	
Soy milk, chocolate, sweetened with sugar, not fortified		☺	Free of lactose.	
Splenda®		☺	Free of lactose.	
Starbucks® Hot Cocoa Double Chocolate, prepared	¼	☕	Cup (150g); 38 mL in total.	+¼
Starbucks® Hot Cocoa Salted Caramel, prepared	¼	☕	Cup (150g); 38 mL in total.	+¼
Sugar, white granulated		☺	Free of lactose.	
Sweetened condensed milk	½	🥣	Portion (38g); 19g in total.	+½
Sweetened condensed milk, reduced fat	½	🥣	Portion (39g); 20g in total.	+½

Hot beverages	IBS	Standard amount	F+G	amount
Jasmine tea		Free of triggers.		☺
Light cream	5¼	Portion (15g); 79g in total.	30¼	
Milk, lactose reduced Lactaid®, skim (fat free)		Free of triggers.		☺
Milk, lactose reduced Lactaid®, whole		Free of triggers.		☺
Milk, unprepared dry powder, nonfat, instant	¼	Portion (22.64g); 6g in total.	1¼	
Mocha, without flavored syrup	½	Cup (150g); 75 mL in total.	3	
Nestle® Hot Cocoa Dark Chocolate, prepared	¼	Cup (150g); 38 mL in total.	2	
Nestle® Hot Cocoa Rich Milk Chocolate, prepared	¼	Cup (150g); 38 mL in total.	2	
Oolong tea	¾	Glass (200g); 150g in total.	¾	
Soy milk, chocolate, with sugar, not fortified	¼	Cup (150g); 38 mL in total.	¼	
Splenda®		Free of triggers.		☺
Starbucks® Hot Cocoa Double Chocolate, prepared	¼	Cup (150g); 38 mL in total.	2	
Starbucks® Hot Cocoa Salted Caramel, prepared	¼	Cup (150g); 38 mL in total.	2	
Sugar, white granulated		Free of triggers.		☺
Sweetened condensed milk	½	Portion (38g); 19g in total.	3¾	
Sweetened condensed milk, reduced fat	½	Portion (39g); 20g in total.	3½	

Hot beverages	FRUCTOSE		Standard amount
Jasmine tea		🙂	Free of fructose.
Light cream		🙂	Free of fructose.
Milk, lactose reduced Lactaid®, skim (fat free)	B ×7½	🙂+	Free of fructose. Per Cup (150 mL) you drink with it, add B-no × F-limit.
Milk, lactose reduced Lactaid®, whole	B ×7½	🙂+	Free of fructose. Per Cup (150 mL) you drink with it, add B-no × F-limit.
Milk, unprepared dry powder, nonfat, instant		🙂	Free of fructose.
Mocha, without flavored syrup	B ×1¾	🙂+	Free of fructose. Per Cup (150 mL) you drink with it, add B-no × F-limit.
Nestle® Hot Cocoa Dark Chocolate, prepared	B ×½	🙂+	Free of fructose. Per Cup (150 mL) you drink with it, add B-no × F-limit.
Nestle® Hot Cocoa Rich Milk Chocolate, prepared		🙂	Free of fructose.
Oolong tea		🙂	Free of fructose.
Soy milk, chocolate, with sugar, not fortified		🙂	Free of fructose.
Splenda®		🙂	Free of fructose.
Starbucks® Hot Cocoa Double Chocolate, prepared	33¼	☕	Cup (150g); 4,988 mL in total.
Starbucks® Hot Cocoa Salted Caramel, prepared	30¼	☕	Cup (150g); 4,538 mL in total.
Sugar, white granulated		🙂	Free of fructose.
Sweetened condensed milk		🙂	Free of fructose.
Sweetened condensed milk, reduced fat		🙂	Free of fructose.

Hot beverages	SORBITOL Stand.		SORBITOL Low sensitivity amount	
Jasmine tea	☺	Free	☺	Free of sorbitol.
Light cream	☺	Free	☺	Free of sorbitol.
Milk, lactose reduced Lactaid®, skim (fat free)	☺	Free	☺	Free of sorbitol.
Milk, lactose reduced Lactaid®, whole	☺	Free	☺	Free of sorbitol.
Milk, unprepared dry powder, nonfat, instant	☺	Free	☺	Free of sorbitol.
Mocha, without flavored syrup	☺	Free	☺	Free of sorbitol.
Nestle® Hot Cocoa Dark Chocolate, prepared	☺	Nearly free	☺	Nearly free of sorbitol
Nestle® Hot Cocoa Rich Milk Chocolate, prepared	☺	Free	☺	Free of sorbitol.
Oolong tea	☺	Free	☺	Free of sorbitol.
Soy milk, chocolate, sugar, not fortified, ready-to-drink	☹	Avoid	4¼ ☕	Cup (150g); 638 mL in total.
Splenda®	☺	Free	☺	Free of sorbitol.
Starbucks® Hot Cocoa Double Chocolate, prepared	☹	Avoid	66½ ☕	Cup (150g); 9,975 mL in total.
Starbucks® Hot Cocoa Salted Caramel, prepared	☹	Avoid	66½ ☕	Cup (150g); 9,975 mL in total.
Sugar, white granulated	☺	Free	☺	Free of sorbitol.
Sweetened condensed milk	☺	Free	☺	Free of sorbitol.
Sweetened condensed milk, reduced fat	☺	Free	☺	Free of sorbitol.

Hot beverages	LACTOSE	Standard amount	⊕
Swiss Miss® Hot Cocoa Sensible Sweets Diet, sugar free, prepared	¼	Cup (150g); 38 mL in total.	+¼
Whipped cream, aerosol	☺	Nearly free of lactose	
Whipped cream, aerosol, fat free	18¾	Portion (5g); 94g in total.	+15¾
White tea	☺	Free of lactose.	
Zsweet®	☺	Free of lactose.	

Hot beverages	IBS	Standard amount	F+G	amount
Swiss Miss® Hot Cocoa Sensible Sweets Diet, sugar free, prepared	¼	Cup (150g); 38 mL in total.	2	
Whipped cream, aerosol		Nearly free of triggers.		☺
Whipped cream, aerosol, fat free	18¾	Portion (5g); 94g in total.		☺
White tea	☺	Free of triggers.		☺
Zsweet®	☹	Avoid consumption!!		☺

Hot beverages	FRUCTOSE		Standard amount
Swiss Miss® Hot Cocoa Sensible Sweets Diet, sugar free, prepared		☺	Nearly free of fructose, avoid at hereditary fructose intolerance.
Whipped cream, aerosol		☺	Free of fructose.
Whipped cream, aerosol, fat free	B ×¼	☺	Free of fructose. Per Portion (5g) you eat with it, add B-no × F-limit.
White tea		☺	Free of fructose.
Zsweet®		☺	Free of fructose.

Hot beverages	SORBITOL Stand.		SORBITOL Low sensitivity amount	
Swiss Miss® Hot Cocoa Sensible Sweets Diet, sugar free, prepared	☺	Free	☺	Free of sorbitol.
Whipped cream, aerosol	☺	Free	☺	Free of sorbitol.
Whipped cream, aerosol, fat free	☺	Free	☺	Free of sorbitol.
White tea	☺	Free	☺	Free of sorbitol.
Zsweet®	☹	Avoid	☹	Avoid consumption!!

3.3.3 Juices

Juices	LACTOSE	Standard amount	➕
Apple banana strawberry juice	🙂	Free of lactose.	
Apple grape juice	🙂	Free of lactose.	
Apricot nectar	🙂	Free of lactose.	
Arby's® orange juice	🙂	Free of lactose.	
Black cherry juice	🙂	Free of lactose.	
Black currant juice	🙂	Free of lactose.	
Blackberry juice	🙂	Free of lactose.	
Capri Sun®, all flavors	🙂	Free of lactose.	
Carrot juice	🙂	Free of lactose.	
Cranberry juice cocktail, with apple juice	🙂	Free of lactose.	
Cranberry juice cocktail, with blueberry juice	🙂	Free of lactose.	
Fruit drink or punch, ready to drink	🙂	Free of lactose.	
Grapefruit juice, unsweetened, white	🙂	Free of lactose.	
Kern's® Mango-Orange Nectar	🙂	Free of lactose.	
Kern's® Strawberry Nectar	🙂	Free of lactose.	

Juices	IBS Standard amount		F+G amount	
Apple banana strawberry juice	☹	Avoid consumption.	¾ 🥛	
Apple grape juice	☹	Avoid consumption!	1½ 🥛	
Apricot nectar	¼ 🥛	Glass (200g); 50 mL in total.	☺	
Arby's® orange juice	¼ 🥛	Glass (200g); 50 mL in total.	☺	
Black cherry juice	¼ 🥛	Glass (200g); 50 mL in total.	☺	
Black currant juice	1½ 🥛	Glass (200g); 300 mL in total.	☺	
Blackberry juice	¼ 🥛	Glass (200g); 50 mL in total.	☺	
Capri Sun®, all flavors	2 🥛	Glass (200g); 400 mL in total.	☺	
Carrot juice	4 🥛	Glass (200g); 800 mL in total.	☺	
Cranberry juice cocktail, with apple juice	☹	Avoid consumption.	1½ 🥛	
Cranberry juice cocktail, with blueberry juice	☹	Avoid consumption.	☺	
Fruit drink or punch, ready to drink	1½ 🥛	Glass (200g); 300 mL in total.	1½ 🥛	
Grapefruit juice, unsweetened, white	¼ 🥛	Glass (200g); 50 mL in total.	1 🥛	
Kern's® Mango-Orange Nectar	☹	Avoid consumption.	3 🥛	
Kern's® Strawberry Nectar	☹	Avoid consumption.	☺	

Juices	FRUCTOSE		Standard amount
Apple banana strawberry juice		😞	Avoid consumption.
Apple grape juice		😞	Avoid consumption!
Apricot nectar	B ×5	😊+	Free of fructose. Per Glass (200 mL) you drink with it, add B-no × F-limit.
Arby's® orange juice	¾	🥛	Glass (200g); 150 mL in total.
Black cherry juice	¼	🥛	Glass (200g); 50 mL in total.
Black currant juice	B ×1½	😊+	Free of fructose. Per Glass (200 mL) you drink with it, add B-no × F-limit.
Blackberry juice	¼	🥛	Glass (200g); 50 mL in total.
Capri Sun®, all flavors	B ×1	😊+	Free of fructose. Per Glass (200 mL) you drink with it, add B-no × F-limit.
Carrot juice	B ×1	😊+	Free of fructose. Per Glass (200 mL) you drink with it, add B-no × F-limit.
Cranberry juice cocktail, with apple juice		😞	Avoid consumption.
Cranberry juice cocktail, with blueberry juice		😞	Avoid consumption.
Fruit drink or punch, ready to drink	B ×1	😊+	Free of fructose. Per Glass (200 mL) you drink with it, add B-no × F-limit.
Grapefruit juice, unsweetened, white	B ×5	😊+	Free of fructose. Per Glass (200 mL) you drink with it, add B-no × F-limit.
Kern's® Mango-Orange Nectar		😞	Avoid consumption.
Kern's® Strawberry Nectar		😞	Avoid consumption.

Juices	SORBITOL Stand.	SORBITOL Low sensitivity amount
Apple banana strawberry juice	☹ Avoid	☹ Avoid consumption!
Apple grape juice	☹ Avoid	☹ Avoid consumption!
Apricot nectar	☹ Avoid	¼ 🥛 Glass (200g); 50 mL in total.
Arby's® orange juice	☹ Avoid	¼ 🥛 Glass (200g); 50 mL in total.
Black cherry juice	☹ Avoid	2½ 🥛 Glass (200g); 500 mL in total.
Black currant juice	☹ Avoid	1½ 🥛 Glass (200g); 300 mL in total.
Blackberry juice	☺ Free	☺ Free of sorbitol.
Capri Sun®, all flavors	☹ Avoid	2 🥛 Glass (200g); 400 mL in total.
Carrot juice	☹ Avoid	4 🥛 Glass (200g); 800 mL in total.
Cranberry juice cocktail, with apple juice	☹ Avoid	☹ Avoid consumption!
Cranberry juice cocktail, with blueberry juice	☹ Avoid	☹ Avoid consumption!
Fruit drink or punch, ready to drink	☹ Avoid	2 🥛 Glass (200g); 400 mL in total.
Grapefruit juice, unsweetened, white	☹ Avoid	¼ 🥛 Glass (200g); 50 mL in total.
Kern's® Mango-Orange Nectar	☹ Avoid	2 🥛 Glass (200g); 400 mL in total.
Kern's® Strawberry Nectar	☹ Avoid	¾ 🥛 Glass (200g); 150 mL in total.

Juices	LACTOSE	Standard amount
Lemon juice, fresh	🙂	Free of lactose.
Libby's® Apricot Nectar	🙂	Free of lactose.
Libby's® Banana Nectar	🙂	Free of lactose.
Libby's® Juicy Juice®, Apple Grape	🙂	Free of lactose.
Libby's® Juicy Juice®, Grape	🙂	Free of lactose.
Libby's® Pear Nectar	🙂	Free of lactose.
Lime juice, fresh	🙂	Free of lactose.
Mango nectar	🙂	Free of lactose.
Northland® Cranberry Juice, all flavors	🙂	Free of lactose.
Orange kiwi passion juice	🙂	Free of lactose.
Passion fruit juice	🙂	Free of lactose.
Peach juice	🙂	Free of lactose.
Pear juice	🙂	Free of lactose.
Pineapple juice	🙂	Free of lactose.
Pineapple orange drink	🙂	Free of lactose.
Pomegranate juice	🙂	Free of lactose.

Juices	IBS Standard amount		F+G amount
Lemon juice, fresh	1½ ☺	Glass (200g); 300 mL in total.	2¼ ☺
Libby's® Apricot Nectar	☹	Avoid consumption.	☺
Libby's® Banana Nectar	☹	Avoid consumption.	½ ☺
Libby's® Juicy Juice®, Apple Grape	☹	Avoid consumption!	1½ ☺
Libby's® Juicy Juice®, Grape	☹	Avoid consumption!	1½ ☺
Libby's® Pear Nectar	☹	Avoid consumption!	☺
Lime juice, fresh	2¼ ☺	Glass (200g); 450g in total.	2¼ ☺
Mango nectar	¾ ☺	Glass (200g); 150 mL in total.	☺
Northland® Cranberry Juice, all flavors	25 ☺	Glass (200g); 5,000 mL in total.	☺
Orange kiwi passion juice	¾ ☺	Glass (200g); 150 mL in total.	☺
Passion fruit juice	☺	Free of triggers.	☺
Peach juice	½ ☺	Glass (200g); 100 mL in total.	½ ☺
Pear juice	☹	Avoid consumption!!	1½ ☺
Pineapple juice	1½ ☺	Glass (200g); 300 mL in total.	1½ ☺
Pineapple orange drink	¾ ☺	Glass (200g); 150 mL in total.	1½ ☺
Pomegranate juice	☹	Avoid consumption!	☺

Juices	FRUCTOSE		Standard amount
Lemon juice, fresh	1¾		Glass (200g); 350 mL in total.
Libby's® Apricot Nectar			Avoid consumption.
Libby's® Banana Nectar			Avoid consumption.
Libby's® Juicy Juice®, Apple Grape			Avoid consumption!
Libby's® Juicy Juice®, Grape			Avoid consumption!
Libby's® Pear Nectar			Avoid consumption!
Lime juice, fresh	B ×¾		Free of fructose. Per Glass (200 mL) you drink with it, add B-no × F-limit.
Mango nectar	¾		Glass (200g); 150 mL in total.
Northland® Cranberry Juice, all flavors	B ×7¼		Free of fructose. Per Glass (200 mL) you drink with it, add B-no × F-limit.
Orange kiwi passion juice			Free of fructose.
Passion fruit juice	B ×3¾		Free of fructose. Per Glass (200 mL) you drink with it, add B-no × F-limit.
Peach juice	½		Glass (200g); 100 mL in total.
Pear juice			Avoid consumption!
Pineapple juice	B ×3¼		Free of fructose. Per Glass (200 mL) you drink with it, add B-no × F-limit.
Pineapple orange drink	¾		Glass (200g); 150 mL in total.
Pomegranate juice	1¼		Glass (200g); 250 mL in total.

Juices	SORBITOL Stand.	SORBITOL Low sensitivity amount
Lemon juice, fresh	☹ Avoid	1½ Glass (200g); 300 mL in total.
Libby's® Apricot Nectar	☹ Avoid	¼ Glass (200g); 50 mL in total.
Libby's® Banana Nectar	☹ Avoid	25 Glass (200g); 5,000 mL in total.
Libby's® Juicy Juice®, Apple Grape	☹ Avoid	¼ Glass (200g); 50 mL in total.
Libby's® Juicy Juice®, Grape	☹ Avoid	¼ Glass (200g); 50 mL in total.
Libby's® Pear Nectar	☹ Avoid	☹ Avoid consumption!
Lime juice, fresh	☺ Free	☺ Free of sorbitol.
Mango nectar	☹ Avoid	1¼ Glass (200g); 250 mL in total.
Northland® Cranberry Juice, all flavors	☹ Avoid	25 Glass (200g); 5,000 mL in total.
Orange kiwi passion juice	☹ Avoid	¾ Glass (200g); 150 mL in total.
Passion fruit juice	☺ Free	☺ Free of sorbitol.
Peach juice	☹ Avoid	¾ Glass (200g); 150 mL in total.
Pear juice	☹ Avoid	☹ Avoid consumption!!
Pineapple juice	☹ Avoid	1¾ Glass (200g); 350 mL in total.
Pineapple orange drink	☺ Free	☺ Free of sorbitol.
Pomegranate juice	☹ Avoid	☹ Avoid consumption!

Juices	LACTOSE	Standard amount	
Raspberry juice	🙂	Free of lactose.	
Tomato juice	🙂	Free of lactose.	
V-8® 100% A-C-E Vitamin Rich Vegetable Juice	🙂	Free of lactose.	
Veryfine Cranberry Raspberry	🙂	Free of lactose.	

Juices	IBS	Standard amount	F+G	amount
Raspberry juice	☹	Avoid consumption!	¾	🥛
Tomato juice	¼ 🥛	Glass (200g); 50 mL in total.	2¾	🥛
V-8® 100% A-C-E Vitamin Rich Vegetable Juice	¼ 🥛	Glass (200g); 50 mL in total.	2¾	🥛
Veryfine Cranberry Rasp-berry	☹	Avoid consumption.	¾	🥛

Juices	FRUCTOSE	Standard amount
Raspberry juice	☹	Avoid consumption!
Tomato juice	¾ 🥛	Glass (200g); 150 mL in total.
V-8® 100% A-C-E Vitamin Rich Vegetable Juice	¼ 🥛	Glass (200g); 50 mL in total.
Veryfine Cranberry Raspberry	☹	Avoid consumption.

Juices	SORBITOL Stand.	SORBITOL Low sensitivity amount	
Raspberry juice	☹ Avoid	☹	Avoid consumption!
Tomato juice	☹ Avoid	¼ 🥛	Glass (200g); 50 mL in total.
V-8® 100% A-C-E Vitamin Rich Vegetable Juice	☹ Avoid	3 🥛	Glass (200g); 600 mL in total.
Veryfine Cranberry Raspberry	☹ Avoid	☹	Avoid consumption!

3.3.4 Other beverages

Other beverages	LACTOSE	Standard amount
7 UP®	☺	Free of lactose.
Canfield's® Root Beer	☺	Free of lactose.
Canfield's® Root Beer, diet	☺	Free of lactose.
Cherry Coke®	☺	Free of lactose.
Coke Zero®	☺	Free of lactose.
Coke®	☺	Free of lactose.
Coke® with Lime	☺	Free of lactose.
Diet 7 UP®	☺	Free of lactose.
Diet Coke®	☺	Free of lactose.
Diet Dr. Pepper®	☺	Free of lactose.
Diet Pepsi®, fountain	☺	Free of lactose.
Fanta Zero®, fruit flavors	☺	Free of lactose.
Fanta® Red	☺	Free of lactose.
Fanta®, fruit flavors	☺	Free of lactose.
Ginger ale	☺	Free of lactose.

Other beverages	IBS	Standard amount	F+G	amount
7 UP®	☹	Avoid consumption!	☺	
Canfield's® Root Beer	☺	Free of triggers.	☺	
Canfield's® Root Beer, diet	☺	Free of triggers.	☺	
Cherry Coke®	½ 🥛	Glass (200g); 100 mL in total.	☺	
Coke Zero®	☺	Free of triggers.	☺	
Coke®	½ 🥛	Glass (200g); 100 mL in total.	☺	
Coke® with Lime	½ 🥛	Glass (200g); 100 mL in total.	☺	
Diet 7 UP®	☺	Free of triggers.	☺	
Diet Coke®	☺	Free of triggers.	☺	
Diet Dr. Pepper®	☺	Free of triggers.	☺	
Diet Pepsi®, fountain	☺	Free of triggers.	☺	
Fanta Zero®, fruit flavors	☺	Free of triggers.	☺	
Fanta® Red	☹	Avoid consumption.	☺	
Fanta®, fruit flavors	8¼ 🥛	Glass (200g); 1,650 mL in total.	☺	
Ginger ale	☹	Avoid consumption!	☺	

Other beverages	FRUCTOSE		Standard amount
7 UP®	☹		Avoid consumption!
Canfield's® Root Beer	☺		Free of fructose.
Canfield's® Root Beer, diet	☺		Free of fructose.
Cherry Coke®	½	🥛	Glass (200g); 100 mL in total.
Coke Zero®	☺		Free of fructose.
Coke®	½	🥛	Glass (200g); 100 mL in total.
Coke® with Lime	½	🥛	Glass (200g); 100 mL in total.
Diet 7 UP®	☺		Free of fructose.
Diet Coke®	☺		Free of fructose.
Diet Dr. Pepper®	☺		Free of fructose.
Diet Pepsi®, fountain	☺		Free of fructose.
Fanta Zero®, fruit flavors	☺		Free of fructose.
Fanta® Red	☹		Avoid consumption.
Fanta®, fruit flavors	8¼	🥛	Glass (200g); 1,650 mL in total.
Ginger ale	☹		Avoid consumption!

Other beverages	SORBITOL Stand.	SORBITOL Low sensitivity amount
7 UP®	🙂 Free	🙂 Free of sorbitol.
Canfield's® Root Beer	🙂 Free	🙂 Free of sorbitol.
Canfield's® Root Beer, diet	🙂 Free	🙂 Free of sorbitol.
Cherry Coke®	🙂 Free	🙂 Free of sorbitol.
Coke Zero®	🙂 Free	🙂 Free of sorbitol.
Coke®	🙂 Free	🙂 Free of sorbitol.
Coke® with Lime	🙂 Free	🙂 Free of sorbitol.
Diet 7 UP®	🙂 Free	🙂 Free of sorbitol.
Diet Coke®	🙂 Free	🙂 Free of sorbitol.
Diet Dr. Pepper®	🙂 Free	🙂 Free of sorbitol.
Diet Pepsi®, fountain	🙂 Free	🙂 Free of sorbitol.
Fanta Zero®, fruit flavors	🙂 Free	🙂 Free of sorbitol.
Fanta® Red	🙂 Free	🙂 Free of sorbitol.
Fanta®, fruit flavors	🙂 Free	🙂 Free of sorbitol.
Ginger ale	🙂 Free	🙂 Free of sorbitol.

Other beverages	LACTOSE	Standard amount
Lipton® Iced Tea Mix, sweetened with sugar, prepared	🙂	Free of lactose.
Lipton® Instant 100% Tea, unsweetened, prepared	🙂	Free of lactose.
Mineral Water	🙂	Free of lactose.
Monster® Energy®	🙂	Free of lactose.
Monster® Khaos	🙂	Free of lactose.
Mountain Dew®	🙂	Free of lactose.
Mountain Dew® Code Red	🙂	Free of lactose.
Nestea® 100% Tea, unsweetened, dry	🙂	Free of lactose.
Nestea® Iced Tea, Sugar Free, dry	🙂	Free of lactose.
Nestea® Iced Tea, Sugar Free, prepared	🙂	Free of lactose.
Nestea® Iced Tea, sweetened with sugar, dry	🙂	Free of lactose.
No Fear®	🙂	Free of lactose.
No Fear® Sugar Free	🙂	Free of lactose.
Pepsi®	🙂	Free of lactose.
Pepsi® Max	🙂	Free of lactose.
Pepsi® Twist	🙂	Free of lactose.

Other beverages	IBS	Standard amount	F+G	amount
Lipton® Iced Tea Mix, with sugar, prepared	😊	Free of triggers.	😊	
Lipton® Instant 100% Tea, unsweetened, prepared	😊	Free of triggers.	😊	
Mineral Water	😊	Free of triggers.	😊	
Monster® Energy®	😊	Free of triggers.	😊	
Monster® Khaos	¼ 🥣	Portion (240g); 60g in total.	😊	
Mountain Dew®	☹️	Avoid consumption.	😊	
Mountain Dew® Code Red	☹️	Avoid consumption.	😊	
Nestea® 100% Tea, unsweetened, dry	😊	Free of triggers.	😊	
Nestea® Iced Tea, Sugar Free, dry	😊	Free of triggers.	😊	
Nestea® Iced Tea, Sugar Free, prepared	😊	Free of triggers.	😊	
Nestea® Iced Tea, sweetened with sugar, dry	😊	Free of triggers.	😊	
No Fear®	😊	Free of triggers.	😊	
No Fear® Sugar Free	😊	Free of triggers.	😊	
Pepsi®	½ 🥛	Glass (200g); 100 mL in total.	😊	
Pepsi® Max	😊	Free of triggers.	😊	
Pepsi® Twist	½ 🥛	Glass (200g); 100 mL in total.	😊	

Other beverages	FRUCTOSE		Standard amount
Lipton® Iced Tea Mix, with sugar, prepared		☺	Free of fructose.
Lipton® Instant 100% Tea, unsweetened, prepared		☺	Free of fructose.
Mineral Water		☺	Free of fructose.
Monster® Energy®	B ×17	☺	Free of fructose. Per Glass (200 mL) you drink with it, add B-no × F-limit.
Monster® Khaos	B ×9½	☺	Free of fructose. Per Portion (240g) you eat with it, add B-no × F-limit.
Mountain Dew®		☹	Avoid consumption.
Mountain Dew® Code Red		☹	Avoid consumption.
Nestea® 100% Tea, unsweetened, dry	B ×22	☺	Free of fructose. Per Glass (200 mL) you drink with it, add B-no × F-limit.
Nestea® Iced Tea, Sugar Free, dry	B ×11	☺	Free of fructose. Per Glass (200 mL) you drink with it, add B-no × F-limit.
Nestea® Iced Tea, Sugar Free, prepared		☺	Free of fructose.
Nestea® Iced Tea, sweetened with sugar, dry		☺	Free of fructose.
No Fear®	B ×6¼	☺	Free of fructose. Per Glass (200 mL) you drink with it, add B-no × F-limit.
No Fear® Sugar Free		☺	Free of fructose.
Pepsi®	½	🥛	Glass (200g); 100 mL in total.
Pepsi® Max		☺	Free of fructose.
Pepsi® Twist	½	🥛	Glass (200g); 100 mL in total.

Other beverages	SORBITOL Stand.	SORBITOL Low sensitivity amount
Lipton® Iced Tea Mix, with sugar, prepared	🙂 Free	🙂 Free of sorbitol.
Lipton® Instant 100% Tea, unsweetened, prepared	🙂 Free	🙂 Free of sorbitol.
Mineral Water	🙂 Free	🙂 Free of sorbitol.
Monster® Energy®	🙂 Free	🙂 Free of sorbitol.
Monster® Khaos	☹️ Avoid	¼ 🥣 Portion (240g); 60g in total.
Mountain Dew®	🙂 Free	🙂 Free of sorbitol.
Mountain Dew® Code Red	🙂 Free	🙂 Free of sorbitol.
Nestea® 100% Tea, unsweetened, dry	🙂 Free	🙂 Free of sorbitol.
Nestea® Iced Tea, Sugar Free, dry	🙂 Free	🙂 Free of sorbitol.
Nestea® Iced Tea, Sugar Free, prepared	🙂 Free	🙂 Free of sorbitol.
Nestea® Iced Tea, sweetened with sugar, dry	🙂 Free	🙂 Free of sorbitol.
No Fear®	☹️ Avoid	50 🥤 Glass (200g); 10,000 mL in total.
No Fear® Sugar Free	🙂 Free	🙂 Free of sorbitol.
Pepsi®	🙂 Free	🙂 Free of sorbitol.
Pepsi® Max	🙂 Free	🙂 Free of sorbitol.
Pepsi® Twist	🙂 Free	🙂 Free of sorbitol.

Other beverages	LACTOSE	Standard amount	
Red Bull® Energy Drink	☺	Free of lactose.	
Red Bull® Energy Drink Sugar Free	☺	Free of lactose.	
Rockstar Original®	☺	Free of lactose.	
Rockstar Original® Sugar Free	☺	Free of lactose.	
Schweppes® Bitter Lemon	☺	Free of lactose.	
Spearmint tea	☺	Free of lactose.	
Sprite®	☺	Free of lactose.	
Sprite® Zero	☺	Free of lactose.	
Tap water	☺	Free of lactose.	
Tonic water	☺	Free of lactose.	
Tonic water, diet	☺	Free of lactose.	
Vanilla Coke®	☺	Free of lactose.	
Yerba® Mate tea	☺	Free of lactose.	

Other beverages	IBS	Standard amount	F+G	amount
Red Bull® Energy Drink	🙂	Free of triggers.	😃	
Red Bull® Energy Drink Sugar Free	🙂	Free of triggers.	🙂	
Rockstar Original®	5 🥛	Glass (200g); 1,000 mL in total.	🙂	
Rockstar Original® Sugar Free	5 🥛	Glass (200g); 1,000 mL in total.	😃	
Schweppes® Bitter Lemon	☹️	Avoid consumption!	🙂	
Spearmint tea	🙂	Free of triggers.	😃	
Sprite®	☹️	Avoid consumption!	🙂	
Sprite® Zero	🙂	Free of triggers.	😃	
Tap water	😃	Free of triggers.	😃	
Tonic water	☹️	Avoid consumption!	🙂	
Tonic water, diet	😃	Free of triggers.	🙂	
Vanilla Coke®	½ 🥛	Glass (200g); 100 mL in total.	🙂	
Yerba® Mate tea	🙂	Free of triggers.	😃	

Other beverages	FRUCTOSE		Standard amount
Red Bull® Energy Drink	B ×7¾	☺+	Free of fructose. Per Glass (200 mL) you drink with it, add B-no × F-limit.
Red Bull® Energy Drink Sugar Free		☺	Free of fructose.
Rockstar Original®	B ×23	☺+	Free of fructose. Per Glass (200 mL) you drink with it, add B-no × F-limit.
Rockstar Original® Sugar Free		☺	Free of fructose.
Schweppes® Bitter Lemon		☹	Avoid consumption!
Spearmint tea		☺	Free of fructose.
Sprite®		☹	Avoid consumption!
Sprite® Zero		☺	Free of fructose.
Tap water		☺	Free of fructose.
Tonic water		☹	Avoid consumption!
Tonic water, diet		☺	Free of fructose.
Vanilla Coke®	½	🥛	Glass (200g); 100 mL in total.
Yerba® Mate tea		☺	Free of fructose.

Other beverages	SORBITOL Stand.		SORBITOL Low sensitivity amount	
Red Bull® Energy Drink	😊	Free	😊	Free of sorbitol.
Red Bull® Energy Drink Sugar Free	😊	Free	😊	Free of sorbitol.
Rockstar Original®	😞	Avoid	5 🥛	Glass (200g); 1,000 mL in total.
Rockstar Original® Sugar Free	😞	Avoid	5 🥛	Glass (200g); 1,000 mL in total.
Schweppes® Bitter Lemon	😊	Free	😊	Free of sorbitol.
Spearmint tea	😊	Free	😊	Free of sorbitol.
Sprite®	😊	Free	😊	Free of sorbitol.
Sprite® Zero	😊	Free	😊	Free of sorbitol.
Tap water	😊	Free	😊	Free of sorbitol.
Tonic water	😊	Free	😊	Free of sorbitol.
Tonic water, diet	😊	Free	😊	Free of sorbitol.
Vanilla Coke®	😊	Free	😊	Free of sorbitol.
Yerba® Mate tea	😊	Free	😊	Free of sorbitol.

3.4 Cold dishes

3.4.1 Bread

Bread	LACTOSE	Standard amount	🟢
Baguette	🙂	Free of lactose.	
Cracked wheat bread, with raisins	🙂	Free of lactose.	
English muffin bread	🙂	Free of lactose.	
Focaccia bread	🙂	Free of lactose.	
French or Vienna roll	🙂	Free of lactose.	
GG® Scandinavian Bran Crispbread (Health Valley®)	🙂	Free of lactose.	
Gluten free bread	🙂	Free of lactose.	
Newman's Own® Organic Pretzels, Spelt	🙂	Free of lactose.	
Potato bread	6¼	Slice (34g); 213g in total.	+5¼
Pumpernickel roll	🙂	Free of lactose.	
Rice bread	🙂	Free of lactose.	
Rye bread	🙂	Free of lactose.	
Rye roll	🙂	Free of lactose.	
Sourdough bread	🙂	Free of lactose.	

Bread	IBS Standard amount			F+G amount	
Baguette	1¾		Slice (42g); 74g in total.	1¾	
Cracked wheat bread, with raisins	1¼		Slice (42g); 53g in total.	1¾	
English muffin bread	1¾		Slice (42g); 74g in total.	1¾	
Focaccia bread	1¼		Slice (42g); 53g in total.	1¼	
French or Vienna roll	1¼		Slice (42g); 53g in total.	1¼	
GG® Scandinavian Bran Crispbread (Health Valley®)	¼		Slice (42g); 11g in total.	¼	
Gluten free bread	3½		Slice (42g); 147g in total.	3½	
Newman's Own® Organic Pretzels, Spelt	¾		Slice (42g); 32g in total.	¾	
Potato bread	1½		Slice (34g); 51g in total.	1½	
Pumpernickel roll	½		Slice (42g); 21g in total.	½	
Rice bread		☺	Free of triggers.		☺
Rye bread	¾		Slice (42g); 32g in total.	¾	
Rye roll	¾		Slice (42g); 32g in total.	¾	
Sourdough bread	¾		Slice (42g); 32g in total.	¾	

Bread	FRUCTOSE	Standard amount
Baguette	😊	Free of fructose.
Cracked wheat bread, with raisins	1¼	Slice (42g); 53g in total.
English muffin bread	38¼	Slice (42g); 1,607g in total.
Focaccia bread	😊	Free of fructose.
French or Vienna roll	😊	Free of fructose.
GG® Scandinavian Bran Crispbread (Health Valley®)	🙂	Nearly free of fructose, avoid at hereditary fructose intolerance.
Gluten free bread	😊	Free of fructose.
Newman's Own® Organic Pretzels, Spelt	B × ½ 🙂	Free of fructose. Per Slice (42g) you eat with it, add B-no × F-limit.
Potato bread	😊	Free of fructose.
Pumpernickel roll	😊	Free of fructose.
Rice bread	😊	Free of fructose.
Rye bread	😊	Free of fructose.
Rye roll	😊	Free of fructose.
Sourdough bread	😊	Free of fructose.

Bread	SORBITOL Stand.		SORBITOL Low sensitivity amount
Baguette	🙂 Free		🙂 Free of sorbitol.
Cracked wheat bread, with raisins	☹ Avoid	4¼ 👆	Slice (42g); 179g in total.
English muffin bread	🙂 Free		🙂 Free of sorbitol.
Focaccia bread	🙂 Free		🙂 Free of sorbitol.
French or Vienna roll	🙂 Free		🙂 Free of sorbitol.
GG® Scandinavian Bran Crispbread (Health Valley®)	🙂 Free		🙂 Free of sorbitol.
Gluten free bread	🙂 Free		🙂 Free of sorbitol.
Newman's Own® Organic Pretzels, Spelt	🙂 Free		🙂 Free of sorbitol.
Potato bread	🙂 Nearly free		🙂 Nearly free of sorbitol
Pumpernickel roll	🙂 Free		🙂 Free of sorbitol.
Rice bread	🙂 Free		🙂 Free of sorbitol.
Rye bread	🙂 Free		🙂 Free of sorbitol.
Rye roll	🙂 Free		🙂 Free of sorbitol.
Sourdough bread	🙂 Free		🙂 Free of sorbitol.

Bread	LACTOSE	Standard amount	
Soy bread	3½	Slice (42g); 147g in total.	+3
Toast, cinnamon and sugar, whole wheat bread	49½	Slice (42g); 2,079g in total.	+41¼
Toast, wheat bread, with butter	62½	Slice (42g); 2,625g in total.	+52
Triticale bread	☺	Free of lactose.	
White bread, store bought	☺	Nearly free of lactose	
White whole grain wheat bread	☺	Free of lactose.	
Whole wheat bread, store bought	☺	Free of lactose.	

Bread	IBS	Standard amount	F+G	amount
Soy bread	1	Slice (42g); 42g in total.	1	
Toast, cinnamon and sugar, whole wheat bread	¾	Slice (42g); 32g in total.	¾	
Toast, wheat bread, with butter	1¼	Slice (42g); 53g in total.	1¼	
Triticale bread	1	Slice (42g); 42g in total.	1	
White bread, store bought	1¼	Slice (42g); 53g in total.	1¼	
White whole grain wheat bread	¾	Slice (42g); 32g in total.	¾	
Whole wheat bread, store bought	1	Slice (42g); 42g in total.	1	

Bread	FRUCTOSE		Standard amount
Soy bread	5½		Slice (42g); 231g in total.
Toast, cinnamon and sugar, whole wheat bread	1½		Slice (42g); 63g in total.
Toast, wheat bread, with butter	1¾		Slice (42g); 74g in total.
Triticale bread	2½		Slice (42g); 105g in total.
White bread, store bought	1¼		Slice (42g); 53g in total.
White whole grain wheat bread	¾		Slice (42g); 32g in total.
Whole wheat bread, store bought	1¼		Slice (42g); 53g in total.

Bread	SORBITOL Stand.	SORBITOL Low sensitivity amount	
Soy bread	Avoid	2	Slice (42g); 84g in total.
Toast, cinnamon and sugar, whole wheat bread	Free		Free of sorbitol.
Toast, wheat bread, with butter	Free		Free of sorbitol.
Triticale bread	Free		Free of sorbitol.
White bread, store bought	Free		Free of sorbitol.
White whole grain wheat bread	Avoid	26¼	Slice (42g); 1,103g in total.
Whole wheat bread, store bought	Free		Free of sorbitol.

3.4.2 Cereals

Cereals	LACTOSE	Standard amount	➕
All-Bran® Original (Kellogg's®)	😊	Free of lactose.	
Amaranth Flakes (Arrowhead Mills)	😊	Free of lactose.	
Cascadian Farm® Organic Gran. Bar, Dark Chocolate Cranberry	10 🍰	Piece (35g); 350g in total.	+8¼
Cheerios® Snack Mix, all flavors	😊	Free of lactose.	
Chocolate Chex® (General Mills®)	😊	Free of lactose.	
Cinnamon toast crunch® (General Mills®)	😊	Free of lactose.	
Cinnamon Toasters® (Malt-O-Meal®)	😊	Free of lactose.	
Cocoa Krispies® (Kellogg's®)	😊	Free of lactose.	
Cocoa Puffs® (General Mills®)	😊	Free of lactose.	
Corn Chex® (General Mills®)	😊	Free of lactose.	
Corn Flakes (Kellogg's®)	😊	Free of lactose.	
Crunchy Nut Roasted Nut & Honey (Kellogg's®)	😊	Nearly free of lactose	
Essentials Oat Bran cereal (Quaker®)	😊	Free of lactose.	
Evaporated milk, diluted, skim (fat free)	🥛	Glass (240g); Avoid consumption!!	0.19
Familia Swiss Muesli®, Original Recipe	😊	Free of lactose.	

Cereals	IBS	Standard amount	F+G	amount
All-Bran® Original (Kellogg's®)	¼	Portion (30g); 8g in total.	¼	
Amaranth Flakes (Arrowhead Mills)	¾	Portion (30g); 23g in total.	¾	
Cascadian Farm® Organic Granola Bar, Trail Mix Dark Chocolate Cranberry	½	Piece (35g); 18g in total.	½	
Cheerios® Snack Mix, all flavors	½	Portion (30g); 15g in total.	½	
Chocolate Chex® (General Mills®)	¼	Tbsp. (15g); 4g in total.	1¼	
Cinnamon toast crunch® (General Mills®)	¼	Portion (30g); 8g in total.	1½	
Cinnamon Toasters® (Malt-O-Meal®)	1½	Portion (30g); 45g in total.	1½	
Cocoa Krispies® (Kellogg's®)	1½	Portion (30g); 45g in total.	1½	
Cocoa Puffs® (General Mills®)	½	Portion (30g); 15g in total.	½	
Corn Chex® (General Mills®)	½	Portion (30g); 15g in total.	½	
Corn Flakes (Kellogg's®)	1½	Portion (30g); 45g in total.	1½	
Crunchy Nut Roasted Nut & Honey (Kellogg's®)	1½	Portion (30g); 45g in total.	1½	
Essentials Oat Bran cereal (Quaker®)	1¼	Portion (55g); 69g in total.	1¼	
Evaporated milk, diluted, skim (fat free)	¼	Glass (200g); 50 mL in total.	1¼	
Familia Swiss Muesli®, Original Recipe	¼	Portion (55g); 14g in total.	¼	

Cereals	FRUCTOSE		Standard amount
All-Bran® Original (Kellogg's®)	B ×¼	☺ +	Free of fructose. Per Portion (30g) you eat with it, add B-no × F-limit.
Amaranth Flakes (Arrowhead Mills)	3		Portion (30g); 90g in total.
Cascadian Farm® Organic Granola Bar, Trail Mix Dark Chocolate Cranberry	B ×4¼	☺ +	Free of fructose. Per Piece (35g) you eat with it, add B-no × F-limit.
Cheerios® Snack Mix, all flavors	5		Portion (30g); 150g in total.
Chocolate Chex® (General Mills®)	¼		Tbsp. (15g); 4g in total.
Cinnamon toast crunch® (General Mills®)	¼		Portion (30g); 8g in total.
Cinnamon Toasters® (Malt-O-Meal®)	2		Portion (30g); 60g in total.
Cocoa Krispies® (Kellogg's®)		☺	Free of fructose.
Cocoa Puffs® (General Mills®)	B ×2	☺ +	Free of fructose. Per Portion (30g) you eat with it, add B-no × F-limit.
Corn Chex® (General Mills®)		☺	Free of fructose.
Corn Flakes (Kellogg's®)	B ×1½	☺ +	Free of fructose. Per Portion (30g) you eat with it, add B-no × F-limit.
Crunchy Nut Roasted Nut & Honey (Kellogg's®)	18¼		Portion (30g); 548g in total.
Essentials Oat Bran cereal (Quaker®)		☺	Free of fructose.
Evaporated milk, diluted, skim (fat free)		☺	Free of fructose.
Familia Swiss Muesli®, Original Recipe	¾		Portion (55g); 41g in total.

Cereals	SORBITOL Stand.		SORBITOL Low sensitivity amount
All-Bran® Original (Kellogg's®)	😀 Free		😀 Free of sorbitol.
Amaranth Flakes (Arrowhead Mills)	🙁 Avoid	2½	Portion (30g); 75g in total.
Cascadian Farm® Organic Granola Bar, Trail Mix Dark Chocolate Cranberry	🙁 Avoid	71¼	Piece (35g); 2,494g in total.
Cheerios® Snack Mix, all flavors	🙂 Nearly free		🙂 Nearly free of sorbitol
Chocolate Chex® (General Mills®)	🙂 Nearly free		🙂 Nearly free of sorbitol
Cinnamon toast crunch® (General Mills®)	😀 Free		😀 Free of sorbitol.
Cinnamon Toasters® (Malt-O-Meal®)	😀 Free		😀 Free of sorbitol.
Cocoa Krispies® (Kellogg's®)	🙂 Nearly free		🙂 Nearly free of sorbitol
Cocoa Puffs® (General Mills®)	🙂 Nearly free		🙂 Nearly free of sorbitol
Corn Chex® (General Mills®)	🙂 Nearly free		🙂 Nearly free of sorbitol
Corn Flakes (Kellogg's®)	🙂 Nearly free		🙂 Nearly free of sorbitol
Crunchy Nut Roasted Nut & Honey (Kellogg's®)	🙁 Avoid	15	Portion (30g); 450g in total.
Essentials Oat Bran cereal (Quaker®)	😀 Free		😀 Free of sorbitol.
Evaporated milk, diluted, skim (fat free)	😀 Free		😀 Free of sorbitol.
Familia Swiss Muesli®, Original Recipe	🙁 Avoid	1	Portion (55g); 55g in total.

Cereals	LACTOSE	Standard amount	
Fiber One Original® (General Mills®)	😊	Free of lactose.	
Fiber One® Nutty Clusters & Almonds (General Mills®)	😊	Free of lactose.	
Froot Loops® (Kellogg's®)	😊	Free of lactose.	
Frosted Flakes® (Kellogg's®)	😊	Free of lactose.	
Frosted Flakes® Reduced Sugar (Kellogg's®)	😊	Free of lactose.	
Frosted Mini-Wheats Big Bite® (Kellogg's®)	😊	Free of lactose.	
GoLEAN® Crisp! Cereal, Cinnamon Crumble (Kashi®)	😊	Free of lactose.	
GoLEAN® Crunch! Cereal, Honey Almond Flax (Kashi®)	😊	Free of lactose.	
Health Valley® Multigrain Chewy Granola Bar, Chocolate Chip	12 🍰	Piece (29g); 348g in total.	+10
Honey	😊	Nearly free of lactose	
Honey Nut Chex® (General Mills®)	😊	Free of lactose.	
Honey Smacks® (Kellogg's®)	😊	Free of lactose.	
Kashi® Chewy Granola Bar, Cherry Dark Chocolate	10 🍰	Piece (35g); 350g in total.	+8¼
Maple syrup, pure	😊	Free of lactose.	
Milk, lactose reduced Lactaid®, skim (fat free) fortified with calcium or not	😊	Free of lactose.	

Cereals	IBS	Standard amount	F+G	amount
Fiber One Original® (General Mills®)	½	Portion (30g); 15g in total.	½	
Fiber One® Nutty Clusters & Almonds (General Mills®)	¼	Portion (55g); 14g in total.	¼	
Froot Loops® (Kellogg's®)	½	Portion (30g); 15g in total.	½	
Frosted Flakes® (Kellogg's®)	1½	Portion (30g); 45g in total.	1½	
Frosted Flakes® Reduced Sugar (Kellogg's®)	1½	Portion (30g); 45g in total.	1½	
Frosted Mini-Wheats Big Bite® (Kellogg's®)	¼	Portion (55g); 14g in total.	¼	
GoLEAN® Crisp! Cereal, Cinnamon Crumble (Kashi®)	¼	Portion (55g); 14g in total.	¼	
GoLEAN® Crunch! Cereal, Honey Almond Flax (Kashi®)	¼	Portion (55g); 14g in total.	¼	
Health Valley® Multigrain Granola Bar, Chocolate Chip	½	Piece (29g); 15g in total.	½	
Honey	½	Tbsp. (15g); 8g in total.	☺	
Honey Nut Chex® (General Mills®)	½	Portion (30g); 15g in total.	½	
Honey Smacks® (Kellogg's®)	½	Portion (30g); 15g in total.	½	
Kashi® Chewy Granola Bar, Cherry Dark Chocolate	½	Piece (35g); 18g in total.	½	
Maple syrup, pure	☺	Free of triggers.	☺	
Milk, lactose reduced Lactaid®, skim (fat free) fortified with calcium or not	☺	Free of triggers.	☺	

Cereals	FRUCTOSE		Standard amount
Fiber One Original® (General Mills®)	41½		Portion (30g); 1,245g in total.
Fiber One® Nutty Clusters & Almonds (General Mills®)		☺	Free of fructose.
Froot Loops® (Kellogg's®)		☺	Free of fructose.
Frosted Flakes® (Kellogg's®)		☺	Free of fructose.
Frosted Flakes® Reduced Sugar (Kellogg's®)	B ×¼	☺	Free of fructose. Per Portion (30g) you eat with it, add B-no × F-limit.
Frosted Mini-Wheats Big Bite® (Kellogg's®)	B ×¼	☺	Free of fructose. Per Portion (55g) you eat with it, add B-no × F-limit.
GoLEAN® Crisp! Cereal, Cinnamon Crumble (Kashi®)	B ×1¼	☺	Free of fructose. Per Portion (55g) you eat with it, add B-no × F-limit.
GoLEAN® Crunch! Cereal, Honey Almond Flax (Kashi®)	B ×1	☺	Free of fructose. Per Portion (55g) you eat with it, add B-no × F-limit.
Health Valley® Multigrain Granola Bar, Chocolate Chip	B ×1	☺	Free of fructose. Per Piece (29g) you eat with it, add B-no × F-limit.
Honey	½		Tbsp. (15g); 8g in total.
Honey Nut Chex® (General Mills®)		☺	Free of fructose.
Honey Smacks® (Kellogg's®)	B ×12	☺	Free of fructose. Per Portion (30g) you eat with it, add B-no × F-limit.
Kashi® Chewy Granola Bar, Cherry Dark Chocolate	B ×1	☺	Free of fructose. Per Piece (35g) you eat with it, add B-no × F-limit.
Maple syrup, pure	B ×¼	☺	Free of fructose. Per Tbsp. (15g) you eat with it, add B-no × F-limit.
Milk, lactose reduced Lactaid®, skim (fat free) fortified with calcium or not	B ×10	☺	Free of fructose. Per Glass (200 mL) you drink with it, add B-no × F-limit.

Cereals	SORBITOL Stand.		SORBITOL Low sensitivity amount
Fiber One Original® (General Mills®)	☺ Free		☺ Free of sorbitol.
Fiber One® Nutty Clusters & Almonds (General Mills®)	☺ Free		☺ Free of sorbitol.
Froot Loops® (Kellogg's®)	☺ Free		☺ Free of sorbitol.
Frosted Flakes® (Kellogg's®)	☺ Nearly free		☺ Nearly free of sorbitol
Frosted Flakes® Reduced Sugar (Kellogg's®)	☺ Nearly free		☺ Nearly free of sorbitol
Frosted Mini-Wheats Big Bite® (Kellogg's®)	☺ Free		☺ Free of sorbitol.
GoLEAN® Crisp! Cereal, Cinnamon Crumble (Kashi®)	☹ Avoid	25¾	Portion (55g); 1,416g in total.
GoLEAN® Crunch! Cereal, Honey Almond Flax (Kashi®)	☹ Avoid	18	Portion (55g); 990g in total.
Health Valley® Multigrain Granola Bar, Chocolate Chip	☺ Nearly free		☺ Nearly free of sorbitol
Honey	☹ Avoid	1¾	Tbsp. (15g); 26g in total.
Honey Nut Chex® (General Mills®)	☹ Avoid	37	Portion (30g); 1,110g in total.
Honey Smacks® (Kellogg's®)	☹ Avoid	83¼	Portion (30g); 2,498g in total.
Kashi® Chewy Granola Bar, Cherry Dark Chocolate	☹ Avoid	1	Piece (35g); 35g in total.
Maple syrup, pure	☺ Free		☺ Free of sorbitol.
Milk, lactose reduced Lactaid®, skim (fat free) fortified with calcium or not	☺ Free		☺ Free of sorbitol.

Cereals	LACTOSE	Standard amount	
Mueslix® (Kellogg's®)	☺	Free of lactose.	
Rice Krispies® (Kellogg's®)	☺	Free of lactose.	
Sorghum	☺	Free of lactose.	
Special K® Blueberry cereal (Kellogg's®)	☺	Free of lactose.	
Special K® Cinnamon Pecan cereal (Kellogg's®)	☺	Free of lactose.	
Special K® Original cereal (Kellogg's®)	13	Portion (30g); 390g in total.	+10¾
Special K® Red Berries cereal (Kellogg's®)	☺	Free of lactose.	
Sprinkles Cookie Crisp® (General Mills®)	☺	Free of lactose.	
Sunbelt Bakery® Chewy Granola Bar, Banana Harvest	14	Piece (25g); 350g in total.	+11¾
Sunbelt Bakery® Chewy Granola Bar, Blueberry Harvest	14	Piece (25g); 350g in total.	+11¾
Sunbelt Bakery® Chewy Granola Bar, Golden Almond	4	Piece (28g); 112g in total.	+3¼
Sunbelt Bakery® Chewy Granola Bar, Low Fat Oatmeal Raisin	11¾	Piece (30g); 353g in total.	+9¾
Sunbelt Bakery® Chewy Granola Bar, Oats & Honey	13	Piece (27g); 351g in total.	+10¾
Sunbelt Bakery® Fudge Dipped Chewy Granola Bar, Coconut	12	Piece (29g); 348g in total.	+10
Weetabix® Organic Crispy Flakes&Fiber Barbara's Bakery®	☺	Free of lactose.	
Wheaties® (General Mills®)	☺	Free of lactose.	

Cereals	IBS Standard amount		F+G amount	
Mueslix® (Kellogg's®)	¼	Portion (55g); 14g in total.	¼	
Rice Krispies® (Kellogg's®)	1½	Portion (30g); 45g in total.	1½	
Sorghum	☺	Free of triggers.	☺	
Special K® Blueberry cereal (Kellogg's®)	½	Portion (30g); 15g in total.	½	
Special K® Cinnamon Pecan cereal (Kellogg's®)	½	Portion (30g); 15g in total.	½	
Special K® Original cereal (Kellogg's®)	½	Portion (30g); 15g in total.	½	
Special K® Red Berries cereal (Kellogg's®)	½	Portion (30g); 15g in total.	½	
Sprinkles Cookie Crisp® (General Mills®)	¾	Portion (30g); 23g in total.	¾	
Sunbelt Bakery® Chewy Granola Bar, Banana Harvest	¾	Piece (25g); 19g in total.	¾	
Sunbelt Bakery® Granola Bar, Blueberry Harvest	¾	Piece (25g); 19g in total.	¾	
Sunbelt Bakery® Chewy Granola Bar, Golden Almond	☹	Avoid consumption!	½	
Sunbelt Bakery® Granola Bar, Low Fat Oatmeal Raisin	☹	Avoid consumption!	½	
Sunbelt Bakery® Chewy Granola Bar, Oats & Honey	☹	Avoid consumption!	½	
Sunbelt Bakery® Fudge Dipped Granola Bar, Coconut	☹	Avoid consumption!	½	
Weetabix® Organic Crispy Flakes & Fiber	¼	Portion (55g); 14g in total.	¼	
Wheaties® (General Mills®)	½	Portion (30g); 15g in total.	½	

Cereals	FRUCTOSE		Standard amount
Mueslix® (Kellogg's®)	B ×¾	☺ +	Free of fructose. Per Portion (55g) you eat with it, add B-no × F-limit.
Rice Krispies® (Kellogg's®)		☺	Free of fructose.
Sorghum		☺	Free of fructose.
Special K® Blueberry cereal (Kellogg's®)	B ×½	☺ +	Free of fructose. Per Portion (30g) you eat with it, add B-no × F-limit.
Special K® Cinnamon Pecan cereal (Kellogg's®)		☺	Nearly free of fructose, avoid at hereditary fructose intolerance.
Special K® Original cereal (Kellogg's®)		☺	Free of fructose.
Special K® Red Berries cereal (Kellogg's®)		☺	Free of fructose.
Sprinkles Cookie Crisp® (General Mills®)	B ×¼	☺ +	Free of fructose. Per Portion (30g) you eat with it, add B-no × F-limit.
Sunbelt Bakery® Chewy Granola Bar, Banana Harvest	B ×¾	☺ +	Free of fructose. Per Piece (25g) you eat with it, add B-no × F-limit.
Sunbelt Bakery® Granola Bar, Blueberry Harvest	B ×¾	☺ +	Free of fructose. Per Piece (25g) you eat with it, add B-no × F-limit.
Sunbelt Bakery® Chewy Granola Bar, Golden Almond	B ×¾	☺ +	Free of fructose. Per Piece (28g) you eat with it, add B-no × F-limit.
Sunbelt Bakery® Granola Bar, Low Fat Oatmeal Raisin		☺	Free of fructose.
Sunbelt Bakery® Chewy Granola Bar, Oats & Honey	B ×¾	☺ +	Free of fructose. Per Piece (27g) you eat with it, add B-no × F-limit.
Sunbelt Bakery® Fudge Dipped Granola Bar, Coconut	B ×1¾	☺ +	Free of fructose. Per Piece (29g) you eat with it, add B-no × F-limit.
Weetabix® Organic Crispy Flakes & Fiber	B ×¾	☺ +	Free of fructose. Per Portion (55g) you eat with it, add B-no × F-limit.
Wheaties® (General Mills®)	83¼	😐	Portion (30g); 2,498g in total.

Cereals	SORBITOL Stand.		SORBITOL Low sensitivity amount
Mueslix® (Kellogg's®)	😞 Avoid	2¾	Portion (55g); 151g in total.
Rice Krispies® (Kellogg's®)	😊 Free		Free of sorbitol.
Sorghum	😊 Free		Free of sorbitol.
Special K® Blueberry cereal (Kellogg's®)	😞 Avoid	15	Portion (30g); 450g in total.
Special K® Cinnamon Pecan cereal (Kellogg's®)	😊 Free		Free of sorbitol.
Special K® Original cereal (Kellogg's®)	😊 Free		Free of sorbitol.
Special K® Red Berries cereal (Kellogg's®)	😞 Avoid	41½	Portion (30g); 1,245g in total.
Sprinkles Cookie Crisp® (General Mills®)	😊 Nearly free		Nearly free of sorbitol
Sunbelt Bakery® Chewy Granola Bar, Banana Harvest	😞 Avoid	¾	Piece (25g); 19g in total.
Sunbelt Bakery® Granola Bar, Blueberry Harvest	😞 Avoid	¾	Piece (25g); 19g in total.
Sunbelt Bakery® Chewy Granola Bar, Golden Almond	😞 Avoid		Avoid consumption!
Sunbelt Bakery® Granola Bar, Low Fat Oatmeal Raisin	😞 Avoid		Avoid consumption!
Sunbelt Bakery® Chewy Granola Bar, Oats & Honey	😞 Avoid		Avoid consumption!
Sunbelt Bakery® Fudge Dipped Granola Bar, Coconut	😞 Avoid		Avoid consumption!
Weetabix® Organic Crispy Flakes & Fiber	😊 Free		Free of sorbitol.
Wheaties® (General Mills®)	😊 Free		Free of sorbitol.

3.4.3 Cold cut

Cold cut	LACTOSE	Standard amount	➕
Almond butter, salted	🙂	Free of lactose.	
Almond butter, unsalted	🙂	Free of lactose.	
Alpine Lace 25% Reduced Fat, Mozzarella	37¼	Portion (30g); 1,118g in total.	+31
American cheese, processed	4½	Portion (30g); 135g in total.	+3¾
Blue cheese	20	Portion (30g); 600g in total.	+16½
Bologna, beef ring	🙂	Free of lactose.	
Bologna, combination of meats, light (reduced fat)	🙂	Free of lactose.	
Brie cheese	22	Portion (30g); 660g in total.	+18½
Butter, light, salted	🙂	Nearly free of lactose	
Butter, unsalted	🙂	Nearly free of lactose	
Camembert cheese	21½	Portion (30g); 645g in total.	+18
Cheddar cheese, natural	43¼	Portion (30g); 1,298g in total.	+36
Cheese sauce, store bought	¼	Portion (66g); 17g in total.	+¼
Colby Jack cheese	27¼	Portion (30g); 818g in total.	+22¾
Cottage cheese, 1% fat, lactose reduced	3¼	Portion (110g); 358g in total.	+2¾

Cold cut	IBS Standard amount		F+G amount	
Almond butter, salted	😊	Free of triggers.	😊	
Almond butter, unsalted	😊	Free of triggers.	😊	
Alpine Lace 25% Reduced Fat, Mozzarella	37¼ 🍽	Portion (30g); 1,118g in total.	😊	
American cheese, processed	4½ 🍽	Portion (30g); 135g in total.	25¾	🍽
Blue cheese	20 🍽	Portion (30g); 600g in total.	😊	
Bologna, beef ring	😊	Free of triggers.	😊	
Bologna, combination of meats, light (reduced fat)	😊	Free of triggers.	😊	
Brie cheese	22 🍽	Portion (30g); 660g in total.	😊	
Butter, light, salted	😊	Free of triggers.	😊	
Butter, unsalted	😊	Nearly free of triggers.	😊	
Camembert cheese	21½ 🍽	Portion (30g); 645g in total.	😊	
Cheddar cheese, natural	43¼ 🍽	Portion (30g); 1,298g in total.	😊	
Cheese sauce, store bought	¼ 🍽	Portion (66g); 17g in total.	1¾	🍽
Colby Jack cheese	27¼ 🍽	Portion (30g); 818g in total.	😊	
Cottage cheese, 1% fat, lactose reduced	3¼ 🍽	Portion (110g); 358g in total.	18¾	🍽

Cold cut	FRUCTOSE		Standard amount
Almond butter, salted		☺	Free of fructose.
Almond butter, unsalted		☺	Free of fructose.
Alpine Lace 25% Reduced Fat, Mozzarella		☺	Free of fructose.
American cheese, processed		☺	Free of fructose.
Blue cheese		☺	Free of fructose.
Bologna, beef ring	B ×5¾	☺+	Free of fructose. Per Portion (55g) you eat with it, add B-no × F-limit.
Bologna, combination of meats, light (reduced fat)	B ×½	☺+	Free of fructose. Per Portion (55g) you eat with it, add B-no × F-limit.
Brie cheese		☺	Free of fructose.
Butter, light, salted		☺	Free of fructose.
Butter, unsalted		☺	Free of fructose.
Camembert cheese		☺	Free of fructose.
Cheddar cheese, natural		☺	Free of fructose.
Cheese sauce, store bought		☺	Free of fructose.
Colby Jack cheese		☺	Free of fructose.
Cottage cheese, 1% fat, lactose reduced	B ×1¾	☺+	Free of fructose. Per Portion (110g) you eat with it, add B-no × F-limit.

Cold cut	SORBITOL Stand.		SORBITOL Low sensitivity amount
Almond butter, salted	☺	Free	☺ Free of sorbitol.
Almond butter, unsalted	☺	Free	☺ Free of sorbitol.
Alpine Lace 25% Reduced Fat, Mozzarella	☺	Free	☺ Free of sorbitol.
American cheese, processed	☺	Free	☺ Free of sorbitol.
Blue cheese	☺	Free	☺ Free of sorbitol.
Bologna, beef ring	☺	Free	☺ Free of sorbitol.
Bologna, combination of meats, light (reduced fat)	☺	Free	☺ Free of sorbitol.
Brie cheese	☺	Free	☺ Free of sorbitol.
Butter, light, salted	☺	Free	☺ Free of sorbitol.
Butter, unsalted	☺	Free	☺ Free of sorbitol.
Camembert cheese	☺	Free	☺ Free of sorbitol.
Cheddar cheese, natural	☺	Free	☺ Free of sorbitol.
Cheese sauce, store bought	☺	Free	☺ Free of sorbitol.
Colby Jack cheese	☺	Free	☺ Free of sorbitol.
Cottage cheese, 1% fat, lactose reduced	☺	Free	☺ Free of sorbitol.

Cold cut	LACTOSE		Standard amount	
Cottage cheese, uncreamed dry curd	3½		Portion (55g); 193g in total.	+2¾
Cream cheese spread	2¾		Portion (30g); 83g in total.	+2¼
Cream cheese, whipped, flavored	2½		Portion (30g); 75g in total.	+2
Cream cheese, whipped, plain	3		Portion (30g); 90g in total.	+2½
Edam cheese	6¾		Portion (30g); 203g in total.	+5¾
Fleischmann's® Move Over Butter Margarine, tub, whipped	21¾		Portion (9g); 196g in total.	+18
Goat cheese, hard	4½		Portion (30g); 135g in total.	+3¾
Gorgonzola cheese	20		Portion (30g); 600g in total.	+16½
Gouda cheese	4½		Portion (30g); 135g in total.	+3¾
Honey			Nearly free of lactose	
Hot dog, combination of meats, plain			Free of lactose.	
Jam or preserves			Free of lactose.	
Jam or preserves, reduced sugar			Free of lactose.	
Jam or preserves, sugar free with aspartame			Free of lactose.	
Jam or preserves, sugar free with saccharin			Free of lactose.	
Jam or preserves, sugar free with sucralose			Free of lactose.	

Cold cut	IBS Standard amount			F+G amount	
Cottage cheese, uncreamed dry curd	3½		Portion (55g); 193g in total.	19¾	
Cream cheese spread	2¾		Portion (30g); 83g in total.	15¾	
Cream cheese, whipped, flavored	2½		Portion (30g); 75g in total.	14	
Cream cheese, whipped, plain	3		Portion (30g); 90g in total.	17¼	
Edam cheese	6¾		Portion (30g); 203g in total.	38¾	
Fleischmann's® Move Over Butter Margarine, tub	21¾		Portion (9g); 196g in total.	☺	
Goat cheese, hard	4½		Portion (30g); 135g in total.	25½	
Gorgonzola cheese	20		Portion (30g); 600g in total.	☺	
Gouda cheese	4½		Portion (30g); 135g in total.	25	
Honey	¼		Portion (21, 19g); 5g in total.	☺	
Hot dog, combination of meats, plain	☺		Free of triggers.	☺	
Jam or preserves	1¾		Portion (20g); 35g in total.	☺	
Jam or preserves, reduced sugar	6¾		Portion (20g); 135g in total.	☺	
Jam or preserves, sugar free with aspartame	5¼		Portion (17g); 89g in total.	☺	
Jam or preserves, sugar free with saccharin	2¼		Portion (14g); 32g in total.	☺	
Jam or preserves, sugar free with sucralose	65¼		Portion (17g); 1,109g in total.	☺	

Cold cut	FRUCTOSE	Standard amount
Cottage cheese, uncreamed dry curd	☺	Free of fructose.
Cream cheese spread	☺	Free of fructose.
Cream cheese, whipped, flavored	☺	Free of fructose.
Cream cheese, whipped, plain	☺	Free of fructose.
Edam cheese	☺	Free of fructose.
Fleischmann's® Move Over Butter Margarine, tub	☺	Free of fructose.
Goat cheese, hard	☺	Free of fructose.
Gorgonzola cheese	☺	Free of fructose.
Gouda cheese	☺	Free of fructose.
Honey	¼	Portion (21, 19g); 5g in total.
Hot dog, combination of meats, plain	B ×3 ☺+	Free of fructose. Per Portion (55g) you eat with it, add B-no × F-limit.
Jam or preserves	B ×2¾ ☺+	Free of fructose. Per Portion (20g) you eat with it, add B-no × F-limit.
Jam or preserves, reduced sugar	6¾	Portion (20g); 135g in total.
Jam or preserves, sugar free with aspartame	10½	Portion (17g); 179g in total.
Jam or preserves, sugar free with saccharin	2¼	Portion (14g); 32g in total.
Jam or preserves, sugar free with sucralose	☺	Free of fructose.

Cold cut	SORBITOL Stand.	SORBITOL	Low sensitivity amount
Cottage cheese, uncreamed dry curd	😊 Free	😊	Free of sorbitol.
Cream cheese spread	😊 Free	😊	Free of sorbitol.
Cream cheese, whipped, flavored	😊 Free	😊	Free of sorbitol.
Cream cheese, whipped, plain	😊 Free	😊	Free of sorbitol.
Edam cheese	😊 Free	😊	Free of sorbitol.
Fleischmann's® Move Over Butter Margarine, tub	😊 Free	😊	Free of sorbitol.
Goat cheese, hard	😊 Free	😊	Free of sorbitol.
Gorgonzola cheese	😊 Free	😊	Free of sorbitol.
Gouda cheese	😊 Free	😊	Free of sorbitol.
Honey	☹ Avoid	1¼	Portion (21, 19g); 26g in total.
Hot dog, combination of meats, plain	😊 Free	😊	Free of sorbitol.
Jam or preserves	☹ Avoid	1¾	Portion (20g); 35g in total.
Jam or preserves, reduced sugar	☹ Avoid	41½	Portion (20g); 830g in total.
Jam or preserves, sugar free with aspartame	☹ Avoid	5¼	Portion (17g); 89g in total.
Jam or preserves, sugar free with saccharin	☹ Avoid	19¼	Portion (14g); 270g in total.
Jam or preserves, sugar free with sucralose	☹ Avoid	65¼	Portion (17g); 1,109g in total.

Cold cut	LACTOSE	Standard amount	⊕
Jam or preserves, without sugar or artificial sweetener	☺	Free of lactose.	
Kraft® Cheese Spread, Roka Blue	1¾	Portion (30g); 53g in total.	+1¼
Limburger cheese	20¼	Portion (30g); 608g in total.	+17
Maple syrup, pure	☺	Free of lactose.	
Margarine, diet, fat free	15½	Portion (14g); 217g in total.	+13
Margarine, tub, salted, sunflower oil	30	Portion (14.19g); 426g in total.	+25
Marmalade, sugar free with aspartame	☺	Free of lactose.	
Marmalade, sugar free with saccharin	☺	Free of lactose.	
Marmalade, sugar free with sucralose	☺	Free of lactose.	
Mascarpone	2½	Portion (30g); 75g in total.	+2
Mortadella	☺	Free of lactose.	
Muenster cheese, natural	8¾	Portion (30g); 263g in total.	+7¼
Nutella® (filbert spread)	32¼	Portion (37g); 1,193g in total.	+27
Roquefort cheese	5	Portion (30g); 150g in total.	+4
Smart Balance® Light with Flax Oil Margarine, tub	32¼	Portion (14g); 452g in total.	+27
Smart Balance® Margarine	31	Portion (14g); 434g in total.	+25¾

Cold cut	IBS	Standard amount	F+G	amount
Jam or preserves, without sugar or artificial sweetener	☹	Avoid consumption!	☺	
Kraft® Cheese Spread, Roka Blue	1¾	Portion (30g); 53g in total.	9¾	
Limburger cheese	20¼	Portion (30g); 608g in total.	☺	
Maple syrup, pure	☺	Free of triggers.	☺	
Margarine, diet, fat free	15½	Portion (14g); 217g in total.	86¾	
Margarine, tub, salted, sunflower oil	30	Portion (14.19g); 426g in total.	☺	
Marmalade, sugar free with aspartame	5¼	Portion (17g); 89g in total.	☺	
Marmalade, sugar free with saccharin	2	Portion (16g); 32g in total.	☺	
Marmalade, sugar free with sucralose	65¼	Portion (17g); 1,109g in total.	☺	
Mascarpone	2½	Portion (30g); 75g in total.	13¾	
Mortadella	☺	Free of triggers.	☺	
Muenster cheese, natural	8¾	Portion (30g); 263g in total.	49½	
Nutella® (filbert spread)	1¼	Portion (37g); 46g in total.	1¼	
Roquefort cheese	5	Portion (30g); 150g in total.	27¾	
Smart Balance® Light with Flax Oil Margarine, tub	32¼	Portion (14g); 452g in total.	☺	
Smart Balance® Margarine	31	Portion (14g); 434g in total.	☺	

Cold cut	FRUCTOSE		Standard amount
Jam or preserves, without sugar or artificial sweetener	¼		Tbsp. (15g); 4g in total.
Kraft® Cheese Spread, Roka Blue		☺	Free of fructose.
Limburger cheese		☺	Free of fructose.
Maple syrup, pure	B ×¼	☺+	Free of fructose. Per Tbsp. (15g) you eat with it, add B-no × F-limit.
Margarine, diet, fat free		☺	Free of fructose.
Margarine, tub, salted, sunflower oil		☺	Free of fructose.
Marmalade, sugar free with aspartame	10½		Portion (17g); 179g in total.
Marmalade, sugar free with saccharin	2		Portion (16g); 32g in total.
Marmalade, sugar free with sucralose		☺	Free of fructose.
Mascarpone		☺	Free of fructose.
Mortadella	B ×¼	☺+	Free of fructose. Per Portion (55g) you eat with it, add B-no × F-limit.
Muenster cheese, natural		☺	Free of fructose.
Nutella® (filbert spread)	40¾		Portion (37g); 1,508g in total.
Roquefort cheese		☺	Free of fructose.
Smart Balance® Light with Flax Oil Margarine, tub		☺	Free of fructose.
Smart Balance® Margarine		☺	Free of fructose.

Cold cut	SORBITOL Stand.	SORBITOL Low sensitivity amount
Jam or preserves, without sugar or artificial sweetener	☹ Avoid	☹ Avoid consumption!
Kraft® Cheese Spread, Roka Blue	☺ Free	☺ Free of sorbitol.
Limburger cheese	☺ Free	☺ Free of sorbitol.
Maple syrup, pure	☺ Free	☺ Free of sorbitol.
Margarine, diet, fat free	☺ Free	☺ Free of sorbitol.
Margarine, tub, salted, sunflower oil	☺ Free	☺ Free of sorbitol.
Marmalade, sugar free with aspartame	☹ Avoid	5¼ 🍽 Portion (17g); 89g in total.
Marmalade, sugar free with saccharin	☹ Avoid	16¾ 🍽 Portion (16g); 268g in total.
Marmalade, sugar free with sucralose	☹ Avoid	65¼ 🍽 Portion (17g); 1,109g in total.
Mascarpone	☺ Free	☺ Free of sorbitol.
Mortadella	☺ Free	☺ Free of sorbitol.
Muenster cheese, natural	☺ Free	☺ Free of sorbitol.
Nutella® (filbert spread)	☹ Avoid	20¾ 🍽 Portion (37g); 768g in total.
Roquefort cheese	☺ Free	☺ Free of sorbitol.
Smart Balance® Light with Flax Oil Margarine, tub	☺ Free	☺ Free of sorbitol.
Smart Balance® Margarine	☺ Free	☺ Free of sorbitol.

Cold cut	LACTOSE		Standard amount	
Soy Kaas Fat Free, all flavors	9		Portion (30g); 270g in total.	+7½
Swiss cheese, natural		☺	Nearly free of lactose	
Swiss cheese, natural, low sodium		☺	Nearly free of lactose	
Tilsit cheese	5¼		Portion (30g); 158g in total.	+4¼

Cold cut	IBS Standard amount			F+G amount	
Soy Kaas Fat Free, all flavors	1¼		Portion (30g); 38g in total.	1¼	
Swiss cheese, natural		☺	Nearly free of triggers.		☺
Swiss cheese, natural, low sodium		☺	Nearly free of triggers.		☺
Tilsit cheese	5¼		Portion (30g); 158g in total.	29½	

Cold cut	FRUCTOSE		Standard amount
Soy Kaas Fat Free, all flavors	34½	😊	Portion (30g); 1,035g in total.
Swiss cheese, natural	B ×¼	😊+	Free of fructose. Per Portion (30g) you eat with it, add B-no × F-limit.
Swiss cheese, natural, low sodium	B ×¼	😊+	Free of fructose. Per Portion (30g) you eat with it, add B-no × F-limit.
Tilsit cheese		😊	Free of fructose.

Cold cut	SORBITOL Stand.		SORBITOL Low sensitivity amount	
Soy Kaas Fat Free, all flavors	😞 Avoid	18½	😊	Portion (30g); 555g in total.
Swiss cheese, natural	😊 Free		😊	Free of sorbitol.
Swiss cheese, natural, low sodium	😊 Free		😊	Free of sorbitol.
Tilsit cheese	😊 Free		😊	Free of sorbitol.

3.4.4 Dairy products

Dairy products	LACTOSE		Standard amount	
Almond milk, vanilla or other flavors, unsweetened		☺	Free of lactose.	
Breyers® Light! Boosts Immunity Yogurt, all flavors	½		Piece (115g); 58g in total.	+¼
Breyers® No Sugar Added Ice Cream, Vanilla	3¼		Tbsp. (15g); 49g in total.	+2½
Breyers® YoCrunch Light Non-fat Yogurt, with granola	¼		Piece (250g); 63g in total.	0.24
Cabot® Non Fat Yogurt, plain	¼		Piece (150g); 38g in total.	0.22
Cabot® Non Fat Yogurt, vanilla	¼		Piece (150g); 38g in total.	+¼
Chobani® Nonfat Greek Yogurt, Black Cherry	5¼		Tbsp. (15g); 79g in total.	+4½
Chobani® Nonfat Greek Yogurt, Lemon	½		Piece (150g); 75g in total.	+¼
Chobani® Nonfat Greek Yogurt, Peach	¼		Piece (250g); 63g in total.	+¼
Chobani® Nonfat Greek Yogurt, Raspberry	¼		Piece (250g); 63g in total.	+¼
Chobani® Nonfat Greek Yogurt, Strawberry	¼		Piece (250g); 63g in total.	+¼
Chocolate pudding, store bought	¾		Piece (200g); 150g in total.	+½
Chocolate pudding, store bought, sugar free	89¼		Tbsp. (15g); 1,339g in total.	+74¼
Cottage cheese, uncreamed dry curd	3½		Portion (55g); 193g in total.	+2¾

Dairy products	IBS Standard amount		F+G amount	
Almond milk, vanilla or other flavors, unsweetened	☹	Avoid consumption!!	☹	
Breyers® Light! Boosts Immunity Yogurt, all flavors	½	Piece (115g); 58g in total.	3	
Breyers® No Sugar Added Ice Cream, Vanilla	☹	Avoid consumption!	18¼	
Breyers® YoCrunch Light Nonfat Yogurt, with granola	¼	Piece (250g); 63g in total.	1½	
Cabot® Non Fat Yogurt, plain	¼	Piece (150g); 38g in total.	1¼	
Cabot® Non Fat Yogurt, vanilla	¼	Piece (150g); 38g in total.	2¼	
Chobani® Nonfat Greek Yogurt, Black Cherry	3¾	Tbsp. (15g); 56g in total.	30¼	
Chobani® Nonfat Greek Yogurt, Lemon	½	Piece (150g); 75g in total.	3	
Chobani® Nonfat Greek Yogurt, Peach	¼	Piece (250g); 63g in total.	1¾	
Chobani® Nonfat Greek Yogurt, Raspberry	¼	Piece (250g); 63g in total.	1¾	
Chobani® Nonfat Greek Yogurt, Strawberry	¼	Piece (250g); 63g in total.	1¾	
Chocolate pudding, store bought	¾	Piece (200g); 150g in total.	1	
Chocolate pudding, store bought, sugar free	☹	Avoid consumption!	21¼	
Cottage cheese, uncreamed dry curd	3½	Portion (55g); 193g in total.	19¾	

Dairy products	FRUCTOSE	Standard amount
Almond milk, vanilla or other flavors, unsweetened	☺	Free of fructose.
Breyers® Light! Boosts Immunity Yogurt, all flavors	21½ 🍰	Piece (115g); 2,473g in total.
Breyers® No Sugar Added Ice Cream, Vanilla	☺	Free of fructose.
Breyers® YoCrunch Light Nonfat Yogurt, with granola	☺	Free of fructose.
Cabot® Non Fat Yogurt, plain	☺	Free of fructose.
Cabot® Non Fat Yogurt, vanilla	22 🍰	Piece (150g); 3,300g in total.
Chobani® Nonfat Greek Yogurt, Black Cherry	☺	Free of fructose.
Chobani® Nonfat Greek Yogurt, Lemon	B ×½ ☺+	Free of fructose. Per Piece (150g) you eat with it, add B-no × F-limit.
Chobani® Nonfat Greek Yogurt, Peach	B ×1 ☺+	Free of fructose. Per Piece (250g) you eat with it, add B-no × F-limit.
Chobani® Nonfat Greek Yogurt, Raspberry	B ×¾ ☺+	Free of fructose. Per Piece (250g) you eat with it, add B-no × F-limit.
Chobani® Nonfat Greek Yogurt, Strawberry	B ×¾ ☺+	Free of fructose. Per Piece (250g) you eat with it, add B-no × F-limit.
Chocolate pudding, store bought	☺	Free of fructose.
Chocolate pudding, store bought, sugar free	☺	Nearly free of fructose, avoid at hereditary fructose intolerance.
Cottage cheese, uncreamed dry curd	☺	Free of fructose.

Dairy products	SORBITOL Stand.	SORBITOL Low sensitivity amount
Almond milk, vanilla or other flavors, unsweetened	🙂 Free	🙂 Free of sorbitol.
Breyers® Light! Boosts Immunity Yogurt, all flavors	🙁 Avoid	14¼ 🍰 Piece (115g); 1,639g in total.
Breyers® No Sugar Added Ice Cream, Vanilla	🙁 Avoid	🙁 Avoid consumption!
Breyers® YoCrunch Light Nonfat Yogurt, with granola	🙁 Avoid	6½ 🍰 Piece (250g); 1,625g in total.
Cabot® Non Fat Yogurt, plain	🙂 Free	🙂 Free of sorbitol.
Cabot® Non Fat Yogurt, vanilla	🙁 Avoid	13¼ 🍰 Piece (150g); 1,988g in total.
Chobani® Nonfat Greek Yogurt, Black Cherry	🙁 Avoid	3¾ 🥄 Tbsp. (15g); 56g in total.
Chobani® Nonfat Greek Yogurt, Lemon	🙂 Free	🙂 Free of sorbitol.
Chobani® Nonfat Greek Yogurt, Peach	🙁 Avoid	4¼ 🍰 Piece (250g); 1,063g in total.
Chobani® Nonfat Greek Yogurt, Raspberry	🙁 Avoid	20 🍰 Piece (250g); 5,000g in total.
Chobani® Nonfat Greek Yogurt, Strawberry	🙁 Avoid	3½ 🍰 Piece (250g); 875g in total.
Chocolate pudding, store bought	🙁 Avoid	25 🍰 Piece (200g); 5,000g in total.
Chocolate pudding, store bought, sugar free	🙁 Avoid	🙁 Avoid consumption!
Cottage cheese, uncreamed dry curd	🙂 Free	🙂 Free of sorbitol.

Dairy products	LACTOSE		Standard amount	
Dannon® Activia® Light Yogurt, vanilla	¼		Piece (115g); 29g in total.	+¼
Dannon® Activia® Yogurt, plain	½		Piece (115g); 58g in total.	+¼
Dannon® Greek Yogurt, Honey	½		Piece (150g); 75g in total.	+¼
Dannon® Greek Yogurt, Plain	½		Piece (150g); 75g in total.	+¼
Dannon® la Crème Yogurt, fruit flavors	¼		Piece (115g); 29g in total.	+¼
Evaporated milk, diluted, 2% fat (reduced fat)			Glass (240g); Avoid consumption!!	0.19
Evaporated milk, diluted, skim (fat free)			Glass (240g); Avoid consumption!!	0.19
Evaporated milk, diluted, whole			Glass (240g); Avoid consumption!!	0.2
Feta cheese	2¼		Portion (30g); 68g in total.	+2
Feta cheese, fat free	¾		Portion (30g); 23g in total.	+¾
Fondue sauce		☺	Nearly free of lactose	
GO Veggie!™ Rice Slices, all flavors	12		Portion (30g); 360g in total.	+10
Greek yogurt, plain, nonfat,	¼		Piece (250g); 63g in total.	+¼
Half and half	2¼		Portion (30g); 68g in total.	+1¾
Kefir	¼		Portion (220g); 55g in total.	+¼
Laughing Cow® Mini Babybel®, Cheddar		☺	Nearly free of lactose	

Dairy products	IBS	Standard amount	F+G	amount
Dannon® Activia® Light Yogurt, vanilla	¼	Piece (115g); 29g in total.	2	
Dannon® Activia® Yogurt, plain	½	Piece (115g); 58g in total.	2¾	
Dannon® Greek Yogurt, Honey	¼	Piece (150g); 38g in total.	2¾	
Dannon® Greek Yogurt, Plain	½	Piece (150g); 75g in total.	1¼	
Dannon® la Crème Yogurt, fruit flavors	¼	Piece (115g); 29g in total.	2	
Evaporated milk, diluted, 2% fat (reduced fat)	¼	Glass (200g); 50 mL in total.	1½	
Evaporated milk, diluted, skim (fat free)	¼	Glass (200g); 50 mL in total.	1¼	
Evaporated milk, diluted, whole	¼	Glass (200g); 50 mL in total.	1½	
Feta cheese	2¼	Portion (30g); 68g in total.	13½	
Feta cheese, fat free	¾	Portion (30g); 23g in total.	5	
Fondue sauce	5	Portion (53g); 265g in total.	☺	
GO Veggie!™ Rice Slices, all flavors	12	Portion (30g); 360g in total.	67¼	
Greek yogurt, plain, nonfat,	¼	Piece (250g); 63g in total.	2½	
Half and half	2¼	Portion (30g); 68g in total.	12¾	
Kefir	¼	Portion (220g); 55g in total.	1¾	
Laughing Cow® Mini Babybel®, Cheddar	☺	Nearly free of triggers.	☺	

Dairy products	FRUCTOSE		Standard amount
Dannon® Activia® Light Yogurt, vanilla	¼		Piece (115g); 29g in total.
Dannon® Activia® Yogurt, plain		☺	Free of fructose.
Dannon® Greek Yogurt, Honey	¼		Piece (150g); 38g in total.
Dannon® Greek Yogurt, Plain		☺	Free of fructose.
Dannon® la Crème Yogurt, fruit flavors	¼		Piece (115g); 29g in total.
Evaporated milk, diluted, 2% fat (reduced fat)		☺	Free of fructose.
Evaporated milk, diluted, skim (fat free)		☺	Free of fructose.
Evaporated milk, diluted, whole		☺	Free of fructose.
Feta cheese		☺	Free of fructose.
Feta cheese, fat free		☺	Free of fructose.
Fondue sauce	B ×¼	☺+	Free of fructose. Per Portion (53g) you eat with it, add B-no × F-limit.
GO Veggie!™ Rice Slices, all flavors		☺	Free of fructose.
Greek yogurt, plain, nonfat,		☺	Free of fructose.
Half and half		☺	Free of fructose.
Kefir		☺	Free of fructose.
Laughing Cow® Mini Babybel®, Cheddar		☺	Free of fructose.

Dairy products	SORBITOL Stand.		SORBITOL Low sensitivity amount
Dannon® Activia® Light Yogurt, vanilla	☺ Free		☺ Free of sorbitol.
Dannon® Activia® Yogurt, plain	☺ Free		☺ Free of sorbitol.
Dannon® Greek Yogurt, Honey	☹ Avoid	3¼	Piece (150g); 488g in total.
Dannon® Greek Yogurt, Plain	☺ Free		☺ Free of sorbitol.
Dannon® la Crème Yogurt, fruit flavors	☹ Avoid	10¾	Piece (115g); 1,236g in total.
Evaporated milk, diluted, 2% fat (reduced fat)	☺ Free		☺ Free of sorbitol.
Evaporated milk, diluted, skim (fat free)	☺ Free		☺ Free of sorbitol.
Evaporated milk, diluted, whole	☺ Free		☺ Free of sorbitol.
Feta cheese	☺ Free		☺ Free of sorbitol.
Feta cheese, fat free	☺ Free		☺ Free of sorbitol.
Fondue sauce	☹ Avoid	5	Portion (53g); 265g in total.
GO Veggie!™ Rice Slices, all flavors	☺ Free		☺ Free of sorbitol.
Greek yogurt, plain, nonfat,	☺ Free		☺ Free of sorbitol.
Half and half	☺ Free		☺ Free of sorbitol.
Kefir	☺ Free		☺ Free of sorbitol.
Laughing Cow® Mini Babybel®, Cheddar	☺ Free		☺ Free of sorbitol.

Dairy products	LACTOSE		Standard amount	
Laughing Cow® Mini Babybel®, Original	12¾		Piece (21g); 268g in total.	+10½
Licuado, mango	¼		Glass (240g); 60 mL in total.	+¼
Light cream	5¼		Portion (15g); 79g in total.	+4½
Milk, lactose reduced Lactaid®, skim (fat free)			Free of lactose.	
Milk, lactose reduced Lactaid®, whole			Free of lactose.	
Milk, lactose reduced, skim (fat free), with calcium Lactaid®			Free of lactose.	
Mozzarella cheese, fat free	2¾		Portion (30g); 83g in total.	+2¼
Mozzarella cheese, whole milk	2¾		Portion (30g); 83g in total.	+2¼
Oat milk			Free of lactose.	
Parmesan cheese, dry (grated)			Nearly free of lactose	
Parmesan cheese, dry (grated), nonfat			Nearly free of lactose	+75¾
Pudding mix, other flavors, cooked type			Free of lactose.	
Rice milk, plain or original, unsweetened, enriched, ready			Free of lactose.	
Rice pudding (arroz con leche), coconut, raisins	½		Piece (200g); 100g in total.	+¼
Rice pudding (arroz con leche), plain	½		Piece (200g); 100g in total.	+¼
Rice pudding (arroz con leche), raisins	½		Piece (200g); 100g in total.	+¼

Dairy products	IBS	Standard amount	F+G	amount
Laughing Cow® Mini Babybel®, Original	12¾	Piece (21g); 268g in total.	70¾	
Licuado, mango	¼	Glass (200g); 50 mL in total.	2½	
Light cream	5¼	Portion (15g); 79g in total.	30¼	
Milk, lactose reduced Lactaid®, skim (fat free)		Free of triggers.		
Milk, lactose reduced Lactaid®, whole		Free of triggers.		
Milk, lactose reduced, skim (fat free), calcium Lactaid®		Free of triggers.		
Mozzarella cheese, fat free	2¾	Portion (30g); 83g in total.	3½	
Mozzarella cheese, whole milk	2¾	Portion (30g); 83g in total.	55	
Oat milk	¼	Glass (200g); 50g in total.	¼	
Parmesan cheese, dry (grated)		Nearly free of triggers.		
Parmesan cheese, dry (grated), nonfat		Nearly free of triggers.		
Pudding mix, other flavors, cooked type		Free of triggers.		
Rice milk, plain or original, unsweetened, enriched, ready		Free of triggers.		
Rice pudding (arroz con leche), coconut, raisins	½	Piece (200g); 100g in total.	3¼	
Rice pudding (arroz con leche), plain	½	Piece (200g); 100g in total.	2¾	
Rice pudding (arroz con leche), raisins	½	Piece (200g); 100g in total.	3	

Dairy products	FRUCTOSE		Standard amount
Laughing Cow® Mini Ba-bybel®, Original		☺	Free of fructose.
Licuado, mango	¼	🥛	Glass (200g); 50 mL in total.
Light cream		☺	Free of fructose.
Milk, lactose reduced Lac-taid®, skim (fat free)	B ×10	☺+	Free of fructose. Per Glass (200 mL) you drink with it, add B-no × F-limit.
Milk, lactose reduced Lac-taid®, whole	B ×10	☺+	Free of fructose. Per Glass (200 mL) you drink with it, add B-no × F-limit.
Milk, lactose reduced, skim (fat free), calcium Lactaid®	B ×10	☺+	Free of fructose. Per Glass (200 mL) you drink with it, add B-no × F-limit.
Mozzarella cheese, fat free		☺	Free of fructose.
Mozzarella cheese, whole milk		☺	Free of fructose.
Oat milk		☺	Nearly free of fructose, avoid at hered-itary fructose intolerance.
Parmesan cheese, dry (grated)		☺	Free of fructose.
Parmesan cheese, dry (grated), nonfat		☺	Free of fructose.
Pudding mix, other flavors, cooked type		☺	Free of fructose.
Rice milk, plain or original, unsweetened, enriched, ready	B ×¼	☺+	Free of fructose. Per Glass (200 mL) you drink with it, add B-no × F-limit.
Rice pudding (arroz con leche), coconut, raisins	4	🍰	Piece (200g); 800g in total.
Rice pudding (arroz con leche), plain	B ×½	☺+	Free of fructose. Per Piece (200g) you eat with it, add B-no × F-limit.
Rice pudding (arroz con leche), raisins	4	🍰	Piece (200g); 800g in total.

Dairy products	SORBITOL Stand.	SORBITOL Low sensitivity amount
Laughing Cow® Mini Babybel®, Original	☺ Free	☺ Free of sorbitol.
Licuado, mango	☹ Avoid	1 🥛 Glass (200g); 200 mL in total.
Light cream	☺ Free	☺ Free of sorbitol.
Milk, lactose reduced Lactaid®, skim (fat free)	☺ Free	☺ Free of sorbitol.
Milk, lactose reduced Lactaid®, whole	☺ Free	☺ Free of sorbitol.
Milk, lactose reduced, skim (fat free), calcium, Lactaid®	☺ Free	☺ Free of sorbitol.
Mozzarella cheese, fat free	☺ Free	☺ Free of sorbitol.
Mozzarella cheese, whole milk	☺ Free	☺ Free of sorbitol.
Oat milk	☺ Free	☺ Free of sorbitol.
Parmesan cheese, dry (grated)	☺ Free	☺ Free of sorbitol.
Parmesan cheese, dry (grated), nonfat	☺ Free	☺ Free of sorbitol.
Pudding mix, other flavors, cooked type	☺ Free	☺ Free of sorbitol.
Rice milk, plain or original, unsweetened, enriched, ready	☺ Free	☺ Free of sorbitol.
Rice pudding (arroz con leche), coconut, raisins	☹ Avoid	1¼ 🍰 Piece (200g); 250g in total.
Rice pudding (arroz con leche), plain	☺ Free	☺ Free of sorbitol.
Rice pudding (arroz con leche), raisins	☹ Avoid	1¼ 🍰 Piece (200g); 250g in total.

Dairy products	LACTOSE		Standard amount	
Ricotta cheese, part skim milk	17½		Portion (55g); 963g in total.	+14½
Slim-Fast® Easy to Digest, Vanilla, ready-to-drink can	2		Glass (240g); 480 mL in total.	+1¾
Sour cream	3¼		Portion (30g); 98g in total.	+2¾
Soy milk, plain or original, with artificial sweetener, ready			Free of lactose.	
Soy milk, vanilla or other flavors, sugar, fat free, ready			Free of lactose.	
Stonyfield® Oikos Greek Yogurt, Blueberry	¼		Piece (250g); 63g in total.	+¼
Stonyfield® Oikos Greek Yogurt, Caramel	½		Piece (100g); 50g in total.	+½
Stonyfield® Oikos Greek Yogurt, Chocolate	½		Piece (150g); 75g in total.	+¼
Stonyfield® Oikos Greek Yogurt, Strawberry	¼		Piece (250g); 63g in total.	+¼
Strawberry milk, plain, prepared	¼		Glass (240g); 60 mL in total.	0.22
Sweetened condensed milk	½		Portion (38g); 19g in total.	+½
Sweetened condensed milk, reduced fat	½		Portion (39g); 20g in total.	+½
Tofu, raw (not silken), cooked, low fat			Free of lactose.	
Whipped cream, aerosol			Nearly free of lactose	
Whipped cream, aerosol, chocolate	9¾		Portion (5g); 49g in total.	+8
Whipped cream, aerosol, fat free	18¾		Portion (5g); 94g in total.	+15¾

Dairy products	IBS	Standard amount	F+G	amount
Ricotta cheese, part skim milk	17½	Portion (55g); 963g in total.		😊
Slim-Fast® Easy to Digest, Vanilla, ready-to-drink can	2½	Glass (200g); 500 mL in total.	14¼	
Sour cream	3¼	Portion (30g); 98g in total.	19¼	
Soy milk, plain or original, artificial sweetener, ready	☹	Avoid consumption!!	☹	
Soy milk, vanilla or other flavors, sugar, fat free, ready	☹	Avoid consumption!!	☹	
Stonyfield® Oikos Greek Yogurt, Blueberry	¼	Piece (250g); 63g in total.	1¾	
Stonyfield® Oikos Greek Yogurt, Caramel	½	Piece (100g); 50g in total.	4	
Stonyfield® Oikos Greek Yogurt, Chocolate	½	Piece (150g); 75g in total.	3	
Stonyfield® Oikos Greek Yogurt, Strawberry	¼	Piece (250g); 63g in total.	1¾	
Strawberry milk, plain, prepared	¼	Glass (200g); 50 mL in total.	1¾	
Sweetened condensed milk	½	Portion (38g); 19g in total.	3¾	
Sweetened condensed milk, reduced fat	½	Portion (39g); 20g in total.	3½	
Tofu, raw (not silken), cooked, low fat	½	Portion (85g); 43g in total.	½	
Whipped cream, aerosol	😊	Nearly free of triggers.	😊	
Whipped cream, aerosol, chocolate	9¾	Portion (5g); 49g in total.	54½	
Whipped cream, aerosol, fat free	18¾	Portion (5g); 94g in total.	😊	

Dairy products	FRUCTOSE		Standard amount
Ricotta cheese, part skim milk		☺	Free of fructose.
Slim-Fast® Easy to Digest, Vanilla, ready-to-drink can		☺	Free of fructose.
Sour cream		☺	Free of fructose.
Soy milk, plain or original, artificial sweetener, ready	3	🥛	Glass (200g); 600 mL in total.
Soy milk, vanilla or other flavors, sugar, fat free, ready	B ×¾	☺+	Free of fructose. Per Glass (200 mL) you drink with it, add B-no × F-limit.
Stonyfield® Oikos Greek Yogurt, Blueberry	B ×1	☺+	Free of fructose. Per Piece (250g) you eat with it, add B-no × F-limit.
Stonyfield® Oikos Greek Yogurt, Caramel	B ×½	☺+	Free of fructose. Per Piece (100g) you eat with it, add B-no × F-limit.
Stonyfield® Oikos Greek Yogurt, Chocolate	66½	🍰	Piece (150g); 9,975g in total.
Stonyfield® Oikos Greek Yogurt, Strawberry	3	🍰	Piece (250g); 750g in total.
Strawberry milk, plain, prepared		☺	Free of fructose.
Sweetened condensed milk		☺	Free of fructose.
Sweetened condensed milk, reduced fat		☺	Free of fructose.
Tofu, raw (not silken), cooked, low fat	1½	🍳	Portion (85g); 128g in total.
Whipped cream, aerosol		☺	Free of fructose.
Whipped cream, aerosol, chocolate		☺	Free of fructose.
Whipped cream, aerosol, fat free	B ×¼	☺+	Free of fructose. Per Portion (5g) you eat with it, add B-no × F-limit.

Dairy products	SORBITOL Stand.	SORBITOL Low sensitivity amount
Ricotta cheese, part skim milk	😊 Free	😊 Free of sorbitol.
Slim-Fast® Easy to Digest, Vanilla, ready-to-drink can	😊 Free	😊 Free of sorbitol.
Sour cream	😊 Free	😊 Free of sorbitol.
Soy milk, plain or original, artificial sweetener, ready	😞 Avoid	1½ 🥛 Glass (200g); 300 mL in total.
Soy milk, vanilla or other flavors, sugar, fat free, ready	😞 Avoid	7 🥛 Glass (200g); 1,400 mL in total.
Stonyfield® Oikos Greek Yogurt, Blueberry	😊 Free	😊 Free of sorbitol.
Stonyfield® Oikos Greek Yogurt, Caramel	😊 Free	😊 Free of sorbitol.
Stonyfield® Oikos Greek Yogurt, Chocolate	😊 Free	😊 Free of sorbitol.
Stonyfield® Oikos Greek Yogurt, Strawberry	😞 Avoid	2 🍰 Piece (250g); 500g in total.
Strawberry milk, plain, prepared	😊 Free	😊 Free of sorbitol.
Sweetened condensed milk	😊 Free	😊 Free of sorbitol.
Sweetened condensed milk, reduced fat	😊 Free	😊 Free of sorbitol.
Tofu, raw (not silken), cooked, low fat	😞 Avoid	¾ 🐟 Portion (85g); 64g in total.
Whipped cream, aerosol	😊 Free	😊 Free of sorbitol.
Whipped cream, aerosol, chocolate	😊 Nearly free	😊 Nearly free of sorbitol
Whipped cream, aerosol, fat free	😊 Free	😊 Free of sorbitol.

Dairy products	LACTOSE	Standard amount	⊕
Yogurt, chocolate or coffee flavors, nonfat, with aspartame	4	Tbsp. (15g); 60g in total.	+3¼
Yogurt, chocolate or coffee flavors, whole milk, sucralose	¼	Piece (250g); 63g in total.	+¼
Yogurt, fruited, whole milk	2¾	Tbsp. (15g); 41g in total.	+2¼

Dairy products	IBS	Standard amount	F+G	amount
Yogurt, chocolate or coffee flavors, nonfat, aspartame	4	Tbsp. (15g); 60g in total.	22½	
Yogurt, chocolate or coffee flavors, whole milk, sucralose	¼	Piece (250g); 63g in total.	1½	
Yogurt, fruited, whole milk	¾	Tbsp. (15g); 11g in total.	16	

Dairy products	FRUCTOSE		Standard amount
Yogurt, chocolate or coffee flavors, nonfat, aspartame		🙂	Free of fructose.
Yogurt, chocolate or coffee flavors, whole milk, sucralose	40	🍰	Piece (250g); 10,000g in total.
Yogurt, fruited, whole milk	¾	🥄	Tbsp. (15g); 11g in total.

Dairy products	SORBITOL Stand.		SORBITOL Low sensitivity amount	
Yogurt, chocolate or coffee flavors, nonfat, aspartame	🙂	Free	🙂	Free of sorbitol.
Yogurt, chocolate or coffee flavors, whole milk, sucralose	🙂	Free	🙂	Free of sorbitol.
Yogurt, fruited, whole milk	☹️	Avoid 60½	🥄	Tbsp. (15g); 908g in total.

3.4.5 Nuts and snacks

Nuts and snacks	LACTOSE	Standard amount	⊕
Almonds, raw	☺	Free of lactose.	
Baby food, zwieback	☺	Free of lactose.	
Brazil nuts, unsalted	☺	Free of lactose.	
Caramel or sugar coated popcorn, store bought	☺	Nearly free of lactose	
Cashews, raw	☺	Free of lactose.	
Cheese cracker	☺	Free of lactose.	
Chestnuts, roasted	☺	Free of lactose.	
Chia seeds	☺	Free of lactose.	
Coconut cream (liquid from grated meat)	☺	Free of lactose.	
Coconut milk, fresh (liquid from grated meat, water added)	☺	Free of lactose.	
Coconut, dried, shredded or flaked, unsweetened	☺	Free of lactose.	
Coconut, fresh	☺	Free of lactose.	
Doritos® Tortilla Chips, Nacho Cheese	☺	Nearly free of lactose	
Filberts, raw	☺	Free of lactose.	
Flax seeds, not fortified	☺	Free of lactose.	

Nuts and snacks	IBS	Standard amount	F+G	amount
Almonds, raw	½	Hand (30g); 15g in total.	½	
Baby food, zwieback	1½	Portion (7g); 11g in total.	1½	
Brazil nuts, unsalted	☺	Free of triggers.	☺	
Caramel or sugar coated popcorn, store bought	☺	Free of triggers.	☺	
Cashews, raw	¼	Hand (30g); 8g in total.	¼	
Cheese cracker	3½	Piece (3g); 11g in total.	3½	
Chestnuts, roasted	3	Portion (30g); 90g in total.	☺	
Chia seeds	1¼	Hand (30g); 38g in total.	1¼	
Coconut cream (liquid from grated meat)	20¾	Hand (30g); 623g in total.	☺	
Coconut milk, fresh (liquid from grated meat, water added)	1¾	Glass (200g); 350g in total.	1¾	
Coconut, dried, shredded or flaked, unsweetened	12¼	Hand (30g); 368g in total.	12¼	
Coconut, fresh	24½	Portion (15g); 368g in total.	24½	
Doritos® Tortilla Chips, Nacho Cheese	10¾	Hand (21g); 226g in total.	10¾	
Filberts, raw	2¾	Hand (30g); 83g in total.	2¾	
Flax seeds, not fortified	2	Tbsp. (15g); 30g in total.	2	

Nuts and snacks	FRUCTOSE		Standard amount
Almonds, raw		😊	Free of fructose.
Baby food, zwieback		😊	Free of fructose.
Brazil nuts, unsalted		😊	Free of fructose.
Caramel or sugar coated pop-corn, store bought	B ×1	😊+	Free of fructose. Per Hand (21g) you eat with it, add B-no × F-limit.
Cashews, raw		😊	Free of fructose.
Cheese cracker		🙂	Nearly free of fructose, avoid at hereditary fructose intolerance.
Chestnuts, roasted	83¼	🍳	Portion (30g); 2,498g in total.
Chia seeds		😊	Free of fructose.
Coconut cream (liquid from grated meat)	20¾		Hand (30g); 623g in total.
Coconut milk, fresh (liquid from grated meat, water added)	B ×1	😊+	Free of fructose. Per Glass (200 mL) you drink with it, add B-no × F-limit.
Coconut, dried, shredded or flaked, unsweetened	B ×¾	😊+	Free of fructose. Per Hand (30g) you eat with it, add B-no × F-limit.
Coconut, fresh	B ×¼	😊+	Free of fructose. Per Portion (15g) you eat with it, add B-no × F-limit.
Doritos® Tortilla Chips, Nacho Cheese		😊	Free of fructose.
Filberts, raw		😊	Free of fructose.
Flax seeds, not fortified		😊	Free of fructose.

Nuts and snacks	SORBITOL Stand.	SORBITOL Low sensitivity amount
Almonds, raw	☺ Free	☺ Free of sorbitol.
Baby food, zwieback	☺ Free	☺ Free of sorbitol.
Brazil nuts, unsalted	☺ Free	☺ Free of sorbitol.
Caramel or sugar coated pop-corn, store bought	☺ Free	☺ Free of sorbitol.
Cashews, raw	☺ Free	☺ Free of sorbitol.
Cheese cracker	☺ Free	☺ Free of sorbitol.
Chestnuts, roasted	☹ Avoid	3 🍽 Portion (30g); 90g in total.
Chia seeds	☺ Free	☺ Free of sorbitol.
Coconut cream (liquid from grated meat)	☺ Free	☺ Free of sorbitol.
Coconut milk, fresh (liquid from grated meat, water added)	☺ Free	☺ Free of sorbitol.
Coconut, dried, shredded or flaked, unsweetened	☺ Free	☺ Free of sorbitol.
Coconut, fresh	☺ Free	☺ Free of sorbitol.
Doritos® Tortilla Chips, Nacho Cheese	☺ Nearly free	☺ Nearly free of sorbitol
Filberts, raw	☹ Avoid	8¼ 🐀 Hand (30g); 248g in total.
Flax seeds, not fortified	☺ Free	☺ Free of sorbitol.

Nuts and snacks	LACTOSE	Standard amount	
Ginko nuts, dried	🙂	Free of lactose.	
Hickorynuts	🙂	Free of lactose.	
Lay's® Potato Chips, Classic	🙂	Free of lactose.	
Lay's® Potato Chips, Salt & Vinegar	🙂	Free of lactose.	
Lay's® Potato Chips, Sour Cream & Onion	🙂	Free of lactose.	
Lay's® Stax Potato Crisps, Cheddar	🙂	Free of lactose.	
Lay's® Stax Potato Crisps, Hot 'n Spicy Barbecue	🙂	Free of lactose.	
Macadamia nuts, raw	🙂	Free of lactose.	
Melba Toast®, Classic (Old London®)	🙂	Free of lactose.	
Old Dutch® Crunch Curls	4 🍤	Hand (21g); 84g in total.	+3¼
Peanut butter, unsalted	🙂	Free of lactose.	
Peanuts, dry roasted, salted	🙂	Free of lactose.	
Pine nuts, pignolias	🙂	Free of lactose.	
Pistachio nuts, raw	🙂	Free of lactose.	
Poore Brothers® Potato Chips, Salt & Cracked Pepper	🙂	Free of lactose.	
Potato chips, salted	🙂	Free of lactose.	

Nuts and snacks	IBS	Standard amount	F+G	amount
Ginko nuts, dried	☺	Nearly free of fructose.	☺	
Hickorynuts	2¾	Hand (30g); 83g in total.	2¾	
Lay's® Potato Chips, Classic	10¾	Hand (21g); 226g in total.	10¾	
Lay's® Potato Chips, Salt & Vinegar	10¾	Hand (21g); 226g in total.	10¾	
Lay's® Potato Chips, Sour Cream & Onion	10¾	Hand (21g); 226g in total.	10¾	
Lay's® Stax Potato Crisps, Cheddar	10¾	Hand (21g); 226g in total.	10¾	
Lay's® Stax Potato Crisps, Hot 'n Spicy Barbecue	10¾	Hand (21g); 226g in total.	10¾	
Macadamia nuts, raw	☺	Free of triggers.	☺	
Melba Toast®, Classic (Old London®)	½	Portion (15g); 8g in total.	½	
Old Dutch® Crunch Curls	4	Hand (21g); 84g in total.	7¼	
Peanut butter, unsalted	☺	Free of triggers.	☺	
Peanuts, dry roasted, salted	☺	Free of triggers.	☺	
Pine nuts, pignolias	2¾	Hand (30g); 83g in total.	2¾	
Pistachio nuts, raw	¼	Hand (21g); 5g in total.	¼	
Poore Brothers® Potato Chips, Salt & Cracked Pepper	10¾	Hand (21g); 226g in total.	10¾	
Potato chips, salted	10¾	Hand (21g); 226g in total.	10¾	

Nuts and snacks	FRUCTOSE		Standard amount
Ginko nuts, dried		😊	Nearly free of fructose, avoid at hereditary fructose intolerance.
Hickorynuts		😊	Free of fructose.
Lay's® Potato Chips, Classic	37¾	🖐	Hand (21g); 793g in total.
Lay's® Potato Chips, Salt & Vinegar	37¾	🖐	Hand (21g); 793g in total.
Lay's® Potato Chips, Sour Cream & Onion	37¾	🖐	Hand (21g); 793g in total.
Lay's® Stax Potato Crisps, Cheddar	37¾	🖐	Hand (21g); 793g in total.
Lay's® Stax Potato Crisps, Hot 'n Spicy Barbecue	49½	🖐	Hand (21g); 1,040g in total.
Macadamia nuts, raw		😊	Free of fructose.
Melba Toast®, Classic (Old London®)	B ×¼	😊+	Free of fructose. Per Portion (15g) you eat with it, add B-no × F-limit.
Old Dutch® Crunch Curls		😊	Free of fructose.
Peanut butter, unsalted	B ×¼	😊+	Free of fructose. Per Portion (32g) you eat with it, add B-no × F-limit.
Peanuts, dry roasted, salted		😊	Free of fructose.
Pine nuts, pignolias		😊	Free of fructose.
Pistachio nuts, raw		😊	Free of fructose.
Poore Brothers® Potato Chips, Salt & Cracked Pepper	49½	🖐	Hand (21g); 1,040g in total.
Potato chips, salted	37¾	🖐	Hand (21g); 793g in total.

Nuts and snacks	SORBITOL Stand.	SORBITOL Low sensitivity amount
Ginko nuts, dried	🙂 Free	🙂 Free of sorbitol.
Hickorynuts	🙂 Free	🙂 Free of sorbitol.
Lay's® Potato Chips, Classic	☹ Avoid	79¼ Hand (21g); 1,664g in total.
Lay's® Potato Chips, Salt & Vinegar	☹ Avoid	79¼ Hand (21g); 1,664g in total.
Lay's® Potato Chips, Sour Cream & Onion	☹ Avoid	79¼ Hand (21g); 1,664g in total.
Lay's® Stax Potato Crisps, Cheddar	☹ Avoid	79¼ Hand (21g); 1,664g in total.
Lay's® Stax Potato Crisps, Hot 'n Spicy Barbecue	🙂 Nearly free	🙂 Nearly free of sorbitol
Macadamia nuts, raw	🙂 Free	🙂 Free of sorbitol.
Melba Toast®, Classic (Old London®)	🙂 Nearly free	🙂 Nearly free of sorbitol
Old Dutch® Crunch Curls	🙂 Nearly free	🙂 Nearly free of sorbitol
Peanut butter, unsalted	🙂 Free	🙂 Free of sorbitol.
Peanuts, dry roasted, salted	🙂 Free	🙂 Free of sorbitol.
Pine nuts, pignolias	🙂 Free	🙂 Free of sorbitol.
Pistachio nuts, raw	🙂 Free	🙂 Free of sorbitol.
Poore Brothers® Potato Chips, Salt & Cracked Pepper	🙂 Nearly free	🙂 Nearly free of sorbitol
Potato chips, salted	☹ Avoid	79¼ Hand (21g); 1,664g in total.

Nuts and snacks	LACTOSE	Standard amount	⊕
Potato sticks	☺	Free of lactose.	
Pretzels, hard, unsalted, sticks	☺	Free of lactose.	
Pringles® Light Fat Free Potato Crisps, Barbecue	☺	Free of lactose.	
Pringles® Potato Crisps, Loaded Baked Potato	☺	Free of lactose.	
Pringles® Potato Crisps, Original	☺	Free of lactose.	
Pringles® Potato Crisps, Salt & Vinegar	☺	Free of lactose.	
Pumpkin or squash seeds, shelled, unsalted	☺	Free of lactose.	
Rice cake	☺	Free of lactose.	
Ritz Cracker (Nabisco®)	☺	Free of lactose.	
Sesame sticks	☺	Free of lactose.	
Soy chips	5¼	Hand (21g); 110g in total.	+4¼
Sunflower seeds, raw	☺	Free of lactose.	
Taco John's® nachos	28	Hand (21g); 588g in total.	+23¼
Tortilla, white, store bought, fried	☺	Free of lactose.	
Walnuts	☺	Free of lactose.	
Wise Onion Flavored Rings	☺	Free of lactose.	

Nuts and snacks	IBS	Standard amount	F+G	amount
Potato sticks	10¾	Hand (21g); 226g in total.	10¾	
Pretzels, hard, unsalted, sticks	1½	Hand (21g); 32g in total.	1½	
Pringles® Light Fat Free Potato Crisps, Barbecue	10¾	Hand (21g); 226g in total.	10¾	
Pringles® Potato Crisps, Loaded Baked Potato	10¾	Hand (21g); 226g in total.	10¾	
Pringles® Potato Crisps, Original	10¾	Hand (21g); 226g in total.	10¾	
Pringles® Potato Crisps, Salt & Vinegar	10¾	Hand (21g); 226g in total.	10¾	
Pumpkin or squash seeds, shelled, unsalted	2¾	Hand (30g); 83g in total.	2¾	
Rice cake		Free of triggers.		
Ritz Cracker (Nabisco®)	¼	Portion (30g); 8g in total.	¼	
Sesame sticks	1½	Hand (21g); 32g in total.	1½	
Soy chips	1	Hand (21g); 21g in total.	2	
Sunflower seeds, raw	2	Hand (30g); 60g in total.	2	
Taco John's® nachos	10	Hand (21g); 210g in total.	10	
Tortilla, white, store bought, fried	¾	Piece (58g); 44g in total.	¾	
Walnuts	2¾	Hand (30g); 83g in total.	2¾	
Wise Onion Flavored Rings	10¼	Portion (30g); 308g in total.	10¼	

Nuts and snacks	FRUCTOSE	Standard amount
Potato sticks	☺	Free of fructose.
Pretzels, hard, unsalted, sticks	☺	Free of fructose.
Pringles® Light Fat Free Potato Crisps, Barbecue	34	Hand (21g); 714g in total.
Pringles® Potato Crisps, Loaded Baked Potato	37¾	Hand (21g); 793g in total.
Pringles® Potato Crisps, Original	68	Hand (21g); 1,428g in total.
Pringles® Potato Crisps, Salt & Vinegar	37¾	Hand (21g); 793g in total.
Pumpkin or squash seeds, shelled, unsalted	☺	Free of fructose.
Rice cake	☺	Free of fructose.
Ritz Cracker (Nabisco®)	☺	Free of fructose.
Sesame sticks	☺	Free of fructose.
Soy chips	7½	Hand (21g); 158g in total.
Sunflower seeds, raw	☺	Free of fructose.
Taco John's® nachos	☺	Free of fructose.
Tortilla, white, store bought, fried	☺	Free of fructose.
Walnuts	☺	Nearly free of fructose, avoid at hereditary fructose intolerance.
Wise Onion Flavored Rings	☺	Free of fructose.

Nuts and snacks	SORBITOL Stand.	SORBITOL Low sensitivity amount
Potato sticks	😞 Avoid	79¼ Hand (21g); 1,664g in total.
Pretzels, hard, unsalted, sticks	😊 Free	😊 Free of sorbitol.
Pringles® Light Fat Free Potato Crisps, Barbecue	😞 Avoid	79¼ Hand (21g); 1,664g in total.
Pringles® Potato Crisps, Loaded Baked Potato	😞 Avoid	79¼ Hand (21g); 1,664g in total.
Pringles® Potato Crisps, Original	😊 Nearly free	😊 Nearly free of sorbitol
Pringles® Potato Crisps, Salt & Vinegar	😞 Avoid	79¼ Hand (21g); 1,664g in total.
Pumpkin or squash seeds, shelled, unsalted	😊 Free	😊 Free of sorbitol.
Rice cake	😊 Free	😊 Free of sorbitol.
Ritz Cracker (Nabisco®)	😊 Free	😊 Free of sorbitol.
Sesame sticks	😊 Nearly free	😊 Nearly free of sorbitol
Soy chips	😞 Avoid	1 Hand (21g); 21g in total.
Sunflower seeds, raw	😊 Free	😊 Free of sorbitol.
Taco John's® nachos	😊 Nearly free	😊 Nearly free of sorbitol
Tortilla, white, store bought, fried	😊 Free	😊 Free of sorbitol.
Walnuts	😊 Free	😊 Free of sorbitol.
Wise Onion Flavored Rings	😊 Nearly free	😊 Nearly free of sorbitol

3.4.6 Sweet pastries

Sweet pastries	LACTOSE		Standard amount	
Almond cookies		☺	Nearly free of lactose	
Apple cake, glazed		☺	Free of lactose.	
Apple strudel		☺	Nearly free of lactose	
Archway® Ginger Snaps		☺	Free of lactose.	
Archway® Oatmeal Raisin Cookies	23¾	🍰	Piece (26g); 618g in total.	+19¾
Archway® Peanut Butter Cookies	23¾	🍰	Piece (34g); 808g in total.	+19¾
Biscotti, chocolate, nuts		☺	Nearly free of lactose	
Brownie, chocolate, fat free	3	🍰	Piece (44g); 132g in total.	+2½
Butter cracker		☺	Free of lactose.	
Carrot cake, glazed, homemade		☺	Free of lactose.	
Cheesecake, plain or flavored, graham cracker crust, homemade	½	🍰	Piece (220g); 110g in total.	+½
Cherry pie, bottom crust only		☺	Free of lactose.	
Chips Ahoy!® Chewy Gooey Caramel Cookies (Nabisco®)	12¼	🍰	Piece (15.5g); 190g in total.	+10¼
Chocolate cake, glazed, store bought		☺	Free of lactose.	

Sweet pastries	IBS	Standard amount	F+G	amount
Almond cookies	3	Piece (12.4g); 37g in total.	3	
Apple cake, glazed	½	Piece (45g); 23g in total.	1¼	
Apple strudel	¼	Piece (64g); 16g in total.	¾	
Archway® Ginger Snaps	28½	Portion (30g); 855g in total.	☺	
Archway® Oatmeal Raisin Cookies	2¼	Piece (26g); 59g in total.	2¼	
Archway® Peanut Butter Cookies	1½	Piece (34g); 51g in total.	1½	
Biscotti, chocolate, nuts	2½	Piece (20.5g); 51g in total.	2½	
Brownie, chocolate, fat free	1	Piece (44g); 44g in total.	1	
Butter cracker	10	Piece (4g); 40g in total.	10	
Carrot cake, glazed, home-made	2	Piece (27.72g); 55g in total.	2	
Cheesecake, plain or flavored, graham cracker crust, home-made	☹	Avoid consumption!!	☹	
Cherry pie, bottom crust only	☹	Avoid consumption!	¼	
Chips Ahoy!® Chewy Gooey Caramel Cookies (Nabisco®)	½	Piece (15, 5g); 8g in total.	3	
Chocolate cake, glazed, store bought	1¾	Piece (29g); 51g in total.	1¾	

Sweet pastries	FRUCTOSE	Standard amount
Almond cookies	☺	Free of fructose.
Apple cake, glazed	¾	Piece (45g); 34g in total.
Apple strudel	¼	Piece (64g); 16g in total.
Archway® Ginger Snaps	28½	Portion (30g); 855g in total.
Archway® Oatmeal Raisin Cookies	☺	Free of fructose.
Archway® Peanut Butter Cookies	2	Piece (34g); 68g in total.
Biscotti, chocolate, nuts	☺	Free of fructose.
Brownie, chocolate, fat free	66¾	Piece (44g); 2,937g in total.
Butter cracker	☺	Free of fructose.
Carrot cake, glazed, home-made	B ×¼ ☺+	Free of fructose. Per Piece (27.72g) you eat with it, add B-no × F-limit.
Cheesecake, plain or flavored, graham cracker crust, home-made	B ×½ ☺+	Free of fructose. Per Piece (220g) you eat with it, add B-no × F-limit.
Cherry pie, bottom crust only	B ×1½ ☺+	Free of fructose. Per Piece (122g) you eat with it, add B-no × F-limit.
Chips Ahoy!® Chewy Gooey Caramel Cookies (Nabisco®)	½	Piece (15.5g); 8g in total.
Chocolate cake, glazed, store bought	B ×½ ☺+	Free of fructose. Per Piece (29g) you eat with it, add B-no × F-limit.

Sweet pastries	SORBITOL Stand.		SORBITOL Low sensitivity amount
Almond cookies	😊 Free		😊 Free of sorbitol.
Apple cake, glazed	😞 Avoid	½	Piece (45g); 23g in total.
Apple strudel	😞 Avoid	¼	Piece (64g); 16g in total.
Archway® Ginger Snaps	😊 Free		😊 Free of sorbitol.
Archway® Oatmeal Raisin Cookies	😞 Avoid	10¼	Piece (26g); 267g in total.
Archway® Peanut Butter Cookies	😞 Avoid	10¾	Piece (34g); 366g in total.
Biscotti, chocolate, nuts	😊 Nearly free		😊 Nearly free of sorbitol
Brownie, chocolate, fat free	😊 Nearly free		😊 Nearly free of sorbitol
Butter cracker	😊 Free		😊 Free of sorbitol.
Carrot cake, glazed, home-made	😞 Avoid	8	Piece (27, 72g); 222g in total.
Cheesecake, plain or flavored, graham cracker crust, home-made	😊 Free		😊 Free of sorbitol.
Cherry pie, bottom crust only	😞 Avoid		😞 Avoid consumption!
Chips Ahoy!® Chewy Gooey Caramel Cookies (Nabisco®)	😊 Nearly free		😊 Nearly free of sorbitol
Chocolate cake, glazed, store bought	😊 Nearly free		😊 Nearly free of sorbitol

Sweet pastries	LACTOSE	Standard amount	⊕
Chocolate chip cookies, store bought	☺	Free of lactose.	
Chocolate cookies, iced, store bought	☺	Free of lactose.	
Chocolate sandwich cookies, double filling	☺	Free of lactose.	
Chocolate sandwich cookies, sugar free	☺	Nearly free of lactose	
Cinnamon crispas (fried flour tortilla, cinnamon, sugar)	☺	Free of lactose.	
Crepe, plain	1¼	Piece (55g); 69g in total.	+1
Croissant, chocolate	3½	Piece (69g); 242g in total.	+3
Croissant, fruit	3½	Piece (74g); 259g in total.	+3
Danish pastry, frosted or glazed, with cheese filling	3	Piece (125g); 375g in total.	+2½
Dare Breaktime Ginger Cookies	☺	Free of lactose.	
Dare® Lemon Crème Cookies	32½	Piece (19.5g); 634g in total.	+27
Doughnut, raised, glazed, coconut topping	4¾	Piece (79g); 375g in total.	+4
Doughnut, raised, glazed, plain	4¾	Piece (77g); 366g in total.	+4
Doughnut, raised, sugared	4¾	Piece (72.5g); 344g in total.	+4
EGG® bread roll	5¼	Piece (35g); 184g in total.	+4¼
Elephant ear (crispy)	4¼	Piece (59g); 251g in total.	+3½

Sweet pastries	IBS	Standard amount	F+G amount
Chocolate chip cookies, store bought	2½	Piece (10g); 25g in total.	2½
Chocolate cookies, iced, store bought	5	Piece (10g); 50g in total.	5
Chocolate sandwich cookies, double filling	3½	Piece (14.5g); 51g in total.	3½
Chocolate sandwich cookies, sugar free	☹	Avoid consumption!!	4¼
Cinnamon crispas (fried flour tortilla, cinnamon, sugar)	1	Portion (55g); 55g in total.	1
Crepe, plain	¾	Piece (55g); 41g in total.	¾
Croissant, chocolate	¾	Piece (69g); 52g in total.	¾
Croissant, fruit	½	Piece (74g); 37g in total.	½
Danish pastry, frosted or glazed, with cheese filling	¼	Piece (125g); 31g in total.	¼
Dare Breaktime Ginger Cookies	8½	Piece (7.5g); 64g in total.	8½
Dare® Lemon Crème Cookies	2½	Piece (19.5g); 49g in total.	2½
Doughnut, raised, glazed, coconut topping	½	Piece (79g); 40g in total.	½
Doughnut, raised, glazed, plain	½	Piece (77g); 39g in total.	½
Doughnut, raised, sugared	¾	Piece (72.5g); 54g in total.	¾
EGG® bread roll	1½	Piece (35g); 53g in total.	1½
Elephant ear (crispy)	1	Piece (59g); 59g in total.	1

Sweet pastries	FRUCTOSE	Standard amount
Chocolate chip cookies, store bought	☺	Free of fructose.
Chocolate cookies, iced, store bought	☺	Free of fructose.
Chocolate sandwich cookies, double filling	☺	Free of fructose.
Chocolate sandwich cookies, sugar free	☺	Free of fructose.
Cinnamon crispas (fried flour tortilla, cinnamon, sugar)	☺	Free of fructose.
Crepe, plain	☺	Free of fructose.
Croissant, chocolate	B ×1 ☺+	Free of fructose. Per Piece (69g) you eat with it, add B-no × F-limit.
Croissant, fruit	B ×2½ ☺+	Free of fructose. Per Piece (74g) you eat with it, add B-no × F-limit.
Danish pastry, frosted or glazed, with cheese filling	☺	Free of fructose.
Dare Breaktime Ginger Cookies	☺	Nearly free of fructose, avoid at hereditary fructose intolerance.
Dare® Lemon Crème Cookies	☺	Free of fructose.
Doughnut, raised, glazed, coconut topping	☺	Free of fructose.
Doughnut, raised, glazed, plain	☺	Free of fructose.
Doughnut, raised, sugared	☺	Free of fructose.
EGG® bread roll	☺	Free of fructose.
Elephant ear (crispy)	☺	Free of fructose.

Sweet pastries	SORBITOL Stand.	SORBITOL Low sensitivity amount
Chocolate chip cookies, store bought	🙂 Nearly free	🙂 Nearly free of sorbitol
Chocolate cookies, iced, store bought	🙂 Nearly free	🙂 Nearly free of sorbitol
Chocolate sandwich cookies, double filling	🙂 Nearly free	🙂 Nearly free of sorbitol
Chocolate sandwich cookies, sugar free	☹️ Avoid	☹️ Avoid consumption!!
Cinnamon crispas (fried flour tortilla, cinnamon, sugar)	😀 Free	😀 Free of sorbitol.
Crepe, plain	😀 Free	😀 Free of sorbitol.
Croissant, chocolate	🙂 Nearly free	🙂 Nearly free of sorbitol
Croissant, fruit	☹️ Avoid	2 🍰 Piece (74g); 148g in total.
Danish pastry, frosted or glazed, with cheese filling	😀 Free	😀 Free of sorbitol.
Dare Breaktime Ginger Cookies	😀 Free	😀 Free of sorbitol.
Dare® Lemon Crème Cookies	😀 Free	😀 Free of sorbitol.
Doughnut, raised, glazed, coconut topping	😀 Free	😀 Free of sorbitol.
Doughnut, raised, glazed, plain	😀 Free	😀 Free of sorbitol.
Doughnut, raised, sugared	😀 Free	😀 Free of sorbitol.
EGG® bread roll	😀 Free	😀 Free of sorbitol.
Elephant ear (crispy)	😀 Free	😀 Free of sorbitol.

Sweet pastries	LACTOSE		Standard amount	⊕
English muffin, whole wheat, with raisins	1¼		Piece (66g); 83g in total.	+1
French toast, homemade, French bread	1¼		Piece (131g); 164g in total.	+1
Frozen custard, chocolate or coffee flavors	½		Portion (87.5g); 44g in total.	+¼
German chocolate cake, glazed, homemade		☺	Free of lactose.	
Girl Scout® Lemonades		☺	Free of lactose.	
Girl Scout® Peanut Butter Patties		☺	Free of lactose.	
Girl Scout® Samoas®	52¼		Piece (14.5g); 758g in total.	+43½
Girl Scout® Shortbread®	18½		Piece (11.34g); 210g in total.	+15½
Girl Scout® Thin Mints	32½		Piece (8g); 260g in total.	+27
Halvah		☺	Free of lactose.	
Lebkuchen (German ginger bread)		☺	Nearly free of lactose	
Little Debbie® Coffee Cake, Apple Streusel		☺	Free of lactose.	
Little Debbie® Fudge Brownies with Walnuts		☺	Free of lactose.	
Long John or Bismarck, glazed, cream or custard filled & nuts	2¼		Piece (105g); 236g in total.	+2
Molasses cookies, store bought		☺	Free of lactose.	
Muffins, banana	1¼		Piece (113g); 141g in total.	+1

Sweet pastries	IBS	Standard amount	F+G amount
English muffin, whole wheat, with raisins	¾	Piece (66g); 50g in total.	¾
French toast, homemade, French bread	¼	Piece (131g); 33g in total.	¼
Frozen custard, chocolate or coffee flavors	½	Portion (87.5g); 44g in total.	½
German chocolate cake, glazed, homemade	1¾	Piece (29g); 51g in total.	1¾
Girl Scout® Lemonades	4	Piece (15.5g); 62g in total.	4
Girl Scout® Peanut Butter Patties	4	Piece (12.5g); 50g in total.	4
Girl Scout® Samoas®	¾	Piece (14.5g); 11g in total.	3½
Girl Scout® Shortbread®	3¼	Piece (11.34g); 37g in total.	3¼
Girl Scout® Thin Mints	6¼	Piece (8g); 50g in total.	6¼
Halvah	1¼	Portion (40g); 50g in total.	1¼
Lebkuchen (German ginger bread)	2	Piece (32.4g); 65g in total.	2
Little Debbie® Coffee Cake, Apple Streusel	½	Piece (52g); 26g in total.	1
Little Debbie® Fudge Brownies with Walnuts	1¾	Piece (30.5g); 53g in total.	1¾
Long John or Bismarck, glazed, cream or custard filled & nuts	½	Piece (105g); 53g in total.	½
Molasses cookies, store bought	3¼	Piece (15g); 49g in total.	3¼
Muffins, banana	¼	Piece (113g); 28g in total.	¼

Sweet pastries	FRUCTOSE	Standard amount
English muffin, whole wheat, with raisins	2	Piece (66g); 132g in total.
French toast, homemade, French bread	B ×½	Free of fructose. Per Piece (131g) you eat with it, add B-no × F-limit.
Frozen custard, chocolate or coffee flavors	B ×2¼	Free of fructose. Per Portion (87.5g) you eat with it, add B-no × F-limit.
German chocolate cake, glazed, homemade	B ×½	Free of fructose. Per Piece (29g) you eat with it, add B-no × F-limit.
Girl Scout® Lemonades		Free of fructose.
Girl Scout® Peanut Butter Patties		Free of fructose.
Girl Scout® Samoas®		Free of fructose.
Girl Scout® Shortbread®		Free of fructose.
Girl Scout® Thin Mints		Nearly free of fructose, avoid at hereditary fructose intolerance.
Halvah	B ×1½	Free of fructose. Per Portion (40g) you eat with it, add B-no × F-limit.
Lebkuchen (German ginger bread)	5¼	Piece (32.4g); 170g in total.
Little Debbie® Coffee Cake, Apple Streusel	¾	Piece (52g); 39g in total.
Little Debbie® Fudge Brownies with Walnuts	B ×4¼	Free of fructose. Per Piece (30.5g) you eat with it, add B-no × F-limit.
Long John / Bismarck, glazed, cream or custard & nuts		Free of fructose.
Molasses cookies, store bought		Nearly free of fructose, avoid at hereditary fructose intolerance.
Muffins, banana	B ×¼	Free of fructose. Per Piece (113g) you eat with it, add B-no × F-limit.

Sweet pastries	SORBITOL Stand.		SORBITOL Low sensitivity amount
English muffin, whole wheat, with raisins	🙁 Avoid	2¼	Piece (66g); 149g in total.
French toast, homemade, French bread	🙂 Free		Free of sorbitol.
Frozen custard, chocolate or coffee flavors	🙂 Nearly free		Nearly free of sorbitol
German chocolate cake, glazed, homemade	🙂 Nearly free		Nearly free of sorbitol
Girl Scout® Lemonades	🙂 Free		Free of sorbitol.
Girl Scout® Peanut Butter Patties	🙂 Nearly free		Nearly free of sorbitol
Girl Scout® Samoas®	🙁 Avoid	¾	Piece (14.5g); 11g in total.
Girl Scout® Shortbread®	🙂 Free		Free of sorbitol.
Girl Scout® Thin Mints	🙂 Nearly free		Nearly free of sorbitol
Halvah	🙂 Free		Free of sorbitol.
Lebkuchen (German ginger bread)	🙁 Avoid	6½	Piece (32.4g); 211g in total.
Little Debbie® Coffee Cake, Apple Streusel	🙁 Avoid	½	Piece (52g); 26g in total.
Little Debbie® Fudge Brownies with Walnuts	🙂 Nearly free		Nearly free of sorbitol
Long John / Bismarck, glazed, cream or custard filled, nuts	🙂 Free		Free of sorbitol.
Molasses cookies, store bought	🙂 Free		Free of sorbitol.
Muffins, banana	🙁 Avoid	29¼	Piece (113g); 3,305g in total.

Sweet pastries	LACTOSE		Standard amount	⊕
Muffins, blueberry, store bought	1¼		Piece (113g); 141g in total.	+1
Muffins, carrot, homemade, with nuts	1¼		Piece (113g); 141g in total.	+1
Muffins, oat bran or oatmeal, store bought	1¼		Piece (113g); 141g in total.	+1
Muffins, pumpkin, store bought	1¼		Piece (113g); 141g in total.	+1
Murray® Sugar Free Oatmeal Cookies		☺	Free of lactose.	
Murray® Sugar Free Shortbread		☺	Free of lactose.	
Nabisco® 100 Calorie Packs, Honey Maid Cinnamon Roll		☺	Free of lactose.	
Nilla Wafers® (Nabisco®)	32½		Piece (3.75g); 122g in total.	+27
Nutter Butter® Cookies (Nabisco®)		☺	Free of lactose.	
Oatmeal cookies, store bought	45¾		Piece (13g); 595g in total.	+38
Oreo® Brownie Cookies (Nabisco®)		☺	Nearly free of lactose	
Oreo® Cookies (Nabisco®)		☺	Free of lactose.	
Oreo® Cookies, Sugar Free (Nabisco®)		☺	Nearly free of lactose	
Pancake, buckwheat, from mix, add water only		☺	Free of lactose.	
Pancake, whole wheat, homemade	2½		Piece (44g); 110g in total.	+2
Peach pie, bottom crust only		☺	Free of lactose.	

Sweet pastries	IBS	Standard amount	F+G	amount
Muffins, blueberry, store bought	¼	Piece (113g); 28g in total.	¼	
Muffins, carrot, homemade, with nuts	¼	Piece (113g); 28g in total.	¼	
Muffins, oat bran or oatmeal, store bought	½	Piece (113g); 57g in total.	½	
Muffins, pumpkin, store bought	¼	Piece (113g); 28g in total.	¼	
Murray® Sugar Free Oatmeal Cookies	☹	Avoid consumption!	4½	
Murray® Sugar Free Short-bread	☹	Avoid consumption!	10½	
Nabisco® 100 Calorie Packs, Honey Maid Cinnamon Roll	4¾	Piece (13g); 62g in total.	4¾	
Nilla Wafers® (Nabisco®)	12¼	Piece (3.75g); 46g in total.	12¼	
Nutter Butter® Cookies (Nabisco®)	3½	Portion (14g); 49g in total.	3½	
Oatmeal cookies, store bought	3¾	Piece (13g); 49g in total.	3¾	
Oreo® Brownie Cookies (Nabisco®)	¼	Piece (42.5g); 11g in total.	1	
Oreo® Cookies (Nabisco®)	4¼	Piece (12g); 51g in total.	4¼	
Oreo® Cookies, Sugar Free (Nabisco®)	☹	Avoid consumption!!	4¼	
Pancake, buckwheat, from mix, add water only	1¼	Piece (44g); 55g in total.	1¼	
Pancake, whole wheat, home-made	1	Piece (44g); 44g in total.	1	
Peach pie, bottom crust only	¼	Piece (122g); 31g in total.	¼	

Sweet pastries	FRUCTOSE		Standard amount
Muffins, blueberry, store bought	25½		Piece (113g); 2,882g in total.
Muffins, carrot, homemade, with nuts		☺	Free of fructose.
Muffins, oat bran or oatmeal, store bought	B ×¼	☺+	Free of fructose. Per Piece (113g) you eat with it, add B-no × F-limit.
Muffins, pumpkin, store bought	B ×¼	☺+	Free of fructose. Per Piece (113g) you eat with it, add B-no × F-limit.
Murray® Sugar Free Oatmeal Cookies		☺	Free of fructose.
Murray® Sugar Free Short-bread		☺	Free of fructose.
Nabisco® 100 Calorie Packs, Honey Maid Cinnamon Roll		☺	Free of fructose.
Nilla Wafers® (Nabisco®)		☺	Free of fructose.
Nutter Butter® Cookies (Nabisco®)		☺	Free of fructose.
Oatmeal cookies, store bought		☺	Free of fructose.
Oreo® Brownie Cookies (Nabisco®)	¼		Piece (42.5g); 11g in total.
Oreo® Cookies (Nabisco®)		☺	Free of fructose.
Oreo® Cookies, Sugar Free (Nabisco®)		☺	Free of fructose.
Pancake, buckwheat, from mix, add water only		☺	Free of fructose.
Pancake, whole wheat, home-made		☺	Free of fructose.
Peach pie, bottom crust only	2¾		Piece (122g); 336g in total.

Sweet pastries	SORBITOL Stand.		SORBITOL Low sensitivity amount
Muffins, blueberry, store bought	😊 Free	😊	Free of sorbitol.
Muffins, carrot, homemade, with nuts	😞 Avoid	3¼ 🍰	Piece (113g); 367g in total.
Muffins, oat bran or oatmeal, store bought	😊 Free	😊	Free of sorbitol.
Muffins, pumpkin, store bought	😞 Avoid	14½ 🍰	Piece (113g); 1,639g in total.
Murray® Sugar Free Oatmeal Cookies	😞 Avoid	😞	Avoid consumption!
Murray® Sugar Free Shortbread	😞 Avoid	😞	Avoid consumption!
Nabisco® 100 Calorie Packs, Honey Maid Cinnamon Roll	😞 Avoid	42½ 🍰	Piece (13g); 553g in total.
Nilla Wafers® (Nabisco®)	😊 Free	😊	Free of sorbitol.
Nutter Butter® Cookies (Nabisco®)	😊 Free	😊	Free of sorbitol.
Oatmeal cookies, store bought	😊 Free	😊	Free of sorbitol.
Oreo® Brownie Cookies (Nabisco®)	🙂 Nearly free	🙂	Nearly free of sorbitol
Oreo® Cookies (Nabisco®)	🙂 Nearly free	🙂	Nearly free of sorbitol
Oreo® Cookies, Sugar Free (Nabisco®)	😞 Avoid	😞	Avoid consumption!!
Pancake, buckwheat, from mix, add water only	😞 Avoid	3¾ 🍰	Piece (44g); 165g in total.
Pancake, whole wheat, homemade	😊 Free	😊	Free of sorbitol.
Peach pie, bottom crust only	😞 Avoid	1 🍰	Piece (122g); 122g in total.

Sweet pastries	LACTOSE	Standard amount	
Pepperidge Farm® Sweet & Simple, Soft Sugar Cookies	☺	Nearly free of lactose	
Pepperidge Farm® Turnover, Apple	9	Piece (89g); 801g in total.	+7½
Pillsbury® Big White Chunk Macadamia Nut Cookies	6¾	Piece (38g); 257g in total.	+5½
Pillsbury® Cinnamon Roll with Icing, all flavors	9	Piece (44g); 396g in total.	+7½
Popcorn, store bought (prepopped), "buttered"	36¾	Portion (30g); 1,103g in total.	+30¾
Rhubarb pie, bottom crust only	☺	Free of lactose.	
Sandwich cookies, vanilla	9	Piece (15g); 135g in total.	+7½
Sticky bun	8¾	Piece (71g); 621g in total.	+7¼
Strawberry pie, bottom crust only	☺	Free of lactose.	
Sugar cookies, iced, store bought	☺	Nearly free of lactose	
Sweet potato bread	☺	Nearly free of lactose	
Tiramisu	2½	Portion (55g); 138g in total.	+2
Twix®	2	Piece (51g); 102g in total.	+1¾
Waffles, bran	¾	Piece (95g); 71g in total.	+¾
Waffles, whole wheat, from mix, add milk, fat and egg	1	Piece (95g); 95g in total.	+¾
Windmill cookies	☺	Free of lactose.	

Sweet pastries	IBS	Standard amount	F+G	amount
Pepperidge Farm® Sweet & Simple, Soft Sugar Cookies	☹	Avoid consumption.	4¾	
Pepperidge Farm® Turnover, Apple	¼	Piece (89g); 22g in total.	½	
Pillsbury® Big White Chunk Macadamia Nut Cookies	½	Piece (38g); 19g in total.	½	
Pillsbury® Cinnamon Roll with Icing, all flavors	1	Piece (44g); 44g in total.	1	
Popcorn, store bought (prepopped), "buttered"	36¾	Portion (30g); 1,103g in total.	☺	
Rhubarb pie, bottom crust only	¼	Piece (122g); 31g in total.	¼	
Sandwich cookies, vanilla	3	Piece (15g); 45g in total.	3	
Sticky bun	½	Piece (71g); 36g in total.	½	
Strawberry pie, bottom crust only	¼	Piece (122g); 31g in total.	¼	
Sugar cookies, iced, store bought	3¼	Piece (15g); 49g in total.	3¼	
Sweet potato bread	1½	Slice (42g); 63g in total.	1½	
Tiramisu	2½	Portion (55g); 138g in total.	12	
Twix®	1¾	Piece (51g); 89g in total.	1¾	
Waffles, bran	¼	Piece (95g); 24g in total.	¼	
Waffles, whole wheat, from mix, add milk, fat and egg	½	Piece (95g); 48g in total.	½	
Windmill cookies	6¼	Piece (10g); 63g in total.	6¼	

Sweet pastries	FRUCTOSE	Standard amount
Pepperidge Farm® Sweet & Simple, Soft Sugar Cookies	☹	Avoid consumption.
Pepperidge Farm® Turnover, Apple	½ 🍰	Piece (89g); 45g in total.
Pillsbury® Big White Chunk Macadamia Nut Cookies	☺	Nearly free of fructose, avoid at hereditary fructose intolerance.
Pillsbury® Cinnamon Roll with Icing, all flavors	B ×8¼ ☺+	Free of fructose. Per Piece (44g) you eat with it, add B-no × F-limit.
Popcorn, store bought (prepopped), "buttered"	☺	Free of fructose.
Rhubarb pie, bottom crust only	☺	Free of fructose.
Sandwich cookies, vanilla	☺	Free of fructose.
Sticky bun	B ×¾ ☺+	Free of fructose. Per Piece (71g) you eat with it, add B-no × F-limit.
Strawberry pie, bottom crust only	1¼ 🍰	Piece (122g); 153g in total.
Sugar cookies, iced, store bought	☺	Free of fructose.
Sweet potato bread	☺	Free of fructose.
Tiramisu	☺	Free of fructose.
Twix®	B ×1½ ☺+	Free of fructose. Per Piece (51g) you eat with it, add B-no × F-limit.
Waffles, bran	B ×¼ ☺+	Free of fructose. Per Piece (95g) you eat with it, add B-no × F-limit.
Waffles, whole wheat, from mix, add milk, fat and egg	B ×¼ ☺+	Free of fructose. Per Piece (95g) you eat with it, add B-no × F-limit.
Windmill cookies	☺	Nearly free of fructose, avoid at hereditary fructose intolerance.

Sweet pastries	SORBITOL Stand.		SORBITOL Low sensitivity amount
Pepperidge Farm® Sweet & Simple, Soft Sugar Cookies	☺ Free		☺ Free of sorbitol.
Pepperidge Farm® Turnover, Apple	☹ Avoid	¼	Piece (89g); 22g in total.
Pillsbury® Big White Chunk Macadamia Nut Cookies	☺ Free		☺ Free of sorbitol.
Pillsbury® Cinnamon Roll with Icing, all flavors	☺ Free		☺ Free of sorbitol.
Popcorn, store bought (prepopped), "buttered"	☺ Free		☺ Free of sorbitol.
Rhubarb pie, bottom crust only	☺ Free		☺ Free of sorbitol.
Sandwich cookies, vanilla	☺ Free		☺ Free of sorbitol.
Sticky bun	☺ Free		☺ Free of sorbitol.
Strawberry pie, bottom crust only	☹ Avoid	¾	Piece (122g); 92g in total.
Sugar cookies, iced, store bought	☺ Free		☺ Free of sorbitol.
Sweet potato bread	☺ Free		☺ Free of sorbitol.
Tiramisu	☺ Free		☺ Free of sorbitol.
Twix®	☺ Free		☺ Free of sorbitol.
Waffles, bran	☺ Free		☺ Free of sorbitol.
Waffles, whole wheat, from mix, add milk, fat and egg	☺ Free		☺ Free of sorbitol.
Windmill cookies	☺ Free		☺ Free of sorbitol.

3.4.7 Sweets

Sweets	LACTOSE		Standard amount	⊕
3 Musketeers®	1¾		Piece (60.4g); 106g in total.	+1½
After Eight® Thin Chocolate Mints	10¼		Piece (8g); 82g in total.	+8½
Almond paste (Marzipan)		☺	Free of lactose.	
Almonds, honey roasted		☺	Free of lactose.	
Breath mint, regular		☺	Free of lactose.	
Breath mint, sugar free		☺	Free of lactose.	
Brown sugar		☺	Free of lactose.	
Buttermels® (Switzer's®)	8		Piece (6.9g); 55g in total.	+6½
Candy necklace		☺	Free of lactose.	
Chewing gum		☺	Free of lactose.	
Chewing gum, sugar free		☺	Free of lactose.	
Chocolate truffles	2½		Piece (16.2g); 41g in total.	+2
Classic Fruit Chocolates (Liberty Orchards®)	56½		Piece (15g); 848g in total.	+47
Coconut Bars, nuts	45¼		Piece (42g); 1,901g in total.	+37¾
Dark chocolate Bar 45%-59% cacao	1¼		135g Bar (125g); 156g in total.	+1

Sweets	IBS	Standard amount	F+G	amount
3 Musketeers®	1¾	Piece (60.4g); 106g in total.	6¼	
After Eight® Thin Chocolate Mints	10¼	Piece (8g); 82g in total.	57¾	
Almond paste (Marzipan)	½	Portion (28.38g); 14g in total.	½	
Almonds, honey roasted	½	Hand (30g); 15g in total.	½	
Breath mint, regular	☺	Free of triggers.	☺	
Breath mint, sugar free	☹	Avoid consumption!!	☺	
Brown sugar	☺	Free of triggers.	☺	
Buttermels® (Switzer's®)	8	Piece (6.9g); 55g in total.	44¾	
Candy necklace	☺	Free of triggers.	☺	
Chewing gum	☺	Free of triggers.	☺	
Chewing gum, sugar free	☹	Avoid consumption!	☺	
Chocolate truffles	2½	Piece (16.2g); 41g in total.	2¾	
Classic Fruit Chocolates (Liberty Orchards®)	5½	Piece (15g); 83g in total.	5½	
Coconut Bars, nuts	45¼	Piece (42g); 1,901g in total.	☺	
Dark chocolate Bar 45%-59% cacao	¼	135g Bar (125g); 31g in total.	¼	

Sweets	FRUCTOSE		Standard amount
3 Musketeers®	B ×3¾	☺ +	Free of fructose. Per Piece (60.4g) you eat with it, add B-no × F-limit.
After Eight® Thin Chocolate Mints		☺	Free of fructose.
Almond paste (Marzipan)		☺	Nearly free of fructose, avoid at hereditary fructose intolerance.
Almonds, honey roasted	1¾	🖐	Hand (30g); 53g in total.
Breath mint, regular	B ×¼	☺ +	Free of fructose. Per Portion (2g) you eat with it, add B-no × F-limit.
Breath mint, sugar free		☺	Free of fructose.
Brown sugar		☺	Free of fructose.
Buttermels® (Switzer's®)	B ×½	☺ +	Free of fructose. Per Piece (6.9g) you eat with it, add B-no × F-limit.
Candy necklace	B ×3¼	☺ +	Free of fructose. Per Piece (21g) you eat with it, add B-no × F-limit.
Chewing gum		☺	Free of fructose.
Chewing gum, sugar free		☺	Free of fructose.
Chocolate truffles		☺	Free of fructose.
Classic Fruit Chocolates (Liberty Orchards®)	B ×¼	☺ +	Free of fructose. Per Piece (15g) you eat with it, add B-no × F-limit.
Coconut Bars, nuts		☺	Free of fructose.
Dark chocolate Bar 45%-59% cacao		☺	Free of fructose.

Sweets	SORBITOL Stand.	SORBITOL Low sensitivity amount
3 Musketeers®	😊 Free	😊 Free of sorbitol.
After Eight® Thin Chocolate Mints	😊 Free	😊 Free of sorbitol.
Almond paste (Marzipan)	☹ Avoid	20½ Portion (28.38g); 582g in total.
Almonds, honey roasted	☹ Avoid	5½ Hand (30g); 165g in total.
Breath mint, regular	😊 Free	😊 Free of sorbitol.
Breath mint, sugar free	☹ Avoid	☹ Avoid consumption!!
Brown sugar	😊 Free	😊 Free of sorbitol.
Buttermels® (Switzer's®)	😊 Free	😊 Free of sorbitol.
Candy necklace	😊 Free	😊 Free of sorbitol.
Chewing gum	😊 Free	😊 Free of sorbitol.
Chewing gum, sugar free	☹ Avoid	☹ Avoid consumption!
Chocolate truffles	😊 Free	😊 Free of sorbitol.
Classic Fruit Chocolates (Liberty Orchards®)	☹ Avoid	31½ Piece (15g); 473g in total.
Coconut Bars, nuts	😊 Free	😊 Free of sorbitol.
Dark chocolate Bar 45%-59% cacao	☹ Avoid	8 135g Bar (125g); 1,000g in total.

Sweets	LACTOSE		Standard amount	⊕
Dark chocolate Bar 60%-69% cacao	7½		135g Bar (125g); 938g in total.	+6¼
Dark chocolate Bar 70%-85% cacao		☺	Free of lactose.	
Dark chocolate Bar, sugar free	26¾		Piece (12g); 321g in total.	+22¼
Dark Fruit Chocolates (Liberty Orchards®)	56½		Piece (15g); 848g in total.	+47
Dark Fruit Chocolates, Sugar Free (Liberty Orchards®)	37¾		Piece (17g); 642g in total.	+31¼
Fifty 50® Sugar Free Low Glycemic Butterscotch Hard Candy		☺	Free of lactose.	
French Burnt Peanuts		☺	Free of lactose.	
Gelatin (jello) powder, flavored, sugar free		☺	Free of lactose.	
Gelatin (jello) powder, plain		☺	Free of lactose.	
Gum drops		☺	Free of lactose.	
Gum drops, sugar free		☺	Free of lactose.	
Gummi bears		☺	Free of lactose.	
Gummi bears, sugar free		☺	Free of lactose.	
Gummi dinosaurs		☺	Free of lactose.	
Gummi dinosaurs, sugar free		☺	Free of lactose.	
Gummi worms		☺	Free of lactose.	

Sweets	IBS	Standard amount	F+G	amount
Dark chocolate Bar 60%-69% cacao	¼	135g Bar (125g); 31g in total.	¼	
Dark chocolate Bar 70%-85% cacao	¼	135g Bar (125g); 31g in total.	¼	
Dark chocolate Bar, sugar free	☹	Avoid consumption!!	4¼	
Dark Fruit Chocolates (Liberty Orchards®)	5½	Piece (15g); 83g in total.	5½	
Dark Fruit Chocolates, Sugar Free (Liberty Orchards®)	☹	Avoid consumption!!	4¾	
Fifty 50® Sugar Free Low Glycemic Butterscotch Hard Candy	☹	Avoid consumption!!	☺	
French Burnt Peanuts	☺	Free of triggers.	☺	
Gelatin (jello) powder, flavored, sugar free	☺	Free of triggers.	☺	
Gelatin (jello) powder, plain	☺	Free of triggers.	☺	
Gum drops	☺	Free of triggers.	☺	
Gum drops, sugar free	☹	Avoid consumption!!	☺	
Gummi bears	☺	Free of triggers.	☺	
Gummi bears, sugar free	☹	Avoid consumption!!	☺	
Gummi dinosaurs	☺	Free of triggers.	☺	
Gummi dinosaurs, sugar free	☹	Avoid consumption!!	☺	
Gummi worms	☺	Free of triggers.	☺	

Sweets	FRUCTOSE	Standard amount
Dark chocolate Bar 60%-69% cacao	☺	Free of fructose.
Dark chocolate Bar 70%-85% cacao	☺	Free of fructose.
Dark chocolate Bar, sugar free	17 🍰	Piece (12g); 204g in total.
Dark Fruit Chocolates (Liberty Orchards®)	B ×¼ ☺+	Free of fructose. Per Piece (15g) you eat with it, add B-no × F-limit.
Dark Fruit Chocolates, Sugar Free (Liberty Orchards®)	☺	Free of fructose.
Fifty 50® Sugar Free Low Glycemic Butterscotch Hard Candy	☺	Free of fructose.
French Burnt Peanuts	B ×1¾ ☺+	Free of fructose. Per Hand (30g) you eat with it, add B-no × F-limit.
Gelatin (jello) powder, flavored, sugar free	☺	Free of fructose.
Gelatin (jello) powder, plain	☺	Free of fructose.
Gum drops	B ×2¼ ☺+	Free of fructose. Per Hand (30g) you eat with it, add B-no × F-limit.
Gum drops, sugar free	☺	Free of fructose.
Gummi bears	B ×3½ ☺+	Free of fructose. Per Hand (30g) you eat with it, add B-no × F-limit.
Gummi bears, sugar free	☺	Free of fructose.
Gummi dinosaurs	B ×3½ ☺+	Free of fructose. Per Hand (30g) you eat with it, add B-no × F-limit.
Gummi dinosaurs, sugar free	☺	Free of fructose.
Gummi worms	B ×3½ ☺+	Free of fructose. Per Hand (30g) you eat with it, add B-no × F-limit.

Sweets	SORBITOL Stand.		SORBITOL Low sensitivity amount
Dark chocolate Bar 60%-69% cacao	☹ Avoid	6½	135g Bar (125g); 813g in total.
Dark chocolate Bar 70%-85% cacao	☹ Avoid	5	135g Bar (125g); 625g in total.
Dark chocolate Bar, sugar free	☹ Avoid	☹	Avoid consumption!!
Dark Fruit Chocolates (Liberty Orchards®)	☹ Avoid	31½	Piece (15g); 473g in total.
Dark Fruit Chocolates, Sugar Free (Liberty Orchards®)	☹ Avoid	☹	Avoid consumption!!
Fifty 50® Sugar Free Low Glycemic Butterscotch Hard Candy	☹ Avoid	☹	Avoid consumption!!
French Burnt Peanuts	☺ Free	☺	Free of sorbitol.
Gelatin (jello) powder, flavored, sugar free	☺ Free	☺	Free of sorbitol.
Gelatin (jello) powder, plain	☺ Free	☺	Free of sorbitol.
Gum drops	☺ Free	☺	Free of sorbitol.
Gum drops, sugar free	☹ Avoid	☹	Avoid consumption!!
Gummi bears	☺ Nearly free	☺	Nearly free of sorbitol
Gummi bears, sugar free	☹ Avoid	☹	Avoid consumption!!
Gummi dinosaurs	☺ Nearly free	☺	Nearly free of sorbitol
Gummi dinosaurs, sugar free	☹ Avoid	☹	Avoid consumption!!
Gummi worms	☺ Nearly free	☺	Nearly free of sorbitol

Sweets	LACTOSE	Standard amount	
Gummi worms, sugar free	😊	Free of lactose.	
Hard candy	😊	Free of lactose.	
Hard candy, sugar free	😊	Free of lactose.	
Hershey's® Caramel Filled Chocolates Sugar Free	74½	Piece (8.6g); 641g in total.	+62
Hershey's® Milk Chocolate Bar	¼	135g Bar (125g); 31g in total.	+¼
Jelly beans®	😊	Free of lactose.	
Jelly beans®, sugar free	😊	Free of lactose.	
Jujyfruits®	😊	Free of lactose.	
Kashi® Layered Granola Bar, Pumpkin Pecan	😊	Free of lactose.	
Kit Kat®	2	Piece (43g); 86g in total.	+1¾
Kit Kat® White	¾	Piece (42g); 32g in total.	+½
Licorice	😊	Free of lactose.	
Little Debbie® Nutty Bars	😊	Free of lactose.	
M & M's® Peanut	2½	Portion (40g); 100g in total.	+2
Mamba® Fruit Chews	😊	Free of lactose.	
Mamba® Sour Fruit Chews	😊	Free of lactose.	

Sweets	IBS	Standard amount	F+G	amount
Gummi worms, sugar free	☹	Avoid consumption!!	☺	
Hard candy	☺	Free of triggers.	☺	
Hard candy, sugar free	☹	Avoid consumption!!	☺	
Hershey's® Caramel Filled Chocolates Sugar Free	☹	Avoid consumption!!	☺	
Hershey's® Milk Chocolate Bar	¼	135g Bar (125g); 31g in total.	¼	
Jelly beans®	☺	Free of triggers.	☺	
Jelly beans®, sugar free	☹	Avoid consumption!!	☺	
Jujyfruits®	☺	Free of triggers.	☺	
Kashi® Layered Granola Bar, Pumpkin Pecan	25	Piece (40g); 1,000g in total.	☺	
Kit Kat®	2	Piece (43g); 86g in total.	2	
Kit Kat® White	¾	Piece (42g); 32g in total.	1½	
Licorice	☺	Free of triggers.	☺	
Little Debbie® Nutty Bars	4¼	Piece (28.5g); 121g in total.	4¼	
M & M's® Peanut	2½	Portion (40g); 100g in total.	8¾	
Mamba® Fruit Chews	☹	Avoid consumption!!	☺	
Mamba® Sour Fruit Chews	☹	Avoid consumption!!	☺	

Sweets	FRUCTOSE	Standard amount
Gummi worms, sugar free	☺	Free of fructose.
Hard candy	B ×¾ ☺+	Free of fructose. Per Piece (6g) you eat with it, add B-no × F-limit.
Hard candy, sugar free	☺	Free of fructose.
Hershey's® Caramel Filled Chocolates Sugar Free	☺	Free of fructose.
Hershey's® Milk Chocolate Bar	☺	Free of fructose.
Jelly beans®	B ×9¾ ☺+	Free of fructose. Per Hand (30g) you eat with it, add B-no × F-limit.
Jelly beans®, sugar free	☺	Free of fructose.
Jujyfruits®	B ×12 ☺+	Free of fructose. Per Hand (30g) you eat with it, add B-no × F-limit.
Kashi® Layered Granola Bar, Pumpkin Pecan	B ×1½ ☺+	Free of fructose. Per Piece (40g) you eat with it, add B-no × F-limit.
Kit Kat®	☺	Free of fructose.
Kit Kat® White	☺	Free of fructose.
Licorice	B ×1½ ☺+	Free of fructose. Per Piece (11g) you eat with it, add B-no × F-limit.
Little Debbie® Nutty Bars	B ×13 ☺+	Free of fructose. Per Piece (28.5g) you eat with it, add B-no × F-limit.
M & M's® Peanut	☺	Free of fructose.
Mamba® Fruit Chews	B ×22 ☺+	Free of fructose. Per Portion (40g) you eat with it, add B-no × F-limit.
Mamba® Sour Fruit Chews	B ×17 ☺+	Free of fructose. Per Portion (40g) you eat with it, add B-no × F-limit.

Sweets	SORBITOL Stand.		SORBITOL Low sensitivity amount	
Gummi worms, sugar free	☹	Avoid	☹	Avoid consumption!!
Hard candy	☺	Free	☺	Free of sorbitol.
Hard candy, sugar free	☹	Avoid	☹	Avoid consumption!!
Hershey's® Caramel Filled Chocolates Sugar Free	☹	Avoid	☹	Avoid consumption!!
Hershey's® Milk Chocolate Bar	☺	Free	☺	Free of sorbitol.
Jelly beans®	☺	Free	☺	Free of sorbitol.
Jelly beans®, sugar free	☹	Avoid	☹	Avoid consumption!!
Jujyfruits®	☺	Free	☺	Free of sorbitol.
Kashi® Layered Granola Bar, Pumpkin Pecan	☹	Avoid	25 🍰	Piece (40g); 1,000g in total.
Kit Kat®	☺	Nearly free	☺	Nearly free of sorbitol
Kit Kat® White	☺	Free	☺	Free of sorbitol.
Licorice	☺	Free	☺	Free of sorbitol.
Little Debbie® Nutty Bars	☺	Nearly free	☺	Nearly free of sorbitol
M & M's® Peanut	☺	Free	☺	Free of sorbitol.
Mamba® Fruit Chews	☹	Avoid	☹	Avoid consumption!!
Mamba® Sour Fruit Chews	☹	Avoid	☹	Avoid consumption!!

Sweets	LACTOSE		Standard amount	
Marshmallow		☺	Free of lactose.	
Mentos®		☺	Free of lactose.	
Milk chocolate Bar, cereal	½		135g Bar (125g); 63g in total.	+½
Milk chocolate Bar, cereal, sugar free	7½		Piece (12g); 90g in total.	+6¼
Milk chocolate Bar, sugar free	3¼		Piece (12g); 39g in total.	+2½
Milk Chocolate covered raisins	2¾		Hand (30g); 83g in total.	+2¼
Milk Maid® Caramels (Brach's®)	½		Piece (40g); 20g in total.	+¼
Molasses, dark		☺	Free of lactose.	
Nestle® Nesquik®, chocolate flavors, unprepared dry			Glass (240g); Avoid consumption!!	0.19
Nougat		☺	Free of lactose.	
Pecan praline	3½		Piece (55g); 193g in total.	+2¾
Riesen®	12¾		Piece (9g); 115g in total.	+10½
Smarties®		☺	Free of lactose.	
Snickers®	1½		Piece (58.7g); 88g in total.	+1¼
Snickers®, Almond	1¾		Piece (49.9g); 87g in total.	+1½
Splenda®		☺	Free of lactose.	

Sweets	IBS	Standard amount	F+G	amount
Marshmallow	🙂	Free of triggers.	🙂	
Mentos®	🙂	Free of triggers.	🙂	
Milk chocolate Bar, cereal	¼	135g Bar (125g); 31g in total.	¼	
Milk chocolate Bar, cereal, sugar free	☹	Avoid consumption!!	4½	
Milk chocolate Bar, sugar free	☹	Avoid consumption!!	4½	
Milk Chocolate covered raisins	2¾	Hand (30g); 83g in total.	3¼	
Milk Maid® Caramels (Brach's®)	½	Piece (40g); 20g in total.	3	
Molasses, dark	3¾	Tbsp. (15g); 56g in total.	🙂	
Nestle® Nesquik®, chocolate flavors, unprepared dry	¼	Glass (200g); 50 mL in total.	1½	
Nougat	¼	Bar (125g); 31g in total.	¼	
Pecan praline	1¼	Piece (55g); 69g in total.	1¼	
Riesen®	☹	Avoid consumption!!	71	
Smarties®	🙂	Free of triggers.	🙂	
Snickers®	1½	Piece (58.7g); 88g in total.	5¾	
Snickers®, Almond	1¾	Piece (49.9g); 87g in total.	6½	
Splenda®	🙂	Free of triggers.	🙂	

Sweets	FRUCTOSE		Standard amount
Marshmallow	B ×4½	☺ +	Free of fructose. Per Portion (30g) you eat with it, add B-no × F-limit.
Mentos®		☺	Free of fructose.
Milk chocolate Bar, cereal		☺	Free of fructose.
Milk chocolate Bar, cereal, sugar free	40	🍰	Piece (12g); 480g in total.
Milk chocolate Bar, sugar free	40	🍰	Piece (12g); 480g in total.
Milk Chocolate covered raisins	B ×¼	☺ +	Free of fructose. Per Hand (30g) you eat with it, add B-no × F-limit.
Milk Maid® Caramels (Brach's®)	B ×5¾	☺ +	Free of fructose. Per Piece (40g) you eat with it, add B-no × F-limit.
Molasses, dark	3¾	🥄	Tbsp. (15g); 56g in total.
Nestle® Nesquik®, chocolate flavors, unprepared dry	1½	🥛	Glass (200g); 300 mL in total.
Nougat	B ×18	☺ +	Free of fructose. Per Bar (125g) you eat with it, add B-no × F-limit.
Pecan praline	B ×1¼	☺ +	Free of fructose. Per Piece (55g) you eat with it, add B-no × F-limit.
Riesen®	B ×2¾	☺ +	Free of fructose. Per Piece (9g) you eat with it, add B-no × F-limit.
Smarties®	B ×55	☺ +	Free of fructose. Per Hand (30g) you eat with it, add B-no × F-limit.
Snickers®	B ×7	☺ +	Free of fructose. Per Piece (58.7g) you eat with it, add B-no × F-limit.
Snickers®, Almond	B ×8¾	☺ +	Free of fructose. Per Piece (49.9g) you eat with it, add B-no × F-limit.
Splenda®		☺	Free of fructose.

Sweets	SORBITOL Stand.		SORBITOL Low sensitivity amount
Marshmallow	☺ Free		☺ Free of sorbitol.
Mentos®	☺ Free		☺ Free of sorbitol.
Milk chocolate Bar, cereal	☹ Avoid	40	135g Bar (125g); 5,000g in total.
Milk chocolate Bar, cereal, sugar free	☹ Avoid		☹ Avoid consumption!!
Milk chocolate Bar, sugar free	☹ Avoid		☹ Avoid consumption!!
Milk Chocolate covered raisins	☹ Avoid	3¼	Hand (30g); 98g in total.
Milk Maid® Caramels (Brach's®)	☺ Free		☺ Free of sorbitol.
Molasses, dark	☺ Free		☺ Free of sorbitol.
Nestle® Nesquik®, chocolate flavors, unprepared dry	☹ Avoid	5½	Glass (200g); 1,100 mL in total.
Nougat	☺ Free		☺ Free of sorbitol.
Pecan praline	☺ Free		☺ Free of sorbitol.
Riesen®	☹ Avoid		☹ Avoid consumption!!
Smarties®	☺ Free		☺ Free of sorbitol.
Snickers®	☺ Free		☺ Free of sorbitol.
Snickers®, Almond	☺ Free		☺ Free of sorbitol.
Splenda®	☺ Free		☺ Free of sorbitol.

Sweets	LACTOSE	Standard amount	
Starburst®, Original	🙂	Free of lactose.	
Suckers®, sugar free	🙂	Free of lactose.	
Sugar, white granulated	🙂	Free of lactose.	
Taffy	🙂	Free of lactose.	
Tic Tacs®	🙂	Free of lactose.	
Toblerone® Swiss Dark Chocolate with Honey & Almond Nougat	7¼	Piece (25g); 181g in total.	+6
Toblerone® Swiss Milk Chocolate with Honey & Almond Nougat	1½	Piece (25g); 38g in total.	+1¼
Toblerone® Swiss White Confection with Honey & Almond Nougat	1	Piece (25g); 25g in total.	+1
Toffee	40¾	Piece (7g); 285g in total.	+34
Toffifay®	7½	Piece (8.2g); 62g in total.	+6¼
Tootsie Pops®	🙂	Free of lactose.	
Werther's® Original Caramel Coffee Hard Candies	17¾	Piece (4g); 71g in total.	+14¾
White chocolate Bar	2½	Piece (12g); 30g in total.	+2
Wild 'n Fruity Gummi Bears (Brach's®)	🙂	Free of lactose.	
Zsweet®	🙂	Free of lactose.	

Sweets	IBS	Standard amount	F+G	amount
Starburst®, Original	30¼ 🍰	Piece (5g); 151g in total.	☺	
Suckers®, sugar free	☹	Avoid consumption!!	☺	
Sugar, white granulated	☺	Free of triggers.	☺	
Taffy	☺	Free of triggers.	☺	
Tic Tacs®	☺	Free of triggers.	☺	
Toblerone® Swiss Dark Chocolate with Honey & Almond Nougat	1½ 🍰	Piece (25g); 38g in total.	1½ 🍰	
Toblerone® Swiss Milk Chocolate with Honey & Almond Nougat	1½ 🍰	Piece (25g); 38g in total.	1½ 🍰	
Toblerone® Swiss White Confection with Honey & Almond Nougat	1 🍰	Piece (25g); 25g in total.	6¾ 🍰	
Toffee	40¾ 🍰	Piece (7g); 285g in total.	☺	
Toffifay®	☹	Avoid consumption!	42¾ 🍰	
Tootsie Pops®	☺	Free of triggers.	☺	
Werther's® Original Caramel Coffee Hard Candies	17¾ 🍰	Piece (4g); 71g in total.	☺	
White chocolate Bar	2½ 🍰	Piece (12g); 30g in total.	14 🍰	
Wild 'n Fruity Gummi Bears (Brach's®)	☺	Free of triggers.	☺	
Zsweet®	☹	Avoid consumption!!	☺	

Sweets	FRUCTOSE		Standard amount
Starburst®, Original	B ×½	😊 ⊕	Free of fructose. Per Piece (5g) you eat with it, add B-no × F-limit.
Suckers®, sugar free		😊	Free of fructose.
Sugar, white granulated		😊	Free of fructose.
Taffy	B ×4¼	😊 ⊕	Free of fructose. Per Piece (8.6g) you eat with it, add B-no × F-limit.
Tic Tacs®		😊	Free of fructose.
Toblerone® Swiss Dark Chocolate with Honey & Almond Nougat		😊	Free of fructose.
Toblerone® Swiss Milk Chocolate with Honey & Almond Nougat		😊	Free of fructose.
Toblerone® Swiss White Confection with Honey & Almond Nougat		😊	Free of fructose.
Toffee		😊	Free of fructose.
Toffifay®	B ×¼	😊 ⊕	Free of fructose. Per Piece (8.2g) you eat with it, add B-no × F-limit.
Tootsie Pops®	B ×2½	😊 ⊕	Free of fructose. Per Piece (17g) you eat with it, add B-no × F-limit.
Werther's® Original Caramel Coffee Hard Candies	B ×½	😊 ⊕	Free of fructose. Per Piece (4g) you eat with it, add B-no × F-limit.
White chocolate Bar		😊	Free of fructose.
Wild 'n Fruity Gummi Bears (Brach's®)	B ×3½	😊 ⊕	Free of fructose. Per Hand (30g) you eat with it, add B-no × F-limit.
Zsweet®		😊	Free of fructose.

Sweets	SORBITOL Stand.		SORBITOL Low sensitivity amount
Starburst®, Original	😦 Avoid	30¼ 🍰	Piece (5g); 151g in total.
Suckers®, sugar free	😦 Avoid	😦	Avoid consumption!!
Sugar, white granulated	😃 Free	😃	Free of sorbitol.
Taffy	😃 Free	😃	Free of sorbitol.
Tic Tacs®	😃 Free	😃	Free of sorbitol.
Toblerone® Swiss Dark Chocolate with Honey & Almond Nougat	😦 Avoid	40 🍰	Piece (25g); 1,000g in total.
Toblerone® Swiss Milk Chocolate with Honey & Almond Nougat	😃 Free	😃	Free of sorbitol.
Toblerone® Swiss White Confection with Honey & Almond Nougat	😃 Free	😃	Free of sorbitol.
Toffee	😃 Free	😃	Free of sorbitol.
Toffifay®	😦 Avoid	😦	Avoid consumption!
Tootsie Pops®	😃 Free	😃	Free of sorbitol.
Werther's® Original Caramel Coffee Hard Candies	😃 Free	😃	Free of sorbitol.
White chocolate Bar	😃 Free	😃	Free of sorbitol.
Wild 'n Fruity Gummi Bears (Brach's®)	🙂 Nearly free	🙂	Nearly free of sorbitol
Zsweet®	😦 Avoid	😦	Avoid consumption!!

3.5 Warm dishes

3.5.1 Meals

Meals	LACTOSE		Standard amount	⊕
Arby's® macaroni and cheese	21½		Portion (217g); 4,666g in total.	+18
Asian noodle bowl, vegetables only		☺	Free of lactose.	
Baby food, Gerber Graduates® Organic Pasta Pick-Ups Three Cheese Ravioli	1		Portion (170g); 170g in total.	+¾
Beef with noodles soup, condensed		☺	Free of lactose.	
Boston Market® macaroni and cheese	½		Portion (243g); 122g in total.	+½
Butternut squash soup	13½		Portion (245g); 3,308g in total.	+11¼
Calzone, cheese	12¼		Piece (168g); 2,058g in total.	+10¼
Casserole (hot dish), pasta with turkey, gravy base, vegetables other than dark green, cheese	3¾		Portion (228g); 855g in total.	+3
Casserole (hot dish), rice with beef, tomato base, vegetables other than dark green, cheese	9¾		Portion (244g); 2,379g in total.	+8¼
Chicken and dumplings soup, condensed	7¼		Portion (126g); 914g in total.	+6
Chicken noodle soup with vegetables, ready-to-serve can		☺	Free of lactose.	
Chicken wonton soup, prepared from condensed can		☺	Free of lactose.	
Chili with beans, beef, canned		☺	Free of lactose.	

Meals	IBS Standard amount		F+G amount
Arby's® macaroni and cheese	½	Portion (217g); 109g in total.	½
Asian noodle bowl, vegetables only	1½	Portion (200g); 300g in total.	1½
Baby food, Gerber Graduates® Organic Pasta Pick-Ups Three Cheese Ravioli	¾	Portion (170g); 128g in total.	¾
Beef with noodles soup, condensed	4	Portion (126g); 504g in total.	4
Boston Market® macaroni and cheese	½	Portion (243g); 122g in total.	½
Butternut squash soup	½	Portion (245g); 123g in total.	½
Calzone, cheese	¼	Piece (168g); 42g in total.	¼
Casserole (hot dish), pasta with turkey, gravy base, veggies except dark green, cheese	½	Portion (228g); 114g in total.	½
Casserole (hot dish), rice with beef, tomato base, vegetables other than dark green, cheese	¼	Portion (244g); 61g in total.	¼
Chicken and dumplings soup, condensed	2¼	Portion (126g); 284g in total.	2¼
Chicken noodle soup with vegetables, ready-to-serve can	1	Portion (245g); 245g in total.	1¼
Chicken wonton soup, prepared from condensed can	☺	Free of triggers.	☺
Chili with beans, beef, canned	3	Tbsp. (15g); 45g in total.	3

Meals	FRUCTOSE		Standard amount
Arby's® macaroni and cheese		☺	Free of fructose.
Asian noodle bowl, vegetables only	B ×1	☺ +	Free of fructose. Per Portion (200g) you eat with it, add B-no × F-limit.
Baby food, Gerber Graduates® Organic Pasta Pick-Ups Three Cheese Ravioli		☺	Free of fructose.
Beef with noodles soup, condensed		☺	Free of fructose.
Boston Market® macaroni and cheese		☺	Free of fructose.
Butternut squash soup		☺	Free of fructose.
Calzone, cheese		☺	Free of fructose.
Casserole (hot dish), pasta with turkey, gravy base, vegetables other than dark green, with cheese		☺	Free of fructose.
Casserole (hot dish), rice with beef, tomato base, vegetables other than dark green, with cheese	B ×1	☺ +	Free of fructose. Per Portion (244g) you eat with it, add B-no × F-limit.
Chicken and dumplings soup, condensed		☺	Free of fructose.
Chicken noodle soup with vegetables, ready-to-serve can		☺	Free of fructose.
Chicken wonton soup, prepared from condensed can		☺	Free of fructose.
Chili with beans, beef, canned	87½	🥄	Tbsp. (15g); 1,313g in total.

Meals	SORBITOL Stand.		SORBITOL Low sensitivity amount
Arby's® macaroni and cheese	😀 Free		Free of sorbitol.
Asian noodle bowl, vegetables only	😞 Avoid	10	Portion (200g); 2,000g in total.
Baby food, Gerber Graduates® Organic Pasta Pick-Ups Three Cheese Ravioli	😀 Free		Free of sorbitol.
Beef with noodles soup, condensed	😞 Avoid	4¼	Portion (126g); 536g in total.
Boston Market® macaroni and cheese	😀 Free		Free of sorbitol.
Butternut squash soup	😞 Avoid	2½	Portion (245g); 613g in total.
Calzone, cheese	😞 Avoid	2¾	Piece (168g); 462g in total.
Casserole (hot dish), pasta with turkey, gravy base, vegetables other than dark green, with cheese	😞 Avoid	1¼	Portion (228g); 285g in total.
Casserole (hot dish), rice with beef, tomato base, vegetables other than dark green, with cheese	😞 Avoid	¼	Portion (244g); 61g in total.
Chicken and dumplings soup, condensed	😞 Avoid	2¼	Portion (126g); 284g in total.
Chicken noodle soup with vegetables, ready-to-serve can	😞 Avoid	1	Portion (245g); 245g in total.
Chicken wonton soup, prepared from condensed can	😞 Avoid	40¾	Portion (245g); 9,984g in total.
Chili with beans, beef, canned	😞 Avoid	55½	Tbsp. (15g); 833g in total.

Meals	LACTOSE	Standard amount	
Chop suey, chicken, no noodles	☺	Free of lactose.	
Chop suey, tofu, no noodles	☺	Free of lactose.	
Cream of asparagus soup, prepared from condensed can	6½	Tbsp. (15g); 98g in total.	+5½
Cream of broccoli soup, condensed	5	Portion (126g); 630g in total.	+4¼
Cream of celery soup, homemade	½	Portion (245g); 123g in total.	+½
Cream of chicken soup, condensed	6½	Portion (126g); 819g in total.	+5½
Cream of mushroom soup, prepared from condensed can	1½	Portion (245g); 368g in total.	+1¼
Cream of potato soup mix, dry	3¼	Portion (23g); 75g in total.	+2¾
Cream of spinach soup mix, dry	☺	Free of lactose.	
Dairy Queen® Foot Long Hot Dog	☺	Free of lactose.	
Fettuccini Alfredo®, no meat, vegetables except dark green	¾	Portion (200g); 150g in total.	+¾
Fettuccini Alfredo®, no meat, carrots or dark green vegetables	5	Portion (200g); 1,000g in total.	+4
Fruit sauce, jelly-based	☺	Free of lactose.	
German style potato salad, with bacon and vinegar dressing	☺	Free of lactose.	
Green pea soup, prepared from condensed can	☺	Free of lactose.	
Hardee's® Loaded Omelet Biscuit	12	Piece (158g); 1,896g in total.	+10

Meals	IBS	Standard amount	F+G amount
Chop suey, chicken, no noodles	¼	Portion (166g); 42g in total.	¼
Chop suey, tofu, no noodles	¼	Portion (166g); 42g in total.	☺
Cream of asparagus soup, prepared condensed can	1½	Tbsp. (15g); 23g in total.	1½
Cream of broccoli soup, condensed	1	Portion (126g); 126g in total.	1
Cream of celery soup, homemade	¼	Portion (245g); 61g in total.	¼
Cream of chicken soup, condensed	6½	Portion (126g); 819g in total.	37¼
Cream of mushroom soup, prepared condensed can	¼	Portion (245g); 61g in total.	½
Cream of potato soup mix, dry	3	Portion (23g); 69g in total.	5
Cream of spinach soup mix, dry	3¼	Portion (17g); 55g in total.	3¼
Dairy Queen® Foot Long Hot Dog	¼	Piece (199g); 50g in total.	¼
Fettuccini Alfredo®, no meat, vegetables except dark green	¼	Portion (200g); 50g in total.	6
Fettuccini Alfredo®, no meat, carrots or dark green veggies	5	Portion (200g); 1,000g in total.	27¾
Fruit sauce, jelly-based	¾	Portion (40g); 30g in total.	☺
German style potato salad, bacon and vinegar dressing	1	Portion (140g); 140g in total.	1
Green pea soup, prepared from condensed can	3¼	Tbsp. (15g); 49g in total.	3¼
Hardee's® Loaded Omelet Biscuit	¼	Piece (158g); 40g in total.	¼

Meals	FRUCTOSE	Standard amount
Chop suey, chicken, no noodles	☺	Free of fructose.
Chop suey, tofu, no noodles	☺	Free of fructose.
Cream of asparagus soup, prepared condensed can	☺	Nearly free of fructose, avoid at hereditary fructose intolerance.
Cream of broccoli soup, condensed	☺	Free of fructose.
Cream of celery soup, homemade	☺	Free of fructose.
Cream of chicken soup, condensed	☺	Nearly free of fructose, avoid at hereditary fructose intolerance.
Cream of mushroom soup, prepared condensed can	☺	Nearly free of fructose, avoid at hereditary fructose intolerance.
Cream of potato soup mix, dry	☺	Free of fructose.
Cream of spinach soup mix, dry	B ×¼ ☺+	Free of fructose. Per Portion (17g) you eat with it, add B-no × F-limit.
Dairy Queen® Foot Long Hot Dog	B ×1¾ ☺+	Free of fructose. Per Piece (199g) you eat with it, add B-no × F-limit.
Fettuccini Alfredo®, no meat, vegetables except dark green	☺	Free of fructose.
Fettuccini Alfredo®, no meat, carrots / dark green vegetables	☺	Free of fructose.
Fruit sauce, jelly-based	B ×5¼ ☺+	Free of fructose. Per Portion (40g) you eat with it, add B-no × F-limit.
German style potato salad, bacon and vinegar dressing	B ×¼ ☺+	Free of fructose. Per Portion (140g) you eat with it, add B-no × F-limit.
Green pea soup, prepared from condensed can	☺	Free of fructose.
Hardee's® Loaded Omelet Biscuit	B ×9¼ ☺+	Free of fructose. Per Piece (158g) you eat with it, add B-no × F-limit.

Meals	SORBITOL Stand.	SORBITOL Low sensitivity amount	
Chop suey, chicken, no noodles	Avoid	¼	Portion (166g); 42g in total.
Chop suey, tofu, no noodles	Avoid	¼	Portion (166g); 42g in total.
Cream of asparagus soup, prepared from condensed can	Nearly free		Nearly free of sorbitol
Cream of broccoli soup, condensed	Avoid	19¾	Portion (126g); 2,489g in total.
Cream of celery soup, homemade	Avoid	¼	Portion (245g); 61g in total.
Cream of chicken soup, condensed	Avoid	26¼	Portion (126g); 3,308g in total.
Cream of mushroom soup, prepared from condensed can	Avoid	¼	Portion (245g); 61g in total.
Cream of potato soup mix, dry	Avoid	3	Portion (23g); 69g in total.
Cream of spinach soup mix, dry	Avoid	18¼	Portion (17g); 310g in total.
Dairy Queen® Foot Long Hot Dog	Avoid	8¼	Piece (199g); 1,642g in total.
Fettuccini Alfredo®, no meat, vegetables except dark green	Avoid	¼	Portion (200g); 50g in total.
Fettuccini Alfredo®, no meat, carrots / dark green veggies	Free		Free of sorbitol.
Fruit sauce, jelly-based	Avoid	¾	Portion (40g); 30g in total.
German style potato salad, bacon and vinegar dressing	Avoid	4¾	Portion (140g); 665g in total.
Green pea soup, prepared from condensed can	Avoid	20	Tbsp. (15g); 300g in total.
Hardee's® Loaded Omelet Biscuit	Free		Free of sorbitol.

Meals	LACTOSE		Standard amount	⊕
Lasagna, homemade, beef	2		Portion (140g); 280g in total.	+1¾
Lasagna, homemade, cheese, no vegetables	1¼		Portion (140g); 175g in total.	+1
Lasagna, homemade, spinach, no meat	8½		Portion (140g); 1,190g in total.	+7
Lentil soup, condensed	☺		Nearly free of lactose	
Lyonnaise (potatoes and onions)	☺		Free of lactose.	
Macaroni or pasta salad, with meat, egg, mayo dressing	☺		Free of lactose.	
Meat ravioli, with tomato sauce	☺		Nearly free of lactose	
Minestrone soup, condensed	☺		Free of lactose.	
Minestrone soup, homemade	☺		Free of lactose.	
Noodle soup mix, dry	☺		Free of lactose.	
Omelet, made with bacon	34¾		Portion (110g); 3,823g in total.	+29
Omelet, made with sausage, potatoes, onions, cheese	52¼		Portion (110g); 5,748g in total.	+43½
Pad Thai, without meat	☺		Free of lactose.	
Paella	☺		Free of lactose.	
Panda Express® Orange Chicken	6½		Portion (140g); 910g in total.	+5¼
Pasta salad with vegetables, Italian dressing	☺		Nearly free of lactose	

Meals	IBS	Standard amount	F+G	amount
Lasagna, homemade, beef	¾	Portion (140g); 105g in total.	¾	
Lasagna, homemade, cheese, no vegetables	¾	Portion (140g); 105g in total.	¾	
Lasagna, homemade, spinach, no meat	½	Portion (140g); 70g in total.	¾	
Lentil soup, condensed	1	Portion (126g); 126g in total.	5½	
Lyonnaise (potatoes and onions)	15¾	Portion (70g); 1,103g in total.	☺	
Macaroni or pasta salad, with meat, egg, mayo dressing	1¼	Portion (140g); 175g in total.	1½	
Meat ravioli, with tomato sauce	¼	Portion (250g); 63g in total.	¼	
Minestrone soup, condensed	½	Portion (126g); 63g in total.	½	
Minestrone soup, homemade	¼	Portion (245g); 61g in total.	¼	
Noodle soup mix, dry	6¼	Portion (16g); 100g in total.	6¼	
Omelet, made with bacon	34¾	Portion (110g); 3,823g in total.	☺	
Omelet, made with sausage, potatoes, onions, cheese	¼	Portion (110g); 28g in total.	¼	
Pad Thai, without meat	3¾	Portion (140g); 525g in total.	☺	
Paella	1	Portion (240g); 240g in total.	1	
Panda Express® Orange Chicken	¼	Portion (140g); 35g in total.	36¼	
Pasta salad with vegetables, Italian dressing	1½	Portion (140g); 210g in total.	1½	

Meals	FRUCTOSE		Standard amount
Lasagna, homemade, beef	B ×¼	☺+	Free of fructose. Per Portion (140g) you eat with it, add B-no × F-limit.
Lasagna, homemade, cheese, no vegetables	6		Portion (140g); 840g in total.
Lasagna, homemade, spinach, no meat	5½		Portion (140g); 770g in total.
Lentil soup, condensed		☺	Free of fructose.
Lyonnaise (potatoes and onions)		☺	Free of fructose.
Macaroni or pasta salad, with meat, egg, mayo dressing	B ×½	☺+	Free of fructose. Per Portion (140g) you eat with it, add B-no × F-limit.
Meat ravioli, with tomato sauce	B ×½	☺+	Free of fructose. Per Portion (250g) you eat with it, add B-no × F-limit.
Minestrone soup, condensed		☺	Free of fructose.
Minestrone soup, homemade		☺	Free of fructose.
Noodle soup mix, dry	B ×¼	☺+	Free of fructose. Per Portion (16g) you eat with it, add B-no × F-limit.
Omelet, made with bacon	B ×1¾	☺+	Free of fructose. Per Portion (110g) you eat with it, add B-no × F-limit.
Omelet, made with sausage, potatoes, onions, cheese	B ×1	☺+	Free of fructose. Per Portion (110g) you eat with it, add B-no × F-limit.
Pad Thai, without meat		☺	Free of fructose.
Paella	2		Portion (240g); 480g in total.
Panda Express® Orange Chicken	¼		Portion (140g); 35g in total.
Pasta salad with vegetables, Italian dressing	2½		Portion (140g); 350g in total.

Meals	SORBITOL Stand.	SORBITOL Low sensitivity amount	
Lasagna, homemade, beef	☹ Avoid	1	Portion (140g); 140g in total.
Lasagna, homemade, cheese, no vegetables	☹ Avoid	¾	Portion (140g); 105g in total.
Lasagna, homemade, spinach, no meat	☹ Avoid	½	Portion (140g); 70g in total.
Lentil soup, condensed	☹ Avoid	1	Portion (126g); 126g in total.
Lyonnaise (potatoes and onions)	☹ Avoid	15¾	Portion (70g); 1,103g in total.
Macaroni or pasta salad, with meat, egg, mayo dressing	☹ Avoid	1¼	Portion (140g); 175g in total.
Meat ravioli, with tomato sauce	☹ Avoid	½	Portion (250g); 125g in total.
Minestrone soup, condensed	☹ Avoid	¾	Portion (126g); 95g in total.
Minestrone soup, homemade	☹ Avoid	1	Portion (245g); 245g in total.
Noodle soup mix, dry	☺ Free	☺	Free of sorbitol.
Omelet, made with bacon	☺ Free	☺	Free of sorbitol.
Omelet, made with sausage, potatoes, onions, cheese	☹ Avoid	6¾	Portion (110g); 743g in total.
Pad Thai, without meat	☹ Avoid	3¾	Portion (140g); 525g in total.
Paella	☹ Avoid	2¼	Portion (240g); 540g in total.
Panda Express® Orange Chicken	☹ Avoid	23¾	Portion (140g); 3,325g in total.
Pasta salad with vegetables, Italian dressing	☹ Avoid	1½	Portion (140g); 210g in total.

Meals	LACTOSE	Standard amount	
Pho soup (Vietnamese noodle soup)	☺	Free of lactose.	
Pizza Hut® cheese bread stick	61½	Piece (56g); 3,444g in total.	+51¼
Pizza Hut® Pepperoni Lover's pizza, stuffed crust	30	Portion (140g); 4,200g in total.	+25
Pizza Hut® Personal Pan, supreme	16¾	Piece (256g); 4,288g in total.	+14
Pizza, homemade or restaurant, cheese, thin crust	12¼	Piece (209g); 2,560g in total.	+10¼
Potato salad, with egg, mayo dressing	☺	Free of lactose.	
Potato soup with broccoli and cheese	29¾	Portion (245g); 7,289g in total.	+24¾
Ratatouille	☺	Nearly free of lactose	
Red beans and rice soup mix, dry	☺	Free of lactose.	
Scrambled egg, made with bacon	2¼	Portion (110g); 248g in total.	+1¾
Sesame chicken	☺	Free of lactose.	
Soup base	☺	Free of lactose.	
Spaghetti, with carbonara sauce	13½	Portion (201g); 2,714g in total.	+11¼
Spinach ravioli, with tomato sauce	5½	Portion (250g); 1,375g in total.	+4½
Spring roll	☺	Free of lactose.	
Squash or pumpkin ravioli, with cream sauce	½	Portion (250g); 125g in total.	+½

Meals	IBS	Standard amount	F+G	amount
Pho soup (Vietnamese noodle soup)	¾	Portion (245g); 184g in total.	¾	
Pizza Hut® cheese bread stick	1¼	Piece (56g); 70g in total.	1¼	
Pizza Hut® Pepperoni Lover's pizza, stuffed crust	¾	Portion (140g); 105g in total.	¾	
Pizza Hut® Personal Pan, supreme	¼	Piece (256g); 64g in total.	4¾	
Pizza, homemade or restaurant, cheese, thin crust	½	Piece (209g); 105g in total.	½	
Potato salad, with egg, mayo dressing	1	Portion (140g); 140g in total.	1	
Potato soup with broccoli and cheese	½	Portion (245g); 123g in total.	½	
Ratatouille	1¼	Portion (110g); 138g in total.	4	
Red beans and rice soup mix, dry	¼	Portion (51.03g); 13g in total.	1¼	
Scrambled egg, made with bacon	2¼	Portion (110g); 248g in total.	12½	
Sesame chicken	3¾	Portion (252g); 945g in total.	☺	
Soup base	54½	Tbsp. (15g); 818g in total.	☺	
Spaghetti, with carbonara sauce	½	Portion (201g); 101g in total.	½	
Spinach ravioli, with tomato sauce	½	Portion (250g); 125g in total.	½	
Spring roll	¼	Portion (140g); 35g in total.	¼	
Squash or pumpkin ravioli, with cream sauce	½	Portion (250g); 125g in total.	½	

Meals	FRUCTOSE		Standard amount
Pho soup (Vietnamese noodle soup)		🙂	Free of fructose.
Pizza Hut® cheese bread stick	B ×¼	🙂+	Free of fructose. Per Piece (56g) you eat with it, add B-no × F-limit.
Pizza Hut® Pepperoni Lover's pizza, stuffed crust		🙂	Free of fructose.
Pizza Hut® Personal Pan, supreme		🙂	Free of fructose.
Pizza, homemade or restaurant, cheese, thin crust	B ×¾	🙂+	Free of fructose. Per Piece (209g) you eat with it, add B-no × F-limit.
Potato salad, with egg, mayo dressing	B ×½	🙂+	Free of fructose. Per Portion (140g) you eat with it, add B-no × F-limit.
Potato soup with broccoli and cheese		🙂	Free of fructose.
Ratatouille		🙂	Free of fructose.
Red beans and rice soup mix, dry	¼	🍲	Portion (51.03g); 13g in total.
Scrambled egg, made with bacon	B ×1¾	🙂+	Free of fructose. Per Portion (110g) you eat with it, add B-no × F-limit.
Sesame chicken		🙂	Free of fructose.
Soup base	54½	🥄	Tbsp. (15g); 818g in total.
Spaghetti, with carbonara sauce	B ×¾	🙂+	Free of fructose. Per Portion (201g) you eat with it, add B-no × F-limit.
Spinach ravioli, with tomato sauce	B ×¼	🙂+	Free of fructose. Per Portion (250g) you eat with it, add B-no × F-limit.
Spring roll	10½	🍲	Portion (140g); 1,470g in total.
Squash or pumpkin ravioli, with cream sauce	B ×¼	🙂+	Free of fructose. Per Portion (250g) you eat with it, add B-no × F-limit.

Meals	SORBITOL Stand.		SORBITOL Low sensitivity amount
Pho soup (Vietnamese noodle soup)	☹ Avoid	6¾	Portion (245g); 1,654g in total.
Pizza Hut® cheese bread stick	☺ Free	☺	Free of sorbitol.
Pizza Hut® Pepperoni Lover's pizza, stuffed crust	☹ Avoid	1	Portion (140g); 140g in total.
Pizza Hut® Personal Pan, supreme	☹ Avoid	¼	Piece (256g); 64g in total.
Pizza, homemade or restaurant, cheese, thin crust	☹ Avoid	¾	Piece (209g); 157g in total.
Potato salad, with egg, mayo dressing	☹ Avoid	2	Portion (140g); 280g in total.
Potato soup with broccoli and cheese	☹ Avoid	13½	Portion (245g); 3,308g in total.
Ratatouille	☹ Avoid	1¼	Portion (110g); 138g in total.
Red beans and rice soup mix, dry	☹ Avoid	¼	Portion (51.03g); 13g in total.
Scrambled egg, made with bacon	☺ Free	☺	Free of sorbitol.
Sesame chicken	☹ Avoid	3¾	Portion (252g); 945g in total.
Soup base	☹ Avoid	74	Tbsp. (15g); 1,110g in total.
Spaghetti, with carbonara sauce	☹ Avoid	6	Portion (201g); 1,206g in total.
Spinach ravioli, with tomato sauce	☹ Avoid	½	Portion (250g); 125g in total.
Spring roll	☹ Avoid	2¾	Portion (140g); 385g in total.
Squash or pumpkin ravioli, with cream sauce	☹ Avoid	40	Portion (250g); 10,000g in total.

Meals	LACTOSE	Standard amount	⊕
Stewed green peas with sofrito	☺	Free of lactose.	
Sushi, with fish	☺	Free of lactose.	
Sushi, with fish and vegetables in seaweed	☺	Free of lactose.	
Sushi, with vegetables in seaweed	☺	Free of lactose.	
Swedish Meatballs	1½	Portion (140g); 210g in total.	+1¼
Sweet and sour chicken	☺	Free of lactose.	
Taco Bell® 7-Layer Burrito	25½	Portion (140g); 3,570g in total.	+21¼
Taco Bell® Crunchwrap Supreme	4¼	Piece (245g); 1,041g in total.	+3½
Taco Bell® Mexican Pizza	13¾	Piece (213g); 2,929g in total.	+11½
Taco Bell® Nachos Supreme	6¼	Portion (140g); 875g in total.	+5¼
Taco, soft corn shell, with beans, cheese	☺	Nearly free of lactose	+77½
Tomato relish	☺	Free of lactose.	
Tomato soup mix, dry	¼	Portion (34.66g); 9g in total.	0.24
Vegetable soup, condensed	☺	Free of lactose.	
Vichyssoise	¾	Portion (245g); 184g in total.	+½
White bean stew with sofrito	☺	Free of lactose.	

Meals	IBS	Standard amount	F+G	amount
Stewed green peas with sofrito	1¼	Tbsp. (15g); 19g in total.	1¼	
Sushi, with fish	2½	Portion (140g); 350g in total.	☺	
Sushi, with fish and vegetables in seaweed	2	Portion (140g); 280g in total.	☺	
Sushi, with vegetables in seaweed	1½	Portion (140g); 210g in total.	☺	
Swedish Meatballs	1½	Portion (140g); 210g in total.	9	
Sweet and sour chicken	2½	Tbsp. (15g); 38g in total.	☺	
Taco Bell® 7-Layer Burrito	¼	Portion (140g); 35g in total.	¼	
Taco Bell® Crunchwrap Supreme	☹	Avoid consumption!!	☹	
Taco Bell® Mexican Pizza	¼	Piece (213g); 53g in total.	¼	
Taco Bell® Nachos Supreme	6¼	Portion (140g); 875g in total.	35¾	
Taco, soft corn shell, with beans, cheese	¼	Portion (140g); 35g in total.	¼	
Tomato relish	5¼	Portion (15g); 79g in total.	33	
Tomato soup mix, dry	¼	Portion (34.66g); 9g in total.	1¼	
Vegetable soup, condensed	1	Portion (126g); 126g in total.	19¾	
Vichyssoise	¾	Portion (245g); 184g in total.	4¼	
White bean stew with sofrito	3	Tbsp. (15g); 45g in total.	3	

Meals	FRUCTOSE	Standard amount
Stewed green peas with sofrito	☺	Free of fructose.
Sushi, with fish	16	Portion (140g); 2,240g in total.
Sushi, with fish and vegetables in seaweed	☺	Free of fructose.
Sushi, with vegetables in seaweed	☺	Free of fructose.
Swedish Meatballs	☺	Free of fructose.
Sweet and sour chicken	2½	Tbsp. (15g); 38g in total.
Taco Bell® 7-Layer Burrito	☺	Free of fructose.
Taco Bell® Crunchwrap Supreme	☺	Free of fructose.
Taco Bell® Mexican Pizza	14½	Piece (213g); 3,089g in total.
Taco Bell® Nachos Supreme	☺	Free of fructose.
Taco, soft corn shell, with beans, cheese	8¼	Portion (140g); 1,155g in total.
Tomato relish	☺	Free of fructose.
Tomato soup mix, dry	6¾	Portion (34.66g); 234g in total.
Vegetable soup, condensed	B × ¼	Free of fructose. Per Portion (126g) you eat with it, add B-no × F-limit.
Vichyssoise	B × ¼	Free of fructose. Per Portion (245g) you eat with it, add B-no × F-limit.
White bean stew with sofrito	☺	Free of fructose.

Meals	SORBITOL Stand.		SORBITOL Low sensitivity amount	
Stewed green peas with sofrito	☹ Avoid	5½	🥄	Tbsp. (15g); 83g in total.
Sushi, with fish	☹ Avoid	2½		Portion (140g); 350g in total.
Sushi, with fish and vegetables in seaweed	☹ Avoid	2		Portion (140g); 280g in total.
Sushi, with vegetables in seaweed	☹ Avoid	1½		Portion (140g); 210g in total.
Swedish Meatballs	☹ Avoid	71¼		Portion (140g); 9,975g in total.
Sweet and sour chicken	☺ Nearly free		☺	Nearly free of sorbitol
Taco Bell® 7-Layer Burrito	☹ Avoid	5¾		Portion (140g); 805g in total.
Taco Bell® Crunchwrap Supreme	☹ Avoid	5		Piece (245g); 1,225g in total.
Taco Bell® Mexican Pizza	☹ Avoid	1		Piece (213g); 213g in total.
Taco Bell® Nachos Supreme	☹ Avoid	7¾		Portion (140g); 1,085g in total.
Taco, soft corn shell, with beans, cheese	☹ Avoid	4¼		Portion (140g); 595g in total.
Tomato relish	☹ Avoid	5¼		Portion (15g); 79g in total.
Tomato soup mix, dry	☹ Avoid	2		Portion (34.66g); 69g in total.
Vegetable soup, condensed	☹ Avoid	1		Portion (126g); 126g in total.
Vichyssoise	☹ Avoid	1¼		Portion (245g); 306g in total.
White bean stew with sofrito	☺ Nearly free		☺	Nearly free of sorbitol

3.5.2   Meat and fish

Meat and fish	LACTOSE	Standard amount	⊕
Beef bacon (kosher)	☺	Free of lactose.	
Beef steak, chuck, visible fat eaten	☺	Free of lactose.	
Bockwurst	☺	Free of lactose.	
Boston Market® 1/4 white rotisserie chicken, with skin	☺	Free of lactose.	
Boston Market® roasted turkey breast	☺	Free of lactose.	
Bratwurst	☺	Free of lactose.	
Bratwurst, beef	☺	Free of lactose.	
Bratwurst, light (reduced fat)	☺	Free of lactose.	
Bratwurst, made with beer	☺	Free of lactose.	
Bratwurst, made with beer, cheese-filled	☺	Nearly free of lactose	
Bratwurst, turkey	☺	Free of lactose.	
Braunschweiger	☺	Free of lactose.	
Caviar	☺	Free of lactose.	
Chicken fricassee with gravy, American style	☺	Free of lactose.	
Clams, stuffed with mushroom, onions, and bread	24½ 🐟	Portion (140g); 3,430g in total.	+20½

Meat and fish	IBS		Standard amount	F+G	amount
Arby's® Chicken Cordon Bleu Sandwich, crispy	1	😐	Portion (140g); 140g in total.	1	😐
Beef bacon (kosher)		😊	Free of triggers.		😊
Beef steak, chuck, visible fat eaten		😊	Free of triggers.		😊
Bockwurst		😊	Free of triggers.		😊
Boston Market® 1/4 white rotisserie chicken, with skin		😊	Free of triggers.		😊
Boston Market® roasted turkey breast		😊	Free of triggers.		😊
Bratwurst		😊	Free of triggers.		😊
Bratwurst, beef		😊	Free of triggers.		😊
Bratwurst, light (reduced fat)		😊	Free of triggers.		😊
Bratwurst, made with beer		😊	Free of triggers.		😊
Bratwurst, made with beer, cheese-filled		😊	Nearly free of triggers.		😊
Bratwurst, turkey		😊	Free of triggers.		😊
Braunschweiger		😊	Free of triggers.		😊
Caviar		😊	Free of triggers.		😊
Chicken fricassee with gravy, American style	5¾	🍲	Portion (244g); 1,403g in total.	5¾	🍲

Meat and fish	FRUCTOSE	Standard amount
Arby's® Chicken Cordon Bleu Sandwich, crispy	2	Portion (140g); 280g in total.
Beef bacon (kosher)	☺	Free of fructose.
Beef steak, chuck, visible fat eaten	☺	Free of fructose.
Bockwurst	B ×¼ ☺+	Free of fructose. Per Portion (55g) you eat with it, add B-no × F-limit.
Boston Market® 1/4 white rotisserie chicken, with skin	☺	Free of fructose.
Boston Market® roasted turkey breast	☺	Free of fructose.
Bratwurst	B ×¼ ☺+	Free of fructose. Per Portion (55g) you eat with it, add B-no × F-limit.
Bratwurst, beef	B ×1 ☺+	Free of fructose. Per Portion (55g) you eat with it, add B-no × F-limit.
Bratwurst, light (reduced fat)	B ×2¾ ☺+	Free of fructose. Per Portion (55g) you eat with it, add B-no × F-limit.
Bratwurst, made with beer	B ×¼ ☺+	Free of fructose. Per Portion (55g) you eat with it, add B-no × F-limit.
Bratwurst, made with beer, cheese-filled	B ×½ ☺+	Free of fructose. Per Portion (55g) you eat with it, add B-no × F-limit.
Bratwurst, turkey	B ×1½ ☺+	Free of fructose. Per Portion (55g) you eat with it, add B-no × F-limit.
Braunschweiger	☺	Free of fructose.
Caviar	☺	Free of fructose.
Chicken fricassee with gravy, American style	☺	Free of fructose.

Meat and fish	SORBITOL Stand.		SORBITOL Low sensitivity amount	
Arby's® Chicken Cordon Bleu Sandwich, crispy	😊	Free	😊	Free of sorbitol.
Beef bacon (kosher)	😊	Free	😊	Free of sorbitol.
Beef steak, chuck, visible fat eaten	😊	Free	😊	Free of sorbitol.
Bockwurst	😊	Free	😊	Free of sorbitol.
Boston Market® 1/4 white rotisserie chicken, with skin	😊	Free	😊	Free of sorbitol.
Boston Market® roasted turkey breast	😊	Free	😊	Free of sorbitol.
Bratwurst	😊	Free	😊	Free of sorbitol.
Bratwurst, beef	😊	Free	😊	Free of sorbitol.
Bratwurst, light (reduced fat)	😊	Free	😊	Free of sorbitol.
Bratwurst, made with beer	😊	Nearly free	😊	Nearly free of sorbitol
Bratwurst, made with beer, cheese-filled	😊	Nearly free	😊	Nearly free of sorbitol
Bratwurst, turkey	😊	Free	😊	Free of sorbitol.
Braunschweiger	😊	Free	😊	Free of sorbitol.
Caviar	😊	Free	😊	Free of sorbitol.
Chicken fricassee with gravy, American style	😊	Free	😊	Free of sorbitol.

Meat and fish	LACTOSE	Standard amount	
Clams, stuffed with mushroom, onions, and bread	24½	Portion (140g); 3,430g in total.	+20½
Fish croquette	2¼	Portion (85g); 191g in total.	+1¾
Fish sticks, patties, or nuggets, breaded, regular	☺	Free of lactose.	
Fish with breading	☺	Free of lactose.	
Gorton's® Battered Fish Fillets - Lemon Pepper	☺	Free of lactose.	
Gorton's® Popcorn Shrimp, Original	☺	Free of lactose.	
Goulash, with beef, noodles or macaroni, tomato base	☺	Free of lactose.	
Herring, pickled	☺	Free of lactose.	
Herring, pickled	☺	Free of lactose.	
Liver pudding	☺	Free of lactose.	
Mrs. Paul's® Calamari Rings	☺	Nearly free of lactose	
Pickled beef	☺	Free of lactose.	
Pork cutlet (sirloin cutlet), visible fat eaten	☺	Free of lactose.	
Ribs, beef, spare, visible fat eaten	☺	Free of lactose.	
Salami, beer or beerwurst, beef	☺	Free of lactose.	
Salmon, red (sockeye), smoked	☺	Free of lactose.	

Meat and fish	IBS	Standard amount	F+G	amount
Clams, stuffed with mushroom, onions, and bread	½	Portion (140g); 70g in total.	3¼	
Fish croquette	1¾	Portion (85g); 149g in total.	1¾	
Fish sticks, patties, or nuggets, breaded, regular	2	Portion (85g); 170g in total.	2	
Fish with breading	☺	Free of triggers.	☺	
Gorton's® Battered Fish Fillets - Lemon Pepper	☺	Free of triggers.	☺	
Gorton's® Popcorn Shrimp, Original	2	Portion (85g); 170g in total.	2	
Goulash, with beef, noodles or macaroni, tomato base	4	Tbsp. (15g); 60g in total.	☺	
Herring, pickled	☺	Free of triggers.	☺	
Herring, pickled	☺	Free of triggers.	☺	
Liver pudding	☺	Free of triggers.	☺	
Mrs. Paul's® Calamari Rings	2¼	Portion (85g); 191g in total.	2¼	
Pickled beef	☺	Free of triggers.	☺	
Pork cutlet (sirloin cutlet), visible fat eaten	1¼	Portion (85g); 106g in total.	1¼	
Ribs, beef, spare, visible fat eaten	☺	Free of triggers.	☺	
Salami, beer or beerwurst, beef	☺	Free of triggers.	☺	
Salmon, red (sockeye), smoked	☺	Free of triggers.	☺	

Meat and fish	FRUCTOSE	Standard amount
Clams, stuffed with mushroom, onions, and bread	🙂	Free of fructose.
Fish croquette	🙂	Free of fructose.
Fish sticks, patties, or nuggets, breaded, regular	🙂	Free of fructose.
Fish with breading	🙂	Free of fructose.
Gorton's® Battered Fish Fillets - Lemon Pepper	🙂	Free of fructose.
Gorton's® Popcorn Shrimp, Original	🙂	Free of fructose.
Goulash, with beef, noodles or macaroni, tomato base	🙂	Nearly free of fructose, avoid at hereditary fructose intolerance.
Herring, pickled	🙂	Free of fructose.
Herring, pickled	🙂	Free of fructose.
Liver pudding	🙂	Free of fructose.
Mrs. Paul's® Calamari Rings	🙂	Free of fructose.
Pickled beef	🙂	Free of fructose.
Pork cutlet (sirloin cutlet), visible fat eaten	🙂	Free of fructose.
Ribs, beef, spare, visible fat eaten	🙂	Free of fructose.
Salami, beer or beerwurst, beef	B ×1 🙂	Free of fructose. Per Portion (55g) you eat with it, add B-no × F-limit.
Salmon, red (sockeye), smoked	🙂	Free of fructose.

Meat and fish	SORBITOL Stand.		SORBITOL Low sensitivity amount
Clams, stuffed with mush-room, onions, and bread	☹ Avoid	½	Portion (140g); 70g in total.
Fish croquette	☺ Nearly free	☺	Nearly free of sorbitol
Fish sticks, patties, or nuggets, breaded, regular	☺ Free	☺	Free of sorbitol.
Fish with breading	☺ Free	☺	Free of sorbitol.
Gorton's® Battered Fish Fillets - Lemon Pepper	☺ Free	☺	Free of sorbitol.
Gorton's® Popcorn Shrimp, Original	☺ Free	☺	Free of sorbitol.
Goulash, with beef, noodles or macaroni, tomato base	☹ Avoid	4	Tbsp. (15g); 60g in total.
Herring, pickled	☺ Free	☺	Free of sorbitol.
Herring, pickled	☺ Free	☺	Free of sorbitol.
Liver pudding	☺ Free	☺	Free of sorbitol.
Mrs. Paul's® Calamari Rings	☺ Free	☺	Free of sorbitol.
Pickled beef	☺ Free	☺	Free of sorbitol.
Pork cutlet (sirloin cutlet), visible fat eaten	☺ Free	☺	Free of sorbitol.
Ribs, beef, spare, visible fat eaten	☺ Free	☺	Free of sorbitol.
Salami, beer or beerwurst, beef	☺ Free	☺	Free of sorbitol.
Salmon, red (sockeye), smoked	☺ Free	☺	Free of sorbitol.

Meat and fish	LACTOSE	Standard amount	⊕
Sauerbraten	☺	Free of lactose.	
Scallops	☺	Free of lactose.	
Sea Pak® Seasoned Shrimp, Roasted Garlic	☺	Free of lactose.	
Sea Pak® Shrimp Scampi in Italian Parmesan Sauce	☺	Nearly free of lactose	
Spiced ham loaf (e.g. Spam), canned	☺	Free of lactose.	
Tuna, canned, light, oil pack, not drained	☺	Free of lactose.	
Venison or deer, stewed	☺	Free of lactose.	

Meat and fish	IBS	Standard amount	F+G amount
Sauerbraten	34¾	Portion (159g); 5,525g in total.	☺
Scallops	☺	Free of triggers.	☺
Sea Pak® Seasoned Shrimp, Roasted Garlic	☺	Free of triggers.	☺
Sea Pak® Shrimp Scampi in Italian Parmesan Sauce	☺	Free of triggers.	☺
Spiced ham loaf (e.g. Spam), canned	☺	Free of triggers.	☺
Tuna, canned, light, oil pack, not drained	☺	Free of triggers.	☺
Venison or deer, stewed	☺	Free of triggers.	☺

Meat and fish	FRUCTOSE	Standard amount
Sauerbraten	34¾	Portion (159g); 5,525g in total.
Scallops	☺	Free of fructose.
Sea Pak® Seasoned Shrimp, Roasted Garlic	☺	Nearly free of fructose, avoid at hereditary fructose intolerance.
Sea Pak® Shrimp Scampi in Italian Parmesan Sauce	☺	Free of fructose.
Spiced ham loaf (e.g. Spam), canned	☺	Free of fructose.
Tuna, canned, light, oil pack, not drained	☺	Free of fructose.
Venison or deer, stewed	☺	Free of fructose.

Meat and fish	SORBITOL Stand.		SORBITOL Low sensitivity amount	
Sauerbraten	☺	Free	☺	Free of sorbitol.
Scallops	☺	Free	☺	Free of sorbitol.
Sea Pak® Seasoned Shrimp, Roasted Garlic	☺	Free	☺	Free of sorbitol.
Sea Pak® Shrimp Scampi in Italian Parmesan Sauce	☺	Free	☺	Free of sorbitol.
Spiced ham loaf (e.g. Spam), canned	☺	Free	☺	Free of sorbitol.
Tuna, canned, light, oil pack, not drained	☺	Free	☺	Free of sorbitol.
Venison or deer, stewed	☺	Free	☺	Free of sorbitol.

3.5.3 Lactose hideouts

Lactose hideouts	LACTOSE		Standard amount	⊕
Casserole (hot dish), chicken with pasta, cream or white sauce, with cheese	½		Portion (238g); 119g in total.	
Chicken cake or patty	1½		Portion (85g); 128g in total.	3¼
Chicken with cheese sauce, vegetables other than dark green	½		Portion (216g); 108g in total.	
Creamed chicken	½		Portion (241g); 121g in total.	
Fish croquette	1¾		Portion (85g); 149g in total.	1¾
Fish or seafood with cream or white sauce	1½		Portion (181g); 272g in total.	
Ham croquette	2¼		Portion (85g); 191g in total.	
Loaf cold cut, spiced	2¼		Portion (55g); 124g in total.	
Meatloaf, pork	2¼		Portion (85g); 191g in total.	
Meatloaf, tuna	5½		Portion (85g); 468g in total.	
Soufflé, meat	1¼		Portion (110g); 138g in total.	1¾
Swedish Meatballs	1½		Portion (140g); 210g in total.	9

Lactose hideouts	IBS	Standard amount	F+G	amount
Casserole (hot dish), chicken with pasta, cream or white sauce, with cheese	½	Portion (238g); 119g in total.		😊
Chicken cake or patty	1½	Portion (85g); 128g in total.	3¼	
Chicken with cheese sauce, vegetables other than dark green	½	Portion (216g); 108g in total.		😊
Creamed chicken	½	Portion (241g); 121g in total.		😊
Fish croquette	1¾	Portion (85g); 149g in total.	1¾	
Fish or seafood with cream or white sauce	1½	Portion (181g); 272g in total.		😊
Ham croquette	2¼	Portion (85g); 191g in total.		😊
Loaf cold cut, spiced	2¼	Portion (55g); 124g in total.		😊
Meatloaf, pork	2¼	Portion (85g); 191g in total.		😊
Meatloaf, tuna	5½	Portion (85g); 468g in total.		😊
Soufflé, meat	1¼	Portion (110g); 138g in total.	1¾	
Swedish Meatballs	1½	Portion (140g); 210g in total.	9	

Lactose hideouts	FRUCTOSE		Standard amount
Casserole (hot dish), chicken with pasta, cream or white sauce, with cheese		☺	Nearly free of fructose, avoid at hereditary fructose intolerance.
Chicken cake or patty	13¼	🍲	Portion (85g); 1,126g in total.
Chicken with cheese sauce, vegetables other than dark green	11½	🍲	Portion (216g); 2,484g in total.
Creamed chicken		☺	Free of fructose.
Fish croquette		☺	Free of fructose.
Fish or seafood with cream or white sauce		☺	Free of fructose.
Ham croquette		☺	Free of fructose.
Loaf cold cut, spiced	B ×¼	☺+	Free of fructose. Per Portion (55g) you eat with it, add B-no × F-limit.
Meatloaf, pork	B ×¼	☺+	Free of fructose. Per Portion (85g) you eat with it, add B-no × F-limit.
Meatloaf, tuna		☺	Free of fructose.
Soufflé, meat	B ×½	☺+	Free of fructose. Per Portion (110g) you eat with it, add B-no × F-limit.
Swedish Meatballs		☺	Free of fructose.

Lactose hideouts	SORBITOL Stand.		SORBITOL Low sensitivity amount	
Casserole (hot dish), chicken with pasta, cream or white sauce, with cheese	☺ Free		☺	Free of sorbitol.
Chicken cake or patty	☹ Avoid	58¾	🥘	Portion (85g); 4,994g in total.
Chicken with cheese sauce, vegetables other than dark green	☹ Avoid	½	🥘	Portion (216g); 108g in total.
Creamed chicken	☹ Avoid	13¾	🥘	Portion (241g); 3,314g in total.
Fish croquette	☺ Nearly free		☺	Nearly free of sorbitol
Fish or seafood with cream or white sauce	☺ Free		☺	Free of sorbitol.
Ham croquette	☺ Nearly free		☺	Nearly free of sorbitol
Loaf cold cut, spiced	☺ Free		☺	Free of sorbitol.
Meatloaf, pork	☹ Avoid	3½	🥘	Portion (85g); 298g in total.
Meatloaf, tuna	☹ Avoid	14½	🥘	Portion (85g); 1,233g in total.
Soufflé, meat	☺ Nearly free		☺	Nearly free of sorbitol
Swedish Meatballs	☹ Avoid	71¼	🥘	Portion (140g); 9,975g in total.

3.5.4   Side dishes

Side dishes	LACTOSE	Standard amount	
Au gratin potato, prepared from fresh	1	Portion (140g); 140g in total.	+¾
Basmati rice, cooked in unsalted water		Free of lactose.	
Boston Market® sweet corn		Free of lactose.	
Bulgur, home cooked		Free of lactose.	
Cheese gnocchi	3½	Portion (70g); 245g in total.	+2¾
Cornbread, from mix	4¾	Portion (55g); 261g in total.	+3¾
Cornbread, homemade	2¾	Portion (55g); 151g in total.	+2¼
Couscous, cooked		Free of lactose.	
Falafel		Free of lactose.	
Fettuccini noodles, whole wheat, cooked in unsalted water		Free of lactose.	
Garbanzo beans (chickpeas), canned, drained		Free of lactose.	
Green peas, raw		Free of lactose.	
Kidney beans, cooked from dried		Free of lactose.	
Lentils, cooked from dried		Free of lactose.	
Plain dumplings for stew, biscuit type	1¾	Portion (55g); 96g in total.	+1½

Side dishes	IBS	Standard amount	F+G amount
Au gratin potato, prepared from fresh		Portion (140g); 140g in total.	6¼
Basmati rice, cooked in un-salted water	☺	Free of triggers.	☺
Boston Market® sweet corn		Portion (85g); 340g in total.	☺
Bulgur, home cooked	☺	Free of triggers.	☺
Cheese gnocchi		Portion (70g); 70g in total.	1
Cornbread, from mix	4	Portion (55g); 261g in total.	26½
Cornbread, homemade	2	Portion (55g); 151g in total.	16¼
Couscous, cooked		Portion (140g); 35g in total.	¼
Falafel		Portion (55g); 41g in total.	¾
Fettuccini noodles, whole wheat, cooked in unsalted water		Portion (140g); 140g in total.	1
Garbanzo beans (chickpeas), canned, drained		Portion (90g); 90g in total.	1½
Green peas, raw	1	Tbsp. (15g); 19g in total.	1¼
Kidney beans, cooked from dried		Portion (90g); 23g in total.	¼
Lentils, cooked from dried		Portion (90g); 68g in total.	¾
Plain dumplings for stew, biscuit type		Portion (55g); 28g in total.	½

Side dishes	FRUCTOSE		Standard amount
Au gratin potato, prepared from fresh		☺	Free of fructose.
Basmati rice, cooked in un-salted water		☺	Free of fructose.
Boston Market® sweet corn	B ×½	☺+	Free of fructose. Per Portion (85g) you eat with it, add B-no × F-limit.
Bulgur, home cooked		☺	Free of fructose.
Cheese gnocchi		☺	Free of fructose.
Cornbread, from mix	B ×¼	☺+	Free of fructose. Per Portion (55g) you eat with it, add B-no × F-limit.
Cornbread, homemade	B ×¼	☺+	Free of fructose. Per Portion (55g) you eat with it, add B-no × F-limit.
Couscous, cooked		☺	Free of fructose.
Falafel		☺	Free of fructose.
Fettuccini noodles, whole wheat, cooked in unsalted water	B ×¼	☺+	Free of fructose. Per Portion (140g) you eat with it, add B-no × F-limit.
Garbanzo beans (chickpeas), canned, drained		☺	Free of fructose.
Green peas, raw	7¼	🥄	Tbsp. (15g); 109g in total.
Kidney beans, cooked from dried		☺	Free of fructose.
Lentils, cooked from dried		☺	Free of fructose.
Plain dumplings for stew, bis-cuit type		☺	Free of fructose.

Side dishes	SORBITOL Stand.		SORBITOL Low sensitivity amount	
Au gratin potato, prepared from fresh	☹	Avoid	7¾	Portion (140g); 1,085g in total.
Basmati rice, cooked in un-salted water	☺	Free		Free of sorbitol.
Boston Market® sweet corn	☹	Avoid	4	Portion (85g); 340g in total.
Bulgur, home cooked	☺	Free		Free of sorbitol.
Cheese gnocchi	☺	Free		Free of sorbitol.
Cornbread, from mix	☺	Nearly free		Nearly free of sorbitol
Cornbread, homemade	☺	Free		Free of sorbitol.
Couscous, cooked	☺	Free		Free of sorbitol.
Falafel	☹	Avoid	1¾	Portion (55g); 96g in total.
Fettuccini noodles, whole wheat, cooked in unsalted water	☺	Free		Free of sorbitol.
Garbanzo beans (chickpeas), canned, drained	☹	Avoid	1	Portion (90g); 90g in total.
Green peas, raw	☹	Avoid	3½	Tbsp. (15g); 53g in total.
Kidney beans, cooked from dried	☺	Free		Free of sorbitol.
Lentils, cooked from dried	☺	Free		Free of sorbitol.
Plain dumplings for stew, bis-cuit type	☺	Free		Free of sorbitol.

Side dishes	LACTOSE	Standard amount	
Polenta	½	Portion (240g); 120g in total.	+½
Potato dumpling (Kartoffelkloesse)	45½	Portion (140g); 6,370g in total.	+37¾
Potato gnocchi		Free of lactose.	
Potato pancakes		Free of lactose.	
Potato, boiled, with skin		Free of lactose.	
Potato, boiled, without skin		Free of lactose.	
Quinoa, cooked		Free of lactose.	
Rice noodles, fried		Free of lactose.	
Snow peas (edible pea pods), cooked from fresh		Free of lactose.	
Spaetzle (spatzen)	5¼	Portion (140g); 735g in total.	+4¼

Side dishes	IBS	Standard amount	F+G amount
Polenta	½	Portion (240g); 120g in total.	3¼
Potato dumpling (Kartoffelkloesse)	35½	Portion (140g); 4,970g in total.	☺
Potato gnocchi	14	Portion (188g); 2,632g in total.	14
Potato pancakes	12¾	Portion (70g); 893g in total.	☺
Potato, boiled, with skin	45¼	Portion (110g); 4,978g in total.	☺
Potato, boiled, without skin	45¼	Portion (110g); 4,978g in total.	☺
Quinoa, cooked	2½	Portion (140g); 350g in total.	2½
Rice noodles, fried	☺	Free of triggers.	☺
Snow peas (edible pea pods), cooked from fresh	¾	Portion (85g); 64g in total.	¾
Spaetzle (spatzen)	1	Portion (140g); 140g in total.	1

Side dishes	FRUCTOSE		Standard amount
Polenta	B ×¼	🙂+	Free of fructose. Per Portion (240g) you eat with it, add B-no × F-limit.
Potato dumpling (Kartoffelkloesse)	B ×¼	🙂+	Free of fructose. Per Portion (140g) you eat with it, add B-no × F-limit.
Potato gnocchi		🙂	Free of fructose.
Potato pancakes	B ×½	🙂+	Free of fructose. Per Portion (70g) you eat with it, add B-no × F-limit.
Potato, boiled, with skin		🙂	Free of fructose.
Potato, boiled, without skin		🙂	Free of fructose.
Quinoa, cooked	B ×1¾	🙂+	Free of fructose. Per Portion (140g) you eat with it, add B-no × F-limit.
Rice noodles, fried		🙂	Free of fructose.
Snow peas (edible pea pods), cooked from fresh	B ×3½	🙂+	Free of fructose. Per Portion (85g) you eat with it, add B-no × F-limit.
Spaetzle (spatzen)	B ×¼	🙂+	Free of fructose. Per Portion (140g) you eat with it, add B-no × F-limit.

Side dishes	SORBITOL Stand.		SORBITOL Low sensitivity amount	
Polenta	☹	Avoid	20¾	Portion (240g); 4,980g in total.
Potato dumpling (Kartof-felkloesse)	☹	Avoid	35½	Portion (140g); 4,970g in total.
Potato gnocchi	☺	Free	☺	Free of sorbitol.
Potato pancakes	☹	Avoid	12¾	Portion (70g); 893g in total.
Potato, boiled, with skin	☹	Avoid	45¼	Portion (110g); 4,978g in total.
Potato, boiled, without skin	☹	Avoid	45¼	Portion (110g); 4,978g in total.
Quinoa, cooked	☺	Free	☺	Free of sorbitol.
Rice noodles, fried	☺	Free	☺	Free of sorbitol.
Snow peas (edible pea pods), cooked from fresh	☺	Free	☺	Free of sorbitol.
Spaetzle (spatzen)	☺	Free	☺	Free of sorbitol.

3.6 Fast food chains

3.6.1 Burger King®

Burger King®	LACTOSE		Standard amount	⊕
Bacon EGG® and Cheese BK Muffin®	11½		Piece (131g); 1,507g in total.	+9½
Barbecue sauce		☺	Free of lactose.	
BBQ roasted jalapeno sauce		☺	Free of lactose.	
BK Big Fish®		☺	Free of lactose.	
BK Fresh Apple Slices		☺	Free of lactose.	
BLT Salad® with TenderCrisp chicken (no dressing or croutons)	79¼		Portion (140g); 11,095g in total.	+66
Caesar Salad (no dressing or croutons)	26½		Portion (100g); 2,650g in total.	+22
Cheeseburger	11½		Piece (121g); 1,392g in total.	+9½
French fries		☺	Free of lactose.	
Hamburger		☺	Free of lactose.	
Ken's® Apple Cider Vinaigrette salad dressing		☺	Nearly free of lactose	
Onion rings		☺	Free of lactose.	
Original Chicken Crisp® Sandwich		☺	Free of lactose.	

Burger King®	IBS	Standard amount	F+G	amount
Bacon EGG® and Cheese BK Muffin®	¼	Piece (131g); 33g in total.	¼	
Barbecue sauce	2¼	Portion (31g); 70g in total.	☺	
BBQ roasted jalapeno sauce	2¾	Portion (31g); 85g in total.	☺	
BK Big Fish®	☹	Avoid consumption!!	☹	
BK Fresh Apple Slices	☹	Avoid consumption!	☺	
BLT Salad® with TenderCrisp chicken (no dressing or croutons)	3	Portion (140g); 420g in total.	☺	
Caesar Salad (no dressing or croutons)	1½	Portion (100g); 150g in total.	☺	
Cheeseburger	¼	Piece (121g); 30g in total.	¼	
French fries	35½	Portion (70g); 2,485g in total.	☺	
Hamburger	½	Piece (109g); 55g in total.	½	
Ken's® Apple Cider Vinaigrette salad dressing	☺	Nearly free of triggers.	☺	
Onion rings	¼	Portion (70g); 18g in total.	¼	
Original Chicken Crisp® Sandwich	1½	Piece (149g); 224g in total.	5¾	

Burger King®	FRUCTOSE	Standard amount
Bacon EGG® and Cheese BK Muffin®	B ×1 ☺+	Free of fructose. Per Piece (131g) you eat with it, add B-no × F-limit.
Barbecue sauce	B ×1¼ ☺+	Free of fructose. Per Portion (31g) you eat with it, add B-no × F-limit.
BBQ roasted jalapeno sauce	B ×1 ☺+	Free of fructose. Per Portion (31g) you eat with it, add B-no × F-limit.
BK Big Fish®	☺	Free of fructose.
BK Fresh Apple Slices	☹	Avoid consumption!
BLT Salad® with TenderCrisp chicken (no dressing or croutons)	4¼	Portion (140g); 595g in total.
Caesar Salad (no dressing or croutons)	1½	Portion (100g); 150g in total.
Cheeseburger	29½	Piece (121g); 3,570g in total.
French fries	☺	Free of fructose.
Hamburger	32¾	Piece (109g); 3,570g in total.
Ken's® Apple Cider Vinaigrette salad dressing	☺	Free of fructose.
Onion rings	B ×1½ ☺+	Free of fructose. Per Portion (70g) you eat with it, add B-no × F-limit.
Original Chicken Crisp® Sandwich	1½	Piece (149g); 224g in total.

Burger King®	SORBITOL Stand.		SORBITOL Low sensitivity amount
Bacon EGG® and Cheese BK Muffin®	☺ Free	☺	Free of sorbitol.
Barbecue sauce	☹ Avoid	2¼	Portion (31g); 70g in total.
BBQ roasted jalapeno sauce	☹ Avoid	2¾	Portion (31g); 85g in total.
BK Big Fish®	☹ Avoid	21¾	Piece (228g); 4,959g in total.
BK Fresh Apple Slices	☹ Avoid	☹	Avoid consumption!
BLT Salad® with TenderCrisp chicken (no dressing or croutons)	☹ Avoid	3	Portion (140g); 420g in total.
Caesar Salad (no dressing or croutons)	☹ Avoid	4¼	Portion (100g); 425g in total.
Cheeseburger	☹ Avoid	3¼	Piece (121g); 393g in total.
French fries	☹ Avoid	35½	Portion (70g); 2,485g in total.
Hamburger	☹ Avoid	3¼	Piece (109g); 354g in total.
Ken's® Apple Cider Vinaigrette salad dressing	☺ Free	☺	Free of sorbitol.
Onion rings	☹ Avoid	¾	Portion (70g); 53g in total.
Original Chicken Crisp® Sandwich	☹ Avoid	67	Piece (149g); 9,983g in total.

Burger King®	LACTOSE		Standard amount	⊕
Pancakes and syrup	½		Piece (187g); 94g in total.	+½
Picante taco sauce		☺	Free of lactose.	
Ranch Crispy Chicken Wrap	5		Piece (137g); 685g in total.	+4¼
Shake, chocolate			Portion (231g); Avoid consumption!!	0.15
Shake, strawberry			Portion (229g); Avoid consumption!!	0.15
Shake, vanilla or other			Portion (238g); Avoid consumption!!	0.14
Sundaes®, caramel	¼		Portion (141g); 35g in total.	+¼
Sundaes®, chocolate fudge	¼		Portion (141g); 35g in total.	+¼
Sundaes®, mini M & M®	¼		Portion (204g); 51g in total.	0.24
Sundaes®, Oreo®	¼		Portion (204g); 51g in total.	+¼
Sundaes®, strawberry	¼		Portion (141g); 35g in total.	+¼
Sweet and sour sauce		☺	Free of lactose.	
TenderCrisp® Chicken Sandwich		☺	Free of lactose.	
Whopper® with cheese	5¾		Piece (315g); 1,811g in total.	+4¾
Zesty onion ring sauce		☺	Nearly free of lactose	

Burger King®	IBS	Standard amount	F+G	amount
Pancakes and syrup	¼	Piece (187g); 47g in total.	¼	
Picante taco sauce	2¼	Portion (35g); 79g in total.	☺	
Ranch Crispy Chicken Wrap	¼	Piece (137g); 34g in total.	¼	
Shake, chocolate	☹	Avoid consumption!!	½	
Shake, strawberry	☹	Avoid consumption!!	1	
Shake, vanilla or other	☹	Avoid consumption!!	¾	
Sundaes®, caramel	¼	Portion (141g); 35g in total.	2	
Sundaes®, chocolate fudge	¼	Portion (141g); 35g in total.	1½	
Sundaes®, mini M & M®	¼	Portion (204g); 51g in total.	1¼	
Sundaes®, Oreo®	¼	Portion (204g); 51g in total.	1¾	
Sundaes®, strawberry	¼	Portion (141g); 35g in total.	2¼	
Sweet and sour sauce	¼	Portion (30g); 8g in total.	☺	
TenderCrisp® Chicken Sandwich	☹	Avoid consumption!!	☹	
Whopper® with cheese	☹	Avoid consumption!!	☹	
Zesty onion ring sauce	64½	Portion (31g); 2,000g in total.	☺	

Burger King®	FRUCTOSE	Standard amount
Pancakes and syrup	B ×6 ☺+	Free of fructose. Per Piece (187g) you eat with it, add B-no × F-limit.
Picante taco sauce	2¼	Portion (35g); 79g in total.
Ranch Crispy Chicken Wrap	☺	Free of fructose.
Shake, chocolate	B ×7¼ ☺+	Free of fructose. Per Portion (231g) you eat with it, add B-no × F-limit.
Shake, strawberry	B ×5¼ ☺+	Free of fructose. Per Portion (229g) you eat with it, add B-no × F-limit.
Shake, vanilla or other	B ×5¾ ☺+	Free of fructose. Per Portion (238g) you eat with it, add B-no × F-limit.
Sundaes®, caramel	B ×8½ ☺+	Free of fructose. Per Portion (141g) you eat with it, add B-no × F-limit.
Sundaes®, chocolate fudge	B ×6¾ ☺+	Free of fructose. Per Portion (141g) you eat with it, add B-no × F-limit.
Sundaes®, mini M & M®	B ×6¾ ☺+	Free of fructose. Per Portion (204g) you eat with it, add B-no × F-limit.
Sundaes®, Oreo®	B ×7¼ ☺+	Free of fructose. Per Portion (204g) you eat with it, add B-no × F-limit.
Sundaes®, strawberry	B ×2½ ☺+	Free of fructose. Per Portion (141g) you eat with it, add B-no × F-limit.
Sweet and sour sauce	¼	Portion (30g); 8g in total.
TenderCrisp® Chicken Sandwich	5	Piece (264g); 1,320g in total.
Whopper® with cheese	1¾	Piece (315g); 551g in total.
Zesty onion ring sauce	☺	Free of fructose.

Burger King®	SORBITOL Stand.		SORBITOL Low sensitivity amount
Pancakes and syrup	☺ Free	☺	Free of sorbitol.
Picante taco sauce	☹ Avoid	2¾	Portion (35g); 96g in total.
Ranch Crispy Chicken Wrap	☹ Avoid	36¼	Piece (137g); 4,966g in total.
Shake, chocolate	☺ Free	☺	Free of sorbitol.
Shake, strawberry	☹ Avoid	3¼	Portion (229g); 744g in total.
Shake, vanilla or other	☺ Free	☺	Free of sorbitol.
Sundaes®, caramel	☺ Free	☺	Free of sorbitol.
Sundaes®, chocolate fudge	☺ Free	☺	Free of sorbitol.
Sundaes®, mini M & M®	☺ Free	☺	Free of sorbitol.
Sundaes®, Oreo®	☹ Avoid	49	Portion (204g); 9,996g in total.
Sundaes®, strawberry	☹ Avoid	2½	Portion (141g); 353g in total.
Sweet and sour sauce	☹ Avoid	41½	Portion (30g); 1,245g in total.
TenderCrisp® Chicken Sandwich	☹ Avoid	2½	Piece (264g); 660g in total.
Whopper® with cheese	☹ Avoid	1	Piece (315g); 315g in total.
Zesty onion ring sauce	☹ Avoid	64½	Portion (31g); 2,000g in total.

3.6.2   KFC®

KFC®	LACTOSE	Standard amount	
Caesar salad dressing	4¾	Portion (30g); 143g in total.	+3¾
Chicken breast, spicy crispy	☺	Free of lactose.	
Chicken Littles with sauce	☺	Free of lactose.	
Cole slaw	☺	Free of lactose.	
Creamy buffalo sauce	6	Portion (29.4g); 176g in total.	+5
Crispy Chicken Caesar Salad	☺	Nearly free of lactose	
Crispy Twister without sauce	☺	Free of lactose.	
Crispy Twister® with sauce	☺	Free of lactose.	
Extra Crispy Tenders	☺	Free of lactose.	
Honey BBQ sauce	☺	Free of lactose.	
Hot wings	☺	Free of lactose.	
House side salad	☺	Free of lactose.	
Mashed potatoes with gravy	½	Portion (140g); 70g in total.	+½
Sweet and sour sauce	☺	Free of lactose.	
Sweet corn	☺	Free of lactose.	

KFC®	IBS Standard amount			F+G amount	
Caesar salad dressing	4¾		Portion (30g); 143g in total.	26½	
Chicken breast, spicy crispy	¾		Piece (175g); 131g in total.	¾	
Chicken Littles with sauce	½		Piece (101g); 51g in total.	½	
Cole slaw	1		Portion (100g); 100g in total.	1	
Creamy buffalo sauce	6		Portion (29.4g); 176g in total.	34½	
Crispy Chicken Caesar Salad	1		Portion (140g); 140g in total.	1	
Crispy Twister without sauce			Avoid consumption!!		
Crispy Twister® with sauce			Avoid consumption!!		
Extra Crispy Tenders	3¼		Piece (52g); 169g in total.	3¼	
Honey BBQ sauce	2¼		Portion (31g); 70g in total.		
Hot wings			Free of triggers.		
House side salad	1¾		Portion (100g); 175g in total.		
Mashed potatoes with gravy	½		Portion (140g); 70g in total.	4	
Sweet and sour sauce	¼		Portion (30g); 8g in total.		
Sweet corn	1¼		Piece (95g); 119g in total.	1¼	

KFC®	FRUCTOSE	Standard amount
Caesar salad dressing	🙂	Free of fructose.
Chicken breast, spicy crispy	🙂	Free of fructose.
Chicken Littles with sauce	3 🍰	Piece (101g); 303g in total.
Cole slaw	B ×¼ 🙂+	Free of fructose. Per Portion (100g) you eat with it, add B-no × F-limit.
Creamy buffalo sauce	B ×1 🙂+	Free of fructose. Per Portion (29.4g) you eat with it, add B-no × F-limit.
Crispy Chicken Caesar Salad	2 🍽	Portion (140g); 280g in total.
Crispy Twister without sauce	10¼ 🍰	Piece (218g); 2,235g in total.
Crispy Twister® with sauce	9¼ 🍰	Piece (240g); 2,220g in total.
Extra Crispy Tenders	🙂	Free of fructose.
Honey BBQ sauce	B ×1¼ 🙂+	Free of fructose. Per Portion (31g) you eat with it, add B-no × F-limit.
Hot wings	🙂	Free of fructose.
House side salad	1¾ 🍽	Portion (100g); 175g in total.
Mashed potatoes with gravy	🙂	Free of fructose.
Sweet and sour sauce	¼ 🍽	Portion (30g); 8g in total.
Sweet corn	🙂	Free of fructose.

KFC®	SORBITOL Stand.		SORBITOL Low sensitivity amount	
Caesar salad dressing	🙂	Free	🙂	Free of sorbitol.
Chicken breast, spicy crispy	🙂	Free	🙂	Free of sorbitol.
Chicken Littles with sauce	☹️	Avoid	33	Piece (101g); 3,333g in total.
Cole slaw	☹️	Avoid	2¾	Portion (100g); 275g in total.
Creamy buffalo sauce	🙂	Free	🙂	Free of sorbitol.
Crispy Chicken Caesar Salad	☹️	Avoid	17¾	Portion (140g); 2,485g in total.
Crispy Twister without sauce	☹️	Avoid	2	Piece (218g); 436g in total.
Crispy Twister® with sauce	☹️	Avoid	2	Piece (240g); 480g in total.
Extra Crispy Tenders	🙂	Free	🙂	Free of sorbitol.
Honey BBQ sauce	☹️	Avoid	2¼	Portion (31g); 70g in total.
Hot wings	🙂	Free	🙂	Free of sorbitol.
House side salad	☹️	Avoid	4	Portion (100g); 400g in total.
Mashed potatoes with gravy	☹️	Avoid	35½	Portion (140g); 4,970g in total.
Sweet and sour sauce	☹️	Avoid	37	Portion (30g); 1,110g in total.
Sweet corn	☹️	Avoid	2½	Piece (95g); 238g in total.

3.6.3 McDonald's®

McDonald's®	LACTOSE		Standard amount	
McDonald's® apple slices		☺	Free of lactose.	
McDonald's® Barbecue sauce		☺	Free of lactose.	
McDonald's® Big Mac®	9¾		Piece (215g); 2,096g in total.	+8¼
McDonald's® caramel sundae®	¼		Portion (182g); 46g in total.	+¼
McDonald's® Cheeseburger	9¾		Piece (114g); 1,112g in total.	+8¼
McDonald's® Chicken McNuggets®		☺	Free of lactose.	
McDonald's® chocolate chip cookies		☺	Free of lactose.	
McDonald's® chocolate milk	¼		Cup (150g); 38 mL in total.	+¼
McDonald's® Crispy Chicken Snack Wrap with ranch sauce	62		Piece (118g); 7,316g in total.	+51½
McDonald's® Double Cheeseburger	4¾		Piece (165g); 784g in total.	+4
McDonald's® Filet-O-Fish®	19¾		Piece (142g); 2,805g in total.	+16½
McDonald's® French fries		☺	Free of lactose.	
McDonald's® Hamburger		☺	Free of lactose.	
McDonald's® hot fudge sundae®	¼		Portion (179g); 45g in total.	+¼
McDonald's® hot mustard sauce		☺	Nearly free of lactose	

McDonald's®	IBS		Standard amount	F+G	amount
McDonald's® apple slices	¼		Piece (34g); 9g in total.		☺
McDonald's® Barbecue sauce	1¾		Portion (31g); 54g in total.		☺
McDonald's® Big Mac®	¼		Piece (215g); 54g in total.	¼	
McDonald's® caramel sundae®	¼		Portion (182g); 46g in total.	1¾	
McDonald's® Cheeseburger	¼		Piece (114g); 29g in total.	¼	
McDonald's® Chicken McNuggets®	10¾		Piece (16, 25g); 175g in total.	10¾	
McDonald's® chocolate chip cookies	¾		Piece (33g); 25g in total.	¾	
McDonald's® chocolate milk	¼		Cup (150g); 38 mL in total.	2	
McDonald's® Crispy Chicken Snack Wrap with ranch sauce	¼		Piece (118g); 30g in total.	¼	
McDonald's® Double Cheeseburger	¼		Piece (165g); 41g in total.	¼	
McDonald's® Filet-O-Fish®	¼		Piece (142g); 36g in total.	¼	
McDonald's® French fries	35½		Portion (70g); 2,485g in total.		☺
McDonald's® Hamburger	½		Piece (100g); 50g in total.	½	
McDonald's® hot fudge sundae®	¼		Portion (179g); 45g in total.	1¼	
McDonald's® hot mustard sauce	☺		Free of triggers.		☺

McDonald's®	FRUCTOSE	Standard amount
McDonald's® apple Slices	¼	Piece (34g); 9g in total.
McDonald's® Barbecue sauce	B ×1½	Free of fructose. Per Portion (31g) you eat with it, add B-no × F-limit.
McDonald's® Big Mac®	4¼	Piece (215g); 914g in total.
McDonald's® caramel sundae®	B ×6¾	Free of fructose. Per Portion (182g) you eat with it, add B-no × F-limit.
McDonald's® Cheeseburger	3¼	Piece (114g); 371g in total.
McDonald's® Chicken McNuggets®		Free of fructose.
McDonald's® chocolate chip cookies	B ×½	Free of fructose. Per Piece (33g) you eat with it, add B-no × F-limit.
McDonald's® chocolate milk	B ×2	Free of fructose. Per Cup (150 mL) you drink with it, add B-no × F-limit.
McDonald's® Crispy Chicken Snack Wrap with ranch sauce		Free of fructose.
McDonald's® Double Cheeseburger	3½	Piece (165g); 578g in total.
McDonald's® Filet-O-Fish®	1¾	Piece (142g); 249g in total.
McDonald's® French fries		Free of fructose.
McDonald's® Hamburger	3¼	Piece (100g); 325g in total.
McDonald's® hot fudge sundae®	B ×7½	Free of fructose. Per Portion (179g) you eat with it, add B-no × F-limit.
McDonald's® hot mustard sauce	B ×1¼	Free of fructose. Per Portion (20g) you eat with it, add B-no × F-limit.

McDonald's®	SORBITOL Stand.		SORBITOL Low sensitivity amount
McDonald's® apple Slices	☹ Avoid	¼	Piece (34g); 9g in total.
McDonald's® Barbecue sauce	☹ Avoid	1¾	Portion (31g); 54g in total.
McDonald's® Big Mac®	☹ Avoid	6½	Piece (215g); 1,398g in total.
McDonald's® caramel sundae®	☺ Free		Free of sorbitol.
McDonald's® Cheeseburger	☹ Avoid	5	Piece (114g); 570g in total.
McDonald's® Chicken McNuggets®	☺ Free		Free of sorbitol.
McDonald's® chocolate chip cookies	☺ Nearly free		Nearly free of sorbitol
McDonald's® chocolate milk	☺ Free		Free of sorbitol.
McDonald's® Crispy Chicken Snack Wrap with ranch sauce	☹ Avoid	84½	Piece (118g); 9,971g in total.
McDonald's® Double Cheeseburger	☹ Avoid	4¼	Piece (165g); 701g in total.
McDonald's® Filet-O-Fish®	☹ Avoid	70¼	Piece (142g); 9,976g in total.
McDonald's® French fries	☹ Avoid	35½	Portion (70g); 2,485g in total.
McDonald's® Hamburger	☹ Avoid	5	Piece (100g); 500g in total.
McDonald's® hot fudge sundae®	☹ Avoid	55¾	Portion (179g); 9,979g in total.
McDonald's® hot mustard sauce	☺ Free		Free of sorbitol.

McDonald's®	LACTOSE	Standard amount	⊕
McDonald's® M & M McFlurry®		Portion (228g); Avoid consumption!!	0.19
McDonald's® McCafe shakes, chocolate flavors	¼	Portion (210g); 53g in total.	+¼
McDonald's® McCafe shakes, vanilla or other flavors	¼	Portion (206g); 52g in total.	+¼
McDonald's® McChicken®		Free of lactose.	
McDonald's® McDouble®	9¾	Piece (151g); 1,472g in total.	+8¼
McDonald's® McRib®		Free of lactose.	
McDonald's® Newman's Own® Creamy Caesar salad dressing	18¼	Portion (30g); 548g in total.	+15¼
McDonald's® Newman's Own® Low Fat Balsamic Vinaigrette salad dressing		Free of lactose.	
McDonald's® orange juice		Free of lactose.	
McDonald's® Quarter Pounder		Free of lactose.	
McDonald's® Sausage & EGG® McMuffin®	9¾	Piece (164g); 1,599g in total.	+8¼
McDonald's® side salad		Free of lactose.	
McDonald's® smoothies, all flavors	2¼	Glass (240g); 540 mL in total.	+1¾
McDonald's® Southwestern chipotle Barbecue sauce		Free of lactose.	
McDonald's® sweet and sour sauce		Free of lactose.	

McDonald's®	IBS Standard amount		F+G amount
McDonald's® M & M McFlurry®		Portion (228g); Avoid consumption!!	1
McDonald's® McCafe shakes, chocolate flavors	¼	Portion (210g); 53g in total.	1½
McDonald's® McCafe shakes, vanilla or other flavors	¼	Portion (206g); 52g in total.	1½
McDonald's® McChicken®	¼	Piece (143g); 36g in total.	¼
McDonald's® McDouble®	¼	Piece (151g); 38g in total.	¼
McDonald's® McRib®	¼	Piece (208g); 52g in total.	¼
McDonald's® Newman's Own® Creamy Caesar salad dressing	7¼	Portion (30g); 218g in total.	
McDonald's® Newman's Own® Low Fat Balsamic Vinaigrette salad dressing		Free of triggers.	
McDonald's® orange juice	¼	Glass (200g); 50 mL in total.	
McDonald's® Quarter Pounder	¼	Piece (173g); 43g in total.	¼
McDonald's® Sausage & EGG® McMuffin®	¼	Piece (164g); 41g in total.	¼
McDonald's® side salad	2½	Portion (100g); 250g in total.	
McDonald's® smoothies, all flavors	1¼	Glass (200g); 250 mL in total.	15½
McDonald's® Southwestern chipotle Barbecue sauce	2¾	Portion (31g); 85g in total.	
McDonald's® sweet and sour sauce	¼	Portion (30g); 8g in total.	

McDonald's®	FRUCTOSE		Standard amount
McDonald's® M & M McFlurry®	B ×3½	☺ +	Free of fructose. Per Portion (228g) you eat with it, add B-no × F-limit.
McDonald's® McCafe shakes, chocolate flavors	B ×5¾	☺ +	Free of fructose. Per Portion (210g) you eat with it, add B-no × F-limit.
McDonald's® McCafe shakes, vanilla or other flavors	B ×¼	☺ +	Free of fructose. Per Portion (206g) you eat with it, add B-no × F-limit.
McDonald's® McChicken®	1½	🍰	Piece (143g); 215g in total.
McDonald's® McDouble®	3½	🍰	Piece (151g); 529g in total.
McDonald's® McRib®	B ×¾	☺ +	Free of fructose. Per Piece (208g) you eat with it, add B-no × F-limit.
McDonald's® Newman's Own® Creamy Caesar salad dressing	39½	🥣	Portion (30g); 1,185g in total.
McDonald's® Newman's Own® Low Fat Balsamic Vinaigrette salad dressing		☺	Free of fructose.
McDonald's® orange juice	¾	🥛	Glass (200g); 150 mL in total.
McDonald's® Quarter Pounder	28¾	🍰	Piece (173g); 4,974g in total.
McDonald's® Sausage & EGG® McMuffin®	B ×1	☺ +	Free of fructose. Per Piece (164g) you eat with it, add B-no × F-limit.
McDonald's® side salad	2¾	🥣	Portion (100g); 275g in total.
McDonald's® smoothies, all flavors	2½	🥛	Glass (200g); 500 mL in total.
McDonald's® Southwestern chipotle Barbecue sauce	B ×1¾	☺ +	Free of fructose. Per Portion (31g) you eat with it, add B-no × F-limit.
McDonald's® sweet and sour sauce	¼	🥣	Portion (30g); 8g in total.

McDonald's®	SORBITOL Stand.		SORBITOL Low sensitivity amount
McDonald's® M & M McFlurry®	😀 Free	😀	Free of sorbitol.
McDonald's® McCafe shakes, chocolate flavors	😞 Avoid	15¾	Portion (210g); 3,308g in total.
McDonald's® McCafe shakes, vanilla or other flavors	😞 Avoid	12	Portion (206g); 2472g in total.
McDonald's® McChicken®	😞 Avoid	69¾	Piece (143g); 9,974g in total.
McDonald's® McDouble®	😞 Avoid	4¼	Piece (151g); 642g in total.
McDonald's® McRib®	😞 Avoid	1¾	Piece (208g); 364g in total.
McDonald's® Newman's Own® Creamy Caesar salad dressing	😞 Avoid	7¼	Portion (30g); 218g in total.
McDonald's® Newman's Own® Low Fat Balsamic Vinaigrette salad dressing	😀 Free	😀	Free of sorbitol.
McDonald's® orange juice	😞 Avoid	¼	Glass (200g); 50 mL in total.
McDonald's® Quarter Pounder	😞 Avoid	2½	Piece (173g); 433g in total.
McDonald's® Sausage & EGG® McMuffin®	😀 Free	😀	Free of sorbitol.
McDonald's® side salad	😞 Avoid	2½	Portion (100g); 250g in total.
McDonald's® smoothies, all flavors	😞 Avoid	1¼	Glass (200g); 250 mL in total.
McDonald's® Southwestern chipotle Barbecue sauce	😞 Avoid	2¾	Portion (31g); 85g in total.
McDonald's® sweet and sour sauce	😞 Avoid	41½	Portion (30g); 1,245g in total.

3.6.4 Subway®

Subway®	LACTOSE	Standard amount	⊕
9-grain Wheat bread	☺	Free of lactose.	
American cheese	4½	Portion (30g); 135g in total.	+3¾
bacon	☺	Free of lactose.	
Cheddar cheese	43¼	Portion (30g); 1,298g in total.	+36
Chipotle southwest salad dressing	7¼	Portion (30g); 218g in total.	+6
Chocolate chip cookie	6¾	Piece (45g); 304g in total.	+5½
Chocolate chunk cookie	6¾	Piece (45g); 304g in total.	+5½
Ham Sandwich with Veggies, no mayo	12½	Piece (219g); 2,738g in total.	+10½
Honey mustard salad dressing	☺	Free of lactose.	
Honey Oat bread	¾	Piece (89g); 67g in total.	+½
Italian BMT® Sandwich with Veggies, no mayo	12½	Piece (226g); 2,825g in total.	+10½
M & M® cookie	6¾	Piece (45g); 304g in total.	+5½
Mustard	☺	Free of lactose.	
Oven Roasted Chicken Sandwich with Veggies, no mayo	12½	Piece (233g); 2,913g in total.	+10½
Parmesan Oregano bread	☺	Nearly free of lactose	

Subway®	IBS		Standard amount	F+G	amount
9-grain Wheat bread	¼		Piece (78g); 20g in total.	¼	
American cheese	4½		Portion (30g); 135g in total.	25¾	
bacon		☺	Free of triggers.		☺
Cheddar cheese	43¼		Portion (30g); 1,298g in total.		☺
Chipotle southwest salad dressing	7¼		Portion (30g); 218g in total.	40½	
Chocolate chip cookie	½		Piece (45g); 23g in total.	½	
Chocolate chunk cookie	½		Piece (45g); 23g in total.	½	
Ham Sandwich with Veggies, no mayo	¼		Piece (219g); 55g in total.	¼	
Honey mustard salad dressing	4½		Portion (30g); 135g in total.		☺
Honey Oat bread	¼		Piece (89g); 22g in total.	¼	
Italian BMT® Sandwich with Veggies, no mayo	¼		Piece (226g); 57g in total.	¼	
M & M® cookie	½		Piece (45g); 23g in total.	½	
Mustard		☺	Free of triggers.		☺
Oven Roasted Chicken Sandwich with Veggies, no mayo		☹	Avoid consumption!!		☹
Parmesan Oregano bread	¾		Piece (75g); 56g in total.	¾	

Subway®	FRUCTOSE	Standard amount
9-grain Wheat bread	1	Piece (78g); 78g in total.
American cheese	☺	Free of fructose.
bacon	☺	Free of fructose.
Cheddar cheese	☺	Free of fructose.
Chipotle southwest salad dressing	☺	Free of fructose.
Chocolate chip cookie	B ×1 ☺+	Free of fructose. Per Piece (45g) you eat with it, add B-no × F-limit.
Chocolate chunk cookie	B ×1 ☺+	Free of fructose. Per Piece (45g) you eat with it, add B-no × F-limit.
Ham Sandwich with Veggies, no mayo	¾	Piece (219g); 164g in total.
Honey mustard salad dressing	4½	Portion (30g); 135g in total.
Honey Oat bread	2¼	Piece (89g); 200g in total.
Italian BMT® Sandwich with Veggies, no mayo	¾	Piece (226g); 170g in total.
M & M® cookie	B ×½ ☺+	Free of fructose. Per Piece (45g) you eat with it, add B-no × F-limit.
Mustard	☺	Free of fructose.
Oven Roasted Chicken Sandwich with Veggies, no mayo	1½	Piece (233g); 350g in total.
Parmesan Oregano bread	B ×½ ☺+	Free of fructose. Per Piece (75g) you eat with it, add B-no × F-limit.

Subway®	SORBITOL Stand.		SORBITOL Low sensitivity amount	
9-grain Wheat bread	😀	Free	🙂	Free of sorbitol.
American cheese	😀	Free	🙂	Free of sorbitol.
Bacon	😀	Free	🙂	Free of sorbitol.
Cheddar cheese	😀	Free	🙂	Free of sorbitol.
Chipotle southwest salad dressing	😀	Free	🙂	Free of sorbitol.
Chocolate chip cookie	🙂	Nearly free	🙂	Nearly free of sorbitol
Chocolate chunk cookie	🙂	Nearly free	🙂	Nearly free of sorbitol
Ham Sandwich with Veggies, no mayo	☹️	Avoid	1¼ 🍰	Piece (219g); 274g in total.
Honey mustard salad dressing	😀	Free	🙂	Free of sorbitol.
Honey Oat bread	☹️	Avoid	6½ 🍰	Piece (89g); 579g in total.
Italian BMT® Sandwich with Veggies, no mayo	☹️	Avoid	1¼ 🍰	Piece (226g); 283g in total.
M & M® cookie	🙂	Nearly free	🙂	Nearly free of sorbitol
Mustard	😀	Free	🙂	Free of sorbitol.
Oven Roasted Chicken Sandwich with Veggies, no mayo	☹️	Avoid	1¼ 🍰	Piece (233g); 291g in total.
Parmesan Oregano bread	😀	Free	🙂	Free of sorbitol.

Subway®	LACTOSE	Standard amount	⊕
Ranch salad dressing	☺	Nearly free of lactose	
Roast Beef Sandwich with Veggies, no mayo	12½	Piece (233g); 2,913g in total.	+10½
Spicy Italian Sandwich with Veggies, no meat	12½	Piece (222g); 2,775g in total.	+10½
Steak & Cheese Sandwich with Veggies, no mayo	☺	Nearly free of lactose	
Sweet Onion Chicken Teriyaki Sandwich with Veggies, no mayo	12½	Piece (276g); 3,450g in total.	+10½
Sweet onion salad dressing	☺	Free of lactose.	
Tuna Sandwich with Veggies, no mayo	12½	Piece (233g); 2,913g in total.	+10½
Turkey Breast & Ham Sandwich with Veggies, no mayo	12½	Piece (219g); 2,738g in total.	+10½
Turkey Breast Sandwich with Veggies, no mayo	12½	Piece (219g); 2,738g in total.	+10½
Veggie Delite Salad, no dressing	34¼	Portion (100g); 3,425g in total.	+28½
Veggie Delite Sandwich, no mayo	12½	Piece (162g); 2,025g in total.	+10½
Vinegar	☺	Free of lactose.	
White chip macadamia nut cookie	6¾	Piece (45g); 304g in total.	+5½
Wrap bread	☺	Free of lactose.	

Subway®	IBS	Standard amount	F+G	amount
Ranch salad dressing	😊	Nearly free of triggers.		😊
Roast Beef Sandwich with Veggies, no mayo	😞	Avoid consumption!!		😞
Spicy Italian Sandwich with Veggies, no meat	¼ 🍰	Piece (222g); 56g in total.	¼	🍰
Steak & Cheese Sandwich with Veggies, no mayo	😞	Avoid consumption!!		😞
Sweet Onion Chicken Teriyaki Sandwich with Veggies, no mayo	😞	Avoid consumption!!		😞
Sweet onion salad dressing	½ 🥣	Portion (30g); 15g in total.	½	🥣
Tuna Sandwich with Veggies, no mayo	😞	Avoid consumption!!		😞
Turkey Breast & Ham Sandwich with Veggies, no mayo	¼ 🍰	Piece (219g); 55g in total.	¼	🍰
Turkey Breast Sandwich with Veggies, no mayo	¼ 🍰	Piece (219g); 55g in total.	¼	🍰
Veggie Delite Salad, no dressing	2¼ 🥣	Portion (100g); 225g in total.		😊
Veggie Delite Sandwich, no mayo	¼ 🍰	Piece (162g); 41g in total.	¼	🍰
Vinegar	20¼ 🥣	Portion (14.94g); 303g in total.		😊
White chip macadamia nut cookie	½ 🍰	Piece (45g); 23g in total.	½	🍰
Wrap bread	½ 🍰	Piece (103g); 52g in total.	½	🍰

Subway®	FRUCTOSE		Standard amount
Ranch salad dressing		☺	Free of fructose.
Roast Beef Sandwich with Veggies, no mayo	¾	🍰	Piece (233g); 175g in total.
Spicy Italian Sandwich with Veggies, no meat	¾	🍰	Piece (222g); 167g in total.
Steak & Cheese Sandwich with Veggies, no mayo	¾	🍰	Piece (245g); 184g in total.
Sweet Onion Chicken Teriyaki Sandwich with Veggies, no mayo	12¾	🍰	Piece (276g); 3,519g in total.
Sweet onion salad dressing	B ×1	☺+	Free of fructose. Per Portion (30g) you eat with it, add B-no × F-limit.
Tuna Sandwich with Veggies, no mayo	¾	🍰	Piece (233g); 175g in total.
Turkey Breast & Ham Sandwich with Veggies, no mayo	¾	🍰	Piece (219g); 164g in total.
Turkey Breast Sandwich with Veggies, no mayo	¾	🍰	Piece (219g); 164g in total.
Veggie Delite Salad, no dressing	49¾	🪐	Portion (100g); 4,975g in total.
Veggie Delite Sandwich, no mayo	¾	🍰	Piece (162g); 122g in total.
Vinegar		☺	Free of fructose.
White chip macadamia nut cookie		☺	Free of fructose.
Wrap bread		☺	Free of fructose.

Subway®	SORBITOL Stand.		SORBITOL Low sensitivity amount	
Ranch salad dressing	☺	Nearly free	☺	Nearly free of sorbitol
Roast Beef Sandwich with Veggies, no mayo	☹ Avoid	1¼		Piece (233g); 291g in total.
Spicy Italian Sandwich with Veggies, no meat	☹ Avoid	1¼		Piece (222g); 278g in total.
Steak & Cheese Sandwich with Veggies, no mayo	☹ Avoid	1¼		Piece (245g); 306g in total.
Sweet Onion Chicken Teriyaki Sandwich with Veggies, no mayo	☹ Avoid	1¼		Piece (276g); 345g in total.
Sweet onion salad dressing	☹ Avoid	55½		Portion (30g); 1,665g in total.
Tuna Sandwich with Veggies, no mayo	☹ Avoid	1¼		Piece (233g); 291g in total.
Turkey Breast & Ham Sandwich with Veggies, no mayo	☹ Avoid	1¼		Piece (219g); 274g in total.
Turkey Breast Sandwich with Veggies, no mayo	☹ Avoid	1¼		Piece (219g); 274g in total.
Veggie Delite Salad, no dressing	☹ Avoid	2¼		Portion (100g); 225g in total.
Veggie Delite Sandwich, no mayo	☹ Avoid	1½		Piece (162g); 243g in total.
Vinegar	☹ Avoid	20¼		Portion (14.94g); 303g in total.
White chip macadamia nut cookie	☺ Free		☺	Free of sorbitol.
Wrap bread	☺ Free		☺	Free of sorbitol.

3.6.5 Taco Bell®

Taco Bell®	LACTOSE		Standard amount	⊕
Chalupas Supreme® with beef, beans, cheese	49¾		Portion (140g); 6,965g in total.	+41½
Taco Bell® Beef Enchirito	69		Portion (140g); 9,660g in total.	+57½
Taco Bell® Caramel Apple Empanada	10½		Portion (125g); 1,313g in total.	+8¾
Taco Bell® Cheesy Fiesta Potatos	4		Portion (140g); 560g in total.	+3¼
Taco Bell® cheesy gordita crunch	15		Portion (140g); 2,100g in total.	+12½
Taco Bell® Cinnamon Twists		☺	Free of lactose.	
Taco Bell® Combo Burrito		☺	Nearly free of lactose	
Taco Bell® Double Decker Taco Supreme®, beef	61		Portion (140g); 8,540g in total.	+51
Taco Bell® Pintos 'n Cheese	17		Portion (130g); 2,210g in total.	+14

Taco Bell®	IBS		Standard amount	F+G	amount
Chalupas Supreme® with beef, beans, cheese	¼		Portion (140g); 35g in total.	¼	
Taco Bell® Beef Enchirito	¼		Portion (140g); 35g in total.	¼	
Taco Bell® Caramel Apple Empanada		☹	Avoid consumption!	2	
Taco Bell® Cheesy Fiesta Potatos	4		Portion (140g); 560g in total.	22¼	
Taco Bell® cheesy gordita crunch	¼		Portion (140g); 35g in total.	¼	
Taco Bell® Cinnamon Twists	1		Portion (55g); 55g in total.	1	
Taco Bell® Combo Burrito	¼		Portion (140g); 35g in total.	¼	
Taco Bell® Double Decker Taco Supreme®, beef	¼		Portion (140g); 35g in total.	¼	
Taco Bell® Pintos 'n Cheese		☹	Avoid consumption!!		☹

Taco Bell®	FRUCTOSE	Standard amount
Chalupas Supreme® with beef, beans, cheese	29¾	Portion (140g); 4,165g in total.
Taco Bell® Beef Enchirito	2¼	Portion (140g); 315g in total.
Taco Bell® Caramel Apple Empanada	B ×1¼	Free of fructose. Per Portion (125g) you eat with it, add B-no × F-limit.
Taco Bell® Cheesy Fiesta Potatos		Free of fructose.
Taco Bell® cheesy gordita crunch	51	Portion (140g); 7,140g in total.
Taco Bell® Cinnamon Twists		Free of fructose.
Taco Bell® Combo Burrito	8¼	Portion (140g); 1,155g in total.
Taco Bell® Double Decker Taco Supreme®, beef	25½	Portion (140g); 3,570g in total.
Taco Bell® Pintos 'n Cheese	2½	Portion (130g); 325g in total.

Taco Bell®	SORBITOL Stand.		SORBITOL Low sensitivity amount	
Chalupas Supreme® with beef, beans, cheese	😞 Avoid	1¾	🥘	Portion (140g); 245g in total.
Taco Bell® Beef Enchirito	😞 Avoid	2¼	🥘	Portion (140g); 315g in total.
Taco Bell® Caramel Apple Empanada	😞 Avoid		😞	Avoid consumption!
Taco Bell® Cheesy Fiesta Potatos	😞 Avoid	35½	🥘	Portion (140g); 4,970g in total.
Taco Bell® cheesy gordita crunch	😊 Free		😊	Free of sorbitol.
Taco Bell® Cinnamon Twists	😊 Free		😊	Free of sorbitol.
Taco Bell® Combo Burrito	😞 Avoid	4¾	🥘	Portion (140g); 665g in total.
Taco Bell® Double Decker Taco Supreme®, beef	😞 Avoid	7	🥘	Portion (140g); 980g in total.
Taco Bell® Pintos 'n Cheese	😞 Avoid	3¼	🥘	Portion (130g); 423g in total.

3.6.6 Wendy's®

Wendy's®	LACTOSE		Standard amount	⊕
Strawberry Shake	¼		Glass (200g); 50 mL in total.	+¼
Wendys' chili cheese fries	2½		Portion (140g); 350g in total.	+2¼
Wendy's® Baconator®	13		Portion (140g); 1,820g in total.	+10¾
Wendy's® Baked Potato, with sour cream and chives			Nearly free of lactose	
Wendy's® Caesar side salad	9		Portion (100g); 900g in total.	+7½
Wendy's® Chicken Nuggets		☺	Free of lactose.	
Wendy's® French fries		☺	Free of lactose.	
Wendy's® Frosty Float®	¼		Portion (192g); 48g in total.	+¼
Wendy's® Jr. Bacon Cheeseburger	13¾		Portion (140g); 1,925g in total.	+11½
Wendy's® Jr. Cheeseburger Deluxe	14		Portion (140g); 1,960g in total.	+11¾
Wendy's® side salad		☺	Free of lactose.	
Wendy's® Spicy Chicken Go Wrap	31½		Portion (140g); 4,410g in total.	+26¼
Wendy's® Spicy Chicken Sandwich		☺	Free of lactose.	

Wendy's®	IBS		Standard amount	F+G	amount
Strawberry Shake	¼		Glass (200g); 50 mL in total.	1¾	
Wendys' chili cheese fries	2½		Portion (140g); 350g in total.	15	
Wendy's® Baconator®	¼		Portion (140g); 35g in total.	¼	
Wendy's® Baked Potato, with sour cream and chives	35½		Portion (140g); 4,970g in total.		☺
Wendy's® Caesar side salad	1¼		Portion (100g); 125g in total.	50¾	
Wendy's® Chicken Nuggets	2		Portion (85g); 170g in total.	2	
Wendy's® French fries	35½		Portion (70g); 2,485g in total.		☺
Wendy's® Frosty Float®	¼		Portion (192g); 48g in total.	2½	
Wendy's® Jr. Bacon Cheeseburger	¼		Portion (140g); 35g in total.	¼	
Wendy's® Jr. Cheeseburger Deluxe	¼		Portion (140g); 35g in total.	¼	
Wendy's® side salad	2¼		Portion (100g); 225g in total.		☺
Wendy's® Spicy Chicken Go Wrap	¼		Portion (140g); 35g in total.	¼	
Wendy's® Spicy Chicken Sandwich	¼		Portion (140g); 35g in total.	¼	

Wendy's®	FRUCTOSE		Standard amount
Strawberry Shake	B ×4¼	☺+	Free of fructose. Per Glass (200 mL) you drink with it, add B-no × F-limit.
Wendys' chili cheese fries		☺	Free of fructose.
Wendy's® Baconator®		☺	Free of fructose.
Wendy's® Baked Potato, with sour cream and chives	B ×¼	☺+	Free of fructose. Per Portion (140g) you eat with it, add B-no × F-limit.
Wendy's® Caesar side salad	1¼		Portion (100g); 125g in total.
Wendy's® Chicken Nuggets		☺	Free of fructose.
Wendy's® French fries		☺	Free of fructose.
Wendy's® Frosty Float®	¼		Portion (192g); 48g in total.
Wendy's® Jr. Bacon Cheese-burger	1¾		Portion (140g); 245g in total.
Wendy's® Jr. Cheeseburger Deluxe	3		Portion (140g); 420g in total.
Wendy's® side salad	2¼		Portion (100g); 225g in total.
Wendy's® Spicy Chicken Go Wrap	35½		Portion (140g); 4,970g in total.
Wendy's® Spicy Chicken Sandwich	9¾		Portion (140g); 1,365g in total.

Wendy's®	SORBITOL Stand.		SORBITOL Low sensitivity amount	
Strawberry Shake	☹ Avoid	3¼		Glass (200g); 650 mL in total.
Wendys' chili cheese fries	☹ Avoid	2¾		Portion (140g); 385g in total.
Wendy's® Baconator®	☹ Avoid	23¾		Portion (140g); 3,325g in total.
Wendy's® Baked Potato, with sour cream and chives	☹ Avoid	35½		Portion (140g); 4,970g in total.
Wendy's® Caesar side salad	☹ Avoid	4¼		Portion (100g); 425g in total.
Wendy's® Chicken Nuggets	☺ Free		☺	Free of sorbitol.
Wendy's® French fries	☹ Avoid	35½		Portion (70g); 2,485g in total.
Wendy's® Frosty Float®	☺ Free		☺	Free of sorbitol.
Wendy's® Jr. Bacon Cheese-burger	☹ Avoid	3¾		Portion (140g); 525g in total.
Wendy's® Jr. Cheeseburger Deluxe	☹ Avoid	2½		Portion (140g); 350g in total.
Wendy's® side salad	☹ Avoid	2¾		Portion (100g); 275g in total.
Wendy's® Spicy Chicken Go Wrap	☹ Avoid	71¼		Portion (140g); 9,975g in total.
Wendy's® Spicy Chicken Sandwich	☹ Avoid	4¾		Portion (140g); 665g in total.

3.7 Fruits and vegetables

3.7.1 Fruit

Fruit	LACTOSE	Standard amount	
Applesauce, canned, sweetened	😊	Free of lactose.	
Applesauce, canned, unsweetened	😊	Free of lactose.	
Apricot, dried, cooked, sweetened	😊	Free of lactose.	
Apricot, dried, uncooked	😊	Free of lactose.	
Apricot, fresh	😊	Free of lactose.	
Banana, chips	😊	Free of lactose.	
Banana, fresh	😊	Free of lactose.	
Blackberries, fresh	😊	Free of lactose.	
Blueberries, fresh	😊	Free of lactose.	
Boysenberries, fresh	😊	Free of lactose.	
Cantaloupe, fresh	😊	Free of lactose.	
Carambola (starfruit), fresh	😊	Free of lactose.	
Clementine, fresh	😊	Free of lactose.	

Fruit	IBS Standard amount			F+G amount	
Apple, fresh, with skin		☹	Avoid consumption!	1¾	
Applesauce, canned, sweetened	¾	🥄	Tbsp. (15g); 11g in total.	21½	🥄
Applesauce, canned, unsweetened	¾	🥄	Tbsp. (15g); 11g in total.	21½	🥄
Apricot, dried, cooked, sweetened	1¼	🍰	Piece (20g); 25g in total.		☺
Apricot, dried, uncooked	¼	🍰	Piece (20g); 5g in total.		☺
Apricot, fresh	¾	🍰	Piece (35g); 26g in total.		☺
Banana, chips	½	🍛	Portion (40g); 20g in total.	½	🍛
Banana, fresh	¾	🍰	Piece (118g); 89g in total.	¾	🍰
Blackberries, fresh	2¼	🍲	Portion (140g); 315g in total.	2¼	🍲
Blueberries, fresh	¾	🍲	Portion (140g); 105g in total.	¾	🍲
Boysenberries, fresh	69¼	🍲	Portion (8g); 554g in total.		☺
Cantaloupe, fresh	1	🍲	Portion (140g); 140g in total.	2	🍲
Carambola (starfruit), fresh	1¼	🍰	Piece (91g); 114g in total.		☺
Clementine, fresh	2¼	🍲	Portion (140g); 315g in total.	2¼	🍲

Fruit	FRUCTOSE	Standard amount
Apple, fresh, with skin	☹	Avoid consumption!
Applesauce, canned, sweetened	1¼ 🥄	Tbsp. (15g); 19g in total.
Applesauce, canned, un-sweetened	¾ 🥄	Tbsp. (15g); 11g in total.
Apricot, dried, cooked, sweetened	B ×1½ ☺+	Free of fructose. Per Piece (20g) you eat with it, add B-no × F-limit.
Apricot, dried, uncooked	B ×8 ☺+	Free of fructose. Per Piece (20g) you eat with it, add B-no × F-limit.
Apricot, fresh	B ×1 ☺+	Free of fructose. Per Piece (35g) you eat with it, add B-no × F-limit.
Banana, chips	3½ 🍽	Portion (40g); 140g in total.
Banana, fresh	B ×¼ ☺+	Free of fructose. Per Piece (118g) you eat with it, add B-no × F-limit.
Blackberries, fresh	3¾ 🍽	Portion (140g); 525g in total.
Blueberries, fresh	3¾ 🍽	Portion (140g); 525g in total.
Boysenberries, fresh	69¼ 🍽	Portion (8g); 554g in total.
Cantaloupe, fresh	1 🍽	Portion (140g); 140g in total.
Carambola (starfruit), fresh	B ×¼ ☺+	Free of fructose. Per Piece (91g) you eat with it, add B-no × F-limit.
Clementine, fresh	7 🍽	Portion (140g); 980g in total.

Fruit	SORBITOL Stand.		SORBITOL Low sensitivity amount
Apple, fresh, with skin	😞 Avoid		😞 Avoid consumption!
Applesauce, canned, sweetened	😞 Avoid	¾ 🥄	Tbsp. (15g); 11g in total.
Applesauce, canned, unsweetened	😞 Avoid	1 🥄	Tbsp. (15g); 15g in total.
Apricot, dried, cooked, sweetened	😞 Avoid	1¼ 🍰	Piece (20g); 25g in total.
Apricot, dried, uncooked	😞 Avoid	¼ 🍰	Piece (20g); 5g in total.
Apricot, fresh	😞 Avoid	¾ 🍰	Piece (35g); 26g in total.
Banana, chips	😞 Avoid	12½ 🍲	Portion (40g); 500g in total.
Banana, fresh	😞 Avoid	9¼ 🍰	Piece (118g); 1,092g in total.
Blackberries, fresh	😊 Free		😊 Free of sorbitol.
Blueberries, fresh	😊 Free		😊 Free of sorbitol.
Boysenberries, fresh	😊 Free		😊 Free of sorbitol.
Cantaloupe, fresh	😞 Avoid	14¼ 🍲	Portion (140g); 1,995g in total.
Carambola (starfruit), fresh	😞 Avoid	1¼ 🍰	Piece (91g); 114g in total.
Clementine, fresh	😊 Free		😊 Free of sorbitol.

Fruit	LACTOSE	Standard amount
Cranberries, dried (Craisins®)	☺	Free of lactose.
Cranberries, fresh	☺	Free of lactose.
Currants, fresh, black	☺	Free of lactose.
Currants, fresh, red and white	☺	Free of lactose.
Dates	☺	Free of lactose.
Elderberries, fresh	☺	Free of lactose.
Figs, dried, cooked, sweetened	☺	Free of lactose.
Figs, fresh	☺	Free of lactose.
Gooseberries, fresh	☺	Free of lactose.
Grapefruit, fresh, pink or red	☺	Free of lactose.
Grapes, fresh	☺	Free of lactose.
Guava (guayaba), fresh, common	☺	Free of lactose.
Honeydew	☺	Free of lactose.
Jackfruit, fresh	☺	Free of lactose.
Kiwi fruit, gold	☺	Free of lactose.
Kiwi fruit, green	☺	Free of lactose.

Fruit	IBS	Standard amount	F+G	amount
Cranberries, dried (Craisins®)	41½	Portion (40g); 1,660g in total.	☺	
Cranberries, fresh	45¼	Portion (55g); 2,489g in total.	☺	
Currants, fresh, black	1¼	Portion (140g); 175g in total.	☺	
Currants, fresh, red and white	1	Portion (140g); 140g in total.	☺	
Dates	☺	Free of triggers.	☺	
Elderberries, fresh	¼	Portion (140g); 35g in total.	☺	
Figs, dried, cooked, sweetened	☺	Free of triggers.	☺	
Figs, fresh	☺	Free of triggers.	☺	
Gooseberries, fresh	☺	Free of triggers.	☺	
Grapefruit, fresh, pink or red	1½	Portion (140g); 210g in total.	1½	
Grapes, fresh	¼	Portion (140g); 35g in total.	2¼	
Guava (guayaba), fresh, common	½	Piece (250g); 125g in total.	☺	
Honeydew	¾	Portion (140g); 105g in total.	1½	
Jackfruit, fresh	½	Tbsp. (15g); 8g in total.	☺	
Kiwi fruit, gold	1	Piece (86g); 86g in total.	☺	
Kiwi fruit, green	3	Piece (69g); 207g in total.	☺	

Fruit	FRUCTOSE	Standard amount
Cranberries, dried (Craisins®)	B ×3¼ ☺+	Free of fructose. Per Portion (40g) you eat with it, add B-no × F-limit.
Cranberries, fresh	B ×2¾ ☺+	Free of fructose. Per Portion (55g) you eat with it, add B-no × F-limit.
Currants, fresh, black	1¼	Portion (140g); 175g in total.
Currants, fresh, red and white	1	Portion (140g); 140g in total.
Dates	☺	Free of fructose.
Elderberries, fresh	¼	Portion (140g); 35g in total.
Figs, dried, cooked, sweetened	B ×¾ ☺+	Free of fructose. Per Piece (50g) you eat with it, add B-no × F-limit.
Figs, fresh	B ×2 ☺+	Free of fructose. Per Piece (50g) you eat with it, add B-no × F-limit.
Gooseberries, fresh	B ×1 ☺+	Free of fructose. Per Portion (140g) you eat with it, add B-no × F-limit.
Grapefruit, fresh, pink or red	2	Portion (140g); 280g in total.
Grapes, fresh	¼	Portion (140g); 35g in total.
Guava (guayaba), fresh, common	1¼	Piece (250g); 313g in total.
Honeydew	¾	Portion (140g); 105g in total.
Jackfruit, fresh	☺	Free of fructose.
Kiwi fruit, gold	1	Piece (86g); 86g in total.
Kiwi fruit, green	3	Piece (69g); 207g in total.

Fruit	SORBITOL Stand.	SORBITOL Low sensitivity amount
Cranberries, dried (Craisins®)	☹ Avoid	41½ Portion (40g); 1,660g in total.
Cranberries, fresh	☹ Avoid	45¼ Portion (55g); 2,489g in total.
Currants, fresh, black	☺ Free	☺ Free of sorbitol.
Currants, fresh, red and white	☺ Free	☺ Free of sorbitol.
Dates	☺ Free	☺ Free of sorbitol.
Elderberries, fresh	☺ Free	☺ Free of sorbitol.
Figs, dried, cooked, sweetened	☺ Free	☺ Free of sorbitol.
Figs, fresh	☺ Free	☺ Free of sorbitol.
Gooseberries, fresh	☺ Free	☺ Free of sorbitol.
Grapefruit, fresh, pink or red	☺ Free	☺ Free of sorbitol.
Grapes, fresh	☹ Avoid	½ Portion (140g); 70g in total.
Guava (guayaba), fresh, common	☹ Avoid	½ Piece (250g); 125g in total.
Honeydew	☺ Free	☺ Free of sorbitol.
Jackfruit, fresh	☹ Avoid	½ Tbsp. (15g); 8g in total.
Kiwi fruit, gold	☺ Free	☺ Free of sorbitol.
Kiwi fruit, green	☺ Free	☺ Free of sorbitol.

Fruit	LACTOSE	Standard amount
Lemon, fresh	😊	Free of lactose.
Lime, fresh	😊	Free of lactose.
Loganberries, fresh	😊	Free of lactose.
Lowbush cranberries (lin-gonberries)	😊	Free of lactose.
Lychees (litchis), fresh	😊	Free of lactose.
Lycium (wolf or goji berries)	😊	Free of lactose.
Mandarin orange, fresh	😊	Free of lactose.
Mango, fresh	😊	Free of lactose.
Mangosteen, fresh	😊	Free of lactose.
Mulberries	😊	Free of lactose.
Muskmelon	😊	Free of lactose.
Nectarine, fresh	😊	Free of lactose.
Orange, fresh	😊	Free of lactose.
Papaya, fresh	😊	Free of lactose.
Passion fruit (maracuya), fresh	😊	Free of lactose.
Peach, fresh	😊	Free of lactose.

Fruit	IBS	Standard amount	F+G	amount
Lemon, fresh	7¾	Piece (58g); 450g in total.	7¾	
Lime, fresh	6¾	Piece (67g); 452g in total.	6¾	
Loganberries, fresh	☺	Free of triggers.	☺	
Lowbush cranberries (lingonberries)	35½	Portion (140g); 4,970g in total.	☺	
Lychees (litchis), fresh	1	Portion (140g); 140g in total.	☺	
Lycium (wolf or goji berries)	☺	Free of triggers.	☺	
Mandarin orange, fresh	1¼	Portion (140g); 175g in total.	2¼	
Mango, fresh	1	Tbsp. (15g); 15g in total.	☺	
Mangosteen, fresh	35½	Portion (140g); 4,970g in total.	☺	
Mulberries	½	Portion (140g); 70g in total.	☺	
Muskmelon	1¼	Portion (140g); 175g in total.	1½	
Nectarine, fresh	1	Tbsp. (15g); 15g in total.	5½	
Orange, fresh	2¼	Portion (140g); 315g in total.	2¼	
Papaya, fresh	☺	Free of triggers.	☺	
Passion fruit (maracuya), fresh	☺	Free of triggers.	☺	
Peach, fresh	¼	Portion (140g); 35g in total.	2¼	

Fruit	FRUCTOSE		Standard amount
Lemon, fresh		☺	Free of fructose.
Lime, fresh		☺	Free of fructose.
Loganberries, fresh	B ×1½	☺+	Free of fructose. Per Portion (140g) you eat with it, add B-no × F-limit.
Lowbush cranberries (lingonberries)	B ×9¼	☺+	Free of fructose. Per Portion (140g) you eat with it, add B-no × F-limit.
Lychees (litchis), fresh	1	🥄	Portion (140g); 140g in total.
Lycium (wolf or goji berries)	B ×1	☺+	Free of fructose. Per Portion (140g) you eat with it, add B-no × F-limit.
Mandarin orange, fresh	1¼	🥄	Portion (140g); 175g in total.
Mango, fresh	1	🥄	Tbsp. (15g); 15g in total.
Mangosteen, fresh	35½	🥄	Portion (140g); 4,970g in total.
Mulberries	½	🥄	Portion (140g); 70g in total.
Muskmelon	1¼	🥄	Portion (140g); 175g in total.
Nectarine, fresh		☺	Free of fructose.
Orange, fresh	2¼	🥄	Portion (140g); 315g in total.
Papaya, fresh	B ×1	☺+	Free of fructose. Per Portion (140g) you eat with it, add B-no × F-limit.
Passion fruit (maracuya), fresh	B ×2½	☺+	Free of fructose. Per Portion (140g) you eat with it, add B-no × F-limit.
Peach, fresh	B ×1	☺+	Free of fructose. Per Portion (140g) you eat with it, add B-no × F-limit.

Fruit	SORBITOL Stand.	SORBITOL Low sensitivity amount
Lemon, fresh	🙂 Free	🙂 Free of sorbitol.
Lime, fresh	🙂 Free	🙂 Free of sorbitol.
Loganberries, fresh	🙂 Free	🙂 Free of sorbitol.
Lowbush cranberries (lingonberries)	🙁 Avoid	35½ 🥣 Portion (140g); 4,970g in total.
Lychees (litchis), fresh	🙂 Free	🙂 Free of sorbitol.
Lycium (wolf or goji berries)	🙂 Free	🙂 Free of sorbitol.
Mandarin orange, fresh	🙂 Free	🙂 Free of sorbitol.
Mango, fresh	🙁 Avoid	4 🥄 Tbsp. (15g); 60g in total.
Mangosteen, fresh	🙂 Free	🙂 Free of sorbitol.
Mulberries	🙂 Free	🙂 Free of sorbitol.
Muskmelon	🙂 Free	🙂 Free of sorbitol.
Nectarine, fresh	🙁 Avoid	1 🥄 Tbsp. (15g); 15g in total.
Orange, fresh	🙂 Free	🙂 Free of sorbitol.
Papaya, fresh	🙂 Free	🙂 Free of sorbitol.
Passion fruit (maracuya), fresh	🙂 Free	🙂 Free of sorbitol.
Peach, fresh	🙁 Avoid	¼ 🥣 Portion (140g); 35g in total.

Fruit	LACTOSE	Standard amount	
Pear, fresh	☺	Free of lactose.	
Persimmon, fresh	☺	Free of lactose.	
Pineapple, dried	☺	Free of lactose.	
Pineapple, fresh	☺	Free of lactose.	
Plantains, green, boiled	☺	Free of lactose.	
Plum, fresh	☺	Free of lactose.	
Pomegranate, fresh (arils-seed/juice sacs)	☺	Free of lactose.	
Quince, fresh	☺	Free of lactose.	
Raisins, uncooked	☺	Free of lactose.	
Rambutan, canned in syrup	☺	Free of lactose.	
Raspberries, fresh, red	☺	Free of lactose.	
Rhubarb, fresh	☺	Free of lactose.	
Rose hips	☺	Free of lactose.	
Santa Claus melon	☺	Free of lactose.	
Sapodilla, fresh	☺	Free of lactose.	
Sour cherries, fresh	☺	Free of lactose.	

Fruit	IBS	Standard amount	F+G	amount
Pear, fresh	¼	Tbsp. (15g); 4g in total.	☺	
Persimmon, fresh	1	Piece (140g); 140g in total.	1	
Pineapple, dried	½	Portion (40g); 20g in total.	2	
Pineapple, fresh	¾	Portion (140g); 105g in total.	2¼	
Plantains, green, boiled	¼	Piece (223g); 56g in total.	¼	
Plum, fresh	¾	Tbsp. (15g); 11g in total.	21½	
Pomegranate, fresh (arils-seed/juice sacs)	2	Tbsp. (15g); 30g in total.	☺	
Quince, fresh	1¼	Tbsp. (15g); 19g in total.	☺	
Raisins, uncooked	½	Portion (40g); 20g in total.	2	
Rambutan, canned in syrup	¾	Portion (140g); 105g in total.	¾	
Raspberries, fresh, red	½	Portion (140g); 70g in total.	1	
Rhubarb, fresh	☺	Free of triggers.	☺	
Rose hips	☺	Free of triggers.	☺	
Santa Claus melon	1¼	Portion (140g); 175g in total.	☺	
Sapodilla, fresh	☺	Free of triggers.	☺	
Sour cherries, fresh	½	Tbsp. (15g); 8g in total.	☺	

Fruit	FRUCTOSE		Standard amount
Pear, fresh	½		Tbsp. (15g); 8g in total.
Persimmon, fresh	2¾		Piece (140g); 385g in total.
Pineapple, dried	½		Portion (40g); 20g in total.
Pineapple, fresh	¾		Portion (140g); 105g in total.
Plantains, green, boiled	¾		Piece (223g); 167g in total.
Plum, fresh	B ×½		Free of fructose. Per Portion (15g) you eat with it, add B-no × F-limit.
Pomegranate, fresh (arils-seed/juice sacs)	B ×½		Free of fructose. Per Piece (15g) you eat with it, add B-no × F-limit.
Quince, fresh	1¼		Tbsp. (15g); 19g in total.
Raisins, uncooked	½		Portion (40g); 20g in total.
Rambutan, canned in syrup	1¼		Portion (140g); 175g in total.
Raspberries, fresh, red	½		Portion (140g); 70g in total.
Rhubarb, fresh			Free of fructose.
Rose hips	B ×½		Free of fructose. Per Portion (140g) you eat with it, add B-no × F-limit.
Santa Claus melon	1¼		Portion (140g); 175g in total.
Sapodilla, fresh	B ×3½		Free of fructose. Per Portion (140g) you eat with it, add B-no × F-limit.
Sour cherries, fresh			Free of fructose.

Fruit	SORBITOL Stand.	SORBITOL Low sensitivity amount
Pear, fresh	Avoid	¼ Tbsp. (15g); 4g in total.
Persimmon, fresh	Free	Free of sorbitol.
Pineapple, dried	Avoid	½ Portion (40g); 20g in total.
Pineapple, fresh	Avoid	¾ Portion (140g); 105g in total.
Plantains, green, boiled	Free	Free of sorbitol.
Plum, fresh	Avoid	¾ Tbsp. (15g); 11g in total.
Pomegranate, fresh (arils-seed/juice sacs)	Avoid	2 Tbsp. (15g); 30g in total.
Quince, fresh	Free	Free of sorbitol.
Raisins, uncooked	Avoid	½ Portion (40g); 20g in total.
Rambutan, canned in syrup	Free	Free of sorbitol.
Raspberries, fresh, red	Avoid	1½ Portion (140g); 210g in total.
Rhubarb, fresh	Free	Free of sorbitol.
Rose hips	Free	Free of sorbitol.
Santa Claus melon	Free	Free of sorbitol.
Sapodilla, fresh	Free	Free of sorbitol.
Sour cherries, fresh	Avoid	½ Tbsp. (15g); 8g in total.

Fruit	LACTOSE	Standard amount	
Soursop (guanabana), fresh	😊	Free of lactose.	
Strawberries, fresh	😊	Free of lactose.	
Sweet cherries, fresh	😊	Free of lactose.	
Watermelon, fresh	😊	Free of lactose.	

Fruit	IBS	Standard amount	F+G	amount
Soursop (guanabana), fresh	1¼	Portion (140g); 175g in total.		😊
Strawberries, fresh	¼	Portion (140g); 35g in total.		😊
Sweet cherries, fresh	¼	Tbsp. (15g); 4g in total.		😊
Watermelon, fresh	1¾	Tbsp. (15g); 26g in total.	10¼	🥄

Fruit	FRUCTOSE	Standard amount
Soursop (guanabana), fresh	1¼	Portion (140g); 175g in total.
Strawberries, fresh	½	Portion (140g); 70g in total.
Sweet cherries, fresh	B ×¼	Free of fructose. Per Portion (15g) you eat with it, add B-no × F-limit.
Watermelon, fresh	1¾	Tbsp. (15g); 26g in total.

Fruit	SORBITOL Stand.	SORBITOL Low sensitivity amount
Soursop (guanabana), fresh	Free	Free of sorbitol.
Strawberries, fresh	Avoid	¼ Portion (140g); 35g in total.
Sweet cherries, fresh	Avoid	¼ Tbsp. (15g); 4g in total.
Watermelon, fresh	Nearly free	Nearly free of sorbitol

3.7.2   Vegetables

Vegetables	LACTOSE	Standard amount	
Alfalfa sprouts	🙂	Free of lactose.	
Artichoke, globe raw	🙂	Free of lactose.	
Arugula, raw	🙂	Free of lactose.	
Asparagus, raw	🙂	Free of lactose.	
Avocado, green skin, Florida type	🙂	Free of lactose.	
Bamboo shoots, canned and drained	🙂	Free of lactose.	
Beets, raw	🙂	Free of lactose.	
Black beans, cooked from dried	🙂	Free of lactose.	
Black olives	🙂	Free of lactose.	
Bok choy, raw	🙂	Free of lactose.	
Boston Market® sweet corn	🙂	Free of lactose.	
Broccoflower (green cauliflower), cooked from fresh	🙂	Free of lactose.	
Broccoli, raw	🙂	Free of lactose.	
Brown mushrooms (Italian or Crimini mushrooms), raw	🙂	Free of lactose.	
Brussels sprouts, cooked from fresh	🙂	Free of lactose.	

Vegetables	IBS	Standard amount	F+G	amount
Alfalfa sprouts	☹	Avoid consumption!!	☹	
Artichoke, globe raw	1 🥄	Tbsp. (15g); 15g in total.	1 🥄	
Arugula, raw	4¾ 🥣	Portion (85g); 404g in total.	☺	
Asparagus, raw	½ 🥣	Portion (85g); 43g in total.	½ 🥣	
Avocado, green skin, Florida type	☺	Free of triggers.	☺	
Bamboo shoots, canned and drained	19½ 🥣	Portion (85g); 1,658g in total.	☺	
Beets, raw	1¼ 🥣	Portion (85g); 106g in total.	1¼ 🥣	
Black beans, cooked from dried	¼ 🥣	Portion (90g); 23g in total.	¼ 🥣	
Black olives	33¼ 🥣	Portion (15g); 499g in total.	☺	
Bok choy, raw	23½ 🥣	Portion (85g); 1,998g in total.	☺	
Boston Market® sweet corn	4 🥣	Portion (85g); 340g in total.	☺	
Broccoflower (green cauliflower), cooked from fresh	1 🥣	Portion (85g); 85g in total.	☺	
Broccoli, raw	½ 🥣	Portion (85g); 43g in total.	½ 🥣	
Brown mushrooms (Italian or Crimini mushrooms), raw	¾ 🥄	Tbsp. (15g); 11g in total.	12¼ 🥄	
Brussels sprouts, cooked from fresh	1 🥣	Portion (85g); 85g in total.	1 🥣	
Butternut squash	½ 🥣	Portion (130g); 65g in total.	½ 🥣	

Vegetables	FRUCTOSE	Standard amount
Alfalfa sprouts	14½	Portion (85g); 1,233g in total.
Artichoke, globe raw	☺	Free of fructose.
Arugula, raw	4¾	Portion (85g); 404g in total.
Asparagus, raw	1½	Portion (85g); 128g in total.
Avocado, green skin, Florida type	B ×1 ☺+	Free of fructose. Per Portion (30g) you eat with it, add B-no × F-limit.
Bamboo shoots, canned and drained	19½	Portion (85g); 1,658g in total.
Beets, raw	☺	Free of fructose.
Black beans, cooked from dried	☺	Free of fructose.
Black olives	☺	Free of fructose.
Bok choy, raw	B ×¼ ☺+	Free of fructose. Per Portion (85g) you eat with it, add B-no × F-limit.
Boston Market® sweet corn	B ×½ ☺+	Free of fructose. Per Portion (85g) you eat with it, add B-no × F-limit.
Broccoflower (green cauli-flower), cooked from fresh	1	Portion (85g); 85g in total.
Broccoli, raw	3	Portion (85g); 255g in total.
Brown mushrooms (Italian or Crimini mushrooms), raw	B ×¼ ☺+	Free of fructose. Per Portion (15g) you eat with it, add B-no × F-limit.
Brussels sprouts, cooked from fresh	☺	Free of fructose.
Butternut squash	☺	Free of fructose.

Vegetables	SORBITOL Stand.		SORBITOL Low sensitivity amount
Alfalfa sprouts	☺ Free		☺ Free of sorbitol.
Artichoke, globe raw	☹ Avoid	23¾	Tbsp. (15g); 356g in total.
Arugula, raw	☺ Free		☺ Free of sorbitol.
Asparagus, raw	☹ Avoid	9¾	Portion (85g); 829g in total.
Avocado, green skin, Florida type	☺ Free		☺ Free of sorbitol.
Bamboo shoots, canned and drained	☺ Free		☺ Free of sorbitol.
Beets, raw	☹ Avoid	3¼	Portion (85g); 276g in total.
Black beans, cooked from dried	☺ Free		☺ Free of sorbitol.
Black olives	☹ Avoid	33¼	Portion (15g); 499g in total.
Bok choy, raw	☹ Avoid	23½	Portion (85g); 1,998g in total.
Boston Market® sweet corn	☹ Avoid	4	Portion (85g); 340g in total.
Broccoflower (green cauliflower), cooked from fresh	☺ Free		☺ Free of sorbitol.
Broccoli, raw	☺ Free		☺ Free of sorbitol.
Brown mushrooms (Italian or Crimini mushrooms), raw	☹ Avoid	¾	Tbsp. (15g); 11g in total.
Brussels sprouts, cooked from fresh	☺ Free		☺ Free of sorbitol.
Butternut squash	☺ Free		☺ Free of sorbitol.

Vegetables	LACTOSE	Standard amount
Cabbage, green, cooked	🙂	Free of lactose.
Cabbage, red, cooked	🙂	Free of lactose.
Cabbage, savoy, raw	🙂	Free of lactose.
Carrots, cooked from fresh	🙂	Free of lactose.
Carrots, raw	🙂	Free of lactose.
Cauliflower, cooked from frozen	🙂	Free of lactose.
Celeriac (celery root), cooked from fresh	🙂	Free of lactose.
Celery, cooked	🙂	Free of lactose.
Chard, raw or blanched, marinated in oil	🙂	Free of lactose.
Chayote squash, cooked	🙂	Free of lactose.
Chestnuts, boiled, steamed	🙂	Free of lactose.
Chicory coffee powder, unprepared	🙂	Free of lactose.
Chicory greens, raw	🙂	Free of lactose.
Coleslaw, with apples and raisins, mayo dressing	🙂	Free of lactose.
Coleslaw, with pineapple, mayo dressing	🙂	Free of lactose.
Collards, raw	🙂	Free of lactose.

Vegetables	IBS	Standard amount	F+G	amount
Cabbage, green, cooked	1¼	Portion (85g); 106g in total.	1¼	
Cabbage, red, cooked	1¼	Portion (85g); 106g in total.	1¼	
Cabbage, savoy, raw	1½	Portion (85g); 128g in total.	1½	
Carrots, cooked from fresh	½	Portion (85g); 43g in total.	☺	
Carrots, raw	¾	Piece (61g); 46g in total.	☺	
Cauliflower, cooked from frozen	2½	Portion (85g); 213g in total.	☺	
Celeriac (celery root), cooked from fresh	¾	Tbsp. (15g); 11g in total.	☺	
Celery, cooked	1	Tbsp. (15g); 15g in total.	☺	
Chard, raw or blanched, marinated in oil	☺	Free of triggers.	☺	
Chayote squash, cooked	6¼	Portion (130g); 813g in total.	☺	
Chestnuts, boiled, steamed	6	Portion (30g); 180g in total.	☺	
Chicory coffee powder, unprepared	½	Portion (2g); 1g in total.	½	
Chicory greens, raw	2¼	Portion (85g); 191g in total.	2¼	
Coleslaw, with apples and raisins, mayo dressing	½	Portion (100g); 50g in total.	1	
Coleslaw, with pineapple, mayo dressing	3¾	Portion (100g); 375g in total.	☺	
Collards, raw	1¼	Portion (85g); 106g in total.	1¼	

Vegetables	FRUCTOSE		Standard amount
Cabbage, green, cooked	B ×¾	☺ +	Free of fructose. Per Portion (85g) you eat with it, add B-no × F-limit.
Cabbage, red, cooked	B ×¼	☺ +	Free of fructose. Per Portion (85g) you eat with it, add B-no × F-limit.
Cabbage, savoy, raw		☺	Free of fructose.
Carrots, cooked from fresh		☺	Free of fructose.
Carrots, raw		☺	Free of fructose.
Cauliflower, cooked from frozen		☺	Free of fructose.
Celeriac (celery root), cooked from fresh	6½	🥄	Tbsp. (15g); 98g in total.
Celery, cooked		☺	Free of fructose.
Chard, raw or blanched, marinated in oil	B ×½	☺ +	Free of fructose. Per Portion (85g) you eat with it, add B-no × F-limit.
Chayote squash, cooked	6¼	🍽	Portion (130g); 813g in total.
Chestnuts, boiled, steamed		☺	Free of fructose.
Chicory coffee powder, unprepared		☺	Nearly free of fructose, avoid at hereditary fructose intolerance.
Chicory greens, raw	5	🍽	Portion (85g); 425g in total.
Coleslaw, with apples and raisins, mayo dressing	½	🍽	Portion (100g); 50g in total.
Coleslaw, with pineapple, mayo dressing	B ×¼	☺ +	Free of fructose. Per Portion (100g) you eat with it, add B-no × F-limit.
Collards, raw		☺	Free of fructose.

Vegetables	SORBITOL Stand.		SORBITOL Low sensitivity amount
Cabbage, green, cooked	😦 Avoid	58¾	Portion (85g); 4,994g in total.
Cabbage, red, cooked	🙂 Free		Free of sorbitol.
Cabbage, savoy, raw	😦 Avoid	39	Portion (85g); 3,315g in total.
Carrots, cooked from fresh	😦 Avoid	½	Portion (85g); 43g in total.
Carrots, raw	😦 Avoid	¾	Piece (61g); 46g in total.
Cauliflower, cooked from frozen	😦 Avoid	2½	Portion (85g); 213g in total.
Celeriac (celery root), cooked from fresh	😦 Avoid	¾	Tbsp. (15g); 11g in total.
Celery, cooked	😦 Avoid	1	Tbsp. (15g); 15g in total.
Chard, raw or blanched, marinated in oil	🙂 Free		Free of sorbitol.
Chayote squash, cooked	🙂 Free		Free of sorbitol.
Chestnuts, boiled, steamed	😦 Avoid	6	Portion (30g); 180g in total.
Chicory coffee powder, unprepared	😦 Avoid	8¾	Portion (2g); 18g in total.
Chicory greens, raw	😦 Avoid	39	Portion (85g); 3,315g in total.
Coleslaw, with apples and raisins, mayo dressing	😦 Avoid	½	Portion (100g); 50g in total.
Coleslaw, with pineapple, mayo dressing	😦 Avoid	3¾	Portion (100g); 375g in total.
Collards, raw	🙂 Free		Free of sorbitol.

Vegetables	LACTOSE	Standard amount	
Cucumber, raw, with peel	☺	Free of lactose.	
Cucumber, raw, without peel	☺	Free of lactose.	
Eggplant, cooked	☺	Free of lactose.	
Endive, curly, raw	☺	Free of lactose.	
Enoki mushrooms, raw	☺	Free of lactose.	
Fennel bulb, raw	☺	Free of lactose.	
Garbanzo beans (chickpeas), canned, drained	☺	Free of lactose.	
Garlic, fresh	☺	Free of lactose.	
Ginger root, raw	☺	Free of lactose.	
Green beans (string beans), cooked from fresh	☺	Free of lactose.	
Green bell peppers	☺	Free of lactose.	
Green olives	☺	Free of lactose.	
Green tomato, raw	☺	Free of lactose.	
Grits (polenta), regular cooking	☺	Free of lactose.	
Hot chili peppers, green, cooked from fresh	☺	Free of lactose.	
Hot chili peppers, red, cooked from fresh	☺	Free of lactose.	

Vegetables	IBS Standard amount		F+G amount	
Cucumber, raw, with peel	1	Portion (85g); 85g in total.	☺	
Cucumber, raw, without peel	1	Portion (85g); 85g in total.	☺	
Eggplant, cooked	2½	Portion (85g); 213g in total.	☺	
Endive, curly, raw	3	Portion (85g); 255g in total.	3¾	
Enoki mushrooms, raw	¾	Tbsp. (15g); 11g in total.	☺	
Fennel bulb, raw	1¼	Portion (85g); 106g in total.	1¼	
Garbanzo beans (chickpeas), canned, drained	1	Portion (90g); 90g in total.	1½	
Garlic, fresh	¾	Portion (4g); 3g in total.	¾	
Ginger root, raw	89¼	Portion (4g); 357g in total.	☺	
Green beans (string beans), cooked from fresh	¼	Portion (85g); 21g in total.	¼	
Green bell peppers	☺	Free of triggers.	☺	
Green olives	18	Portion (15g); 270g in total.	☺	
Green tomato, raw	¾	Portion (85g); 64g in total.	6½	
Grits (polenta), regular cooking	☺	Free of triggers.	☺	
Hot chili peppers, green, cooked from fresh	2½	Piece (43g); 108g in total.	2½	
Hot chili peppers, red, cooked from fresh	2½	Piece (43g); 108g in total.	2½	

Vegetables	FRUCTOSE		Standard amount
Cucumber, raw, with peel	2¾		Portion (85g); 234g in total.
Cucumber, raw, without peel	2½		Portion (85g); 213g in total.
Eggplant, cooked	2¾		Portion (85g); 234g in total.
Endive, curly, raw			Free of fructose.
Enoki mushrooms, raw			Free of fructose.
Fennel bulb, raw	B ×¾		Free of fructose. Per Portion (85g) you eat with it, add B-no × F-limit.
Garbanzo beans (chickpeas), canned, drained			Free of fructose.
Garlic, fresh			Nearly free of fructose, avoid at hereditary fructose intolerance.
Ginger root, raw	89¼		Portion (4g); 357g in total.
Green beans (string beans), cooked from fresh	4½		Portion (85g); 383g in total.
Green bell peppers			Free of fructose.
Green olives			Nearly free of fructose, avoid at hereditary fructose intolerance.
Green tomato, raw	1¾		Portion (85g); 149g in total.
Grits (polenta), regular cooking			Free of fructose.
Hot chili peppers, green, cooked from fresh	4½		Piece (43g); 194g in total.
Hot chili peppers, red, cooked from fresh	2¾		Piece (43g); 118g in total.

Vegetables	SORBITOL Stand.		SORBITOL Low sensitivity amount	
Cucumber, raw, with peel	🙁	Avoid	1	Portion (85g); 85g in total.
Cucumber, raw, without peel	🙁	Avoid	1	Portion (85g); 85g in total.
Eggplant, cooked	🙁	Avoid	2½	Portion (85g); 213g in total.
Endive, curly, raw	🙁	Avoid	3	Portion (85g); 255g in total.
Enoki mushrooms, raw	🙁	Avoid	¾	Tbsp. (15g); 11g in total.
Fennel bulb, raw	🙁	Avoid	2	Portion (85g); 170g in total.
Garbanzo beans (chickpeas), canned, drained	🙁	Avoid	1	Portion (90g); 90g in total.
Garlic, fresh	🙂	Free	🙂	Free of sorbitol.
Ginger root, raw	🙂	Free	🙂	Free of sorbitol.
Green beans (string beans), cooked from fresh	🙂	Free	🙂	Free of sorbitol.
Green bell peppers	🙂	Free	🙂	Free of sorbitol.
Green olives	🙁	Avoid	18	Portion (15g); 270g in total.
Green tomato, raw	🙁	Avoid	¾	Portion (85g); 64g in total.
Grits (polenta), regular cooking	🙂	Free	🙂	Free of sorbitol.
Hot chili peppers, green, cooked from fresh	🙂	Free	🙂	Free of sorbitol.
Hot chili peppers, red, cooked from fresh	🙂	Free	🙂	Free of sorbitol.

Vegetables	LACTOSE	Standard amount	
Hubbard squash	☺	Free of lactose.	
Jerusalem artichoke (sun-choke), raw	☺	Free of lactose.	
Kale, raw	☺	Free of lactose.	
Kelp, raw	☺	Free of lactose.	
Kidney beans, cooked from dried	☺	Free of lactose.	
Kohlrabi, cooked	☺	Free of lactose.	
Leeks, leafs	☺	Free of lactose.	
Leeks, root	☺	Free of lactose.	
Leeks, whole	☺	Free of lactose.	
Lentils, cooked from dried	☺	Free of lactose.	
Lettuce, Boston, bibb or butter-head	☺	Free of lactose.	
Lettuce, green leaf	☺	Free of lactose.	
Lettuce, iceberg	☺	Free of lactose.	
Lettuce, red leaf	☺	Free of lactose.	
Lettuce, romaine or cos	☺	Free of lactose.	
Lima beans, cooked from dried	☺	Free of lactose.	

Vegetables	IBS	Standard amount	F+G	amount
Hubbard squash		Free of triggers.		
Jerusalem artichoke (sun-choke), raw	3¼	Pinch (1g); 3g in total.	3¼	
Kale, raw	¾	Portion (85g); 64g in total.		
Kelp, raw		Free of triggers.		
Kidney beans, cooked from dried	¼	Portion (90g); 23g in total.	¼	
Kohlrabi, cooked	13	Portion (85g); 1,105g in total.		
Leeks, leafs	¼	Portion (85g); 21g in total.	¾	
Leeks, root	¼	Tbsp. (15g); 4g in total.	¼	
Leeks, whole	¼	Portion (85g); 21g in total.	¼	
Lentils, cooked from dried	¾	Portion (90g); 68g in total.	¾	
Lettuce, Boston, bibb or butterhead	6¾	Portion (85g); 574g in total.		
Lettuce, green leaf	7½	Portion (85g); 638g in total.		
Lettuce, iceberg	6	Portion (85g); 510g in total.		
Lettuce, red leaf	6¾	Portion (85g); 574g in total.		
Lettuce, romaine or cos	1¼	Portion (85g); 106g in total.		
Lima beans, cooked from dried	¼	Portion (90g); 23g in total.	¼	

Vegetables	FRUCTOSE		Standard amount
Hubbard squash		☺	Free of fructose.
Jerusalem artichoke (sun-choke), raw		☺	Free of fructose.
Kale, raw		☺	Free of fructose.
Kelp, raw		☺	Free of fructose.
Kidney beans, cooked from dried		☺	Free of fructose.
Kohlrabi, cooked	B ×¼	☺	Free of fructose. Per Portion (85g) you eat with it, add B-no × F-limit.
Leeks, leafs	1½		Portion (85g); 128g in total.
Leeks, root	9¼		Tbsp. (15g); 139g in total.
Leeks, whole	1½		Portion (85g); 128g in total.
Lentils, cooked from dried		☺	Free of fructose.
Lettuce, Boston, bibb or butterhead	6¾		Portion (85g); 574g in total.
Lettuce, green leaf	7½		Portion (85g); 638g in total.
Lettuce, iceberg	6		Portion (85g); 510g in total.
Lettuce, red leaf	6¾		Portion (85g); 574g in total.
Lettuce, romaine or cos	1¼		Portion (85g); 106g in total.
Lima beans, cooked from dried	½		Portion (90g); 45g in total.

Vegetables	SORBITOL Stand.	SORBITOL Low sensitivity amount
Hubbard squash	🙂 Free	🙂 Free of sorbitol.
Jerusalem artichoke (sunchoke), raw	🙂 Free	🙂 Free of sorbitol.
Kale, raw	🙁 Avoid	¾ Portion (85g); 64g in total.
Kelp, raw	🙂 Free	🙂 Free of sorbitol.
Kidney beans, cooked from dried	🙂 Free	🙂 Free of sorbitol.
Kohlrabi, cooked	🙁 Avoid	13 Portion (85g); 1,105g in total.
Leeks, leafs	🙁 Avoid	¼ Portion (85g); 21g in total.
Leeks, root	🙁 Avoid	2¼ Tbsp. (15g); 34g in total.
Leeks, whole	🙁 Avoid	¼ Portion (85g); 21g in total.
Lentils, cooked from dried	🙂 Free	🙂 Free of sorbitol.
Lettuce, Boston, bibb or butterhead	🙁 Avoid	19½ Portion (85g); 1,658g in total.
Lettuce, green leaf	🙁 Avoid	16¾ Portion (85g); 1,424g in total.
Lettuce, iceberg	🙁 Avoid	19½ Portion (85g); 1,658g in total.
Lettuce, red leaf	🙁 Avoid	19½ Portion (85g); 1,658g in total.
Lettuce, romaine or cos	🙁 Avoid	16¾ Portion (85g); 1,424g in total.
Lima beans, cooked from dried	🙂 Free	🙂 Free of sorbitol.

Vegetables	LACTOSE	Standard amount	
Lotus root, cooked	☺	Free of lactose.	
Maitake mushrooms, raw	☺	Free of lactose.	
Morel mushrooms, raw	☺	Free of lactose.	
Mung bean sprouts, cooked from fresh	☺	Free of lactose.	
Mung beans, cooked from dried	☺	Free of lactose.	
Mushrooms, batter dipped or breaded	☺	Free of lactose.	
Okra, raw	☺	Free of lactose.	
Onion, white, yellow or red, raw	☺	Free of lactose.	
Oyster mushrooms, raw	☺	Free of lactose.	
Parsnip, cooked	☺	Free of lactose.	
Pickled beets	☺	Free of lactose.	
Portabella mushrooms, cooked from fresh	☺	Free of lactose.	
Purslane, raw	☺	Free of lactose.	
Radicchio, raw	☺	Free of lactose.	
Radish, raw	☺	Free of lactose.	
Rutabaga, raw or blanched, marinated in oil mixture	☺	Free of lactose.	

Vegetables	IBS	Standard amount	F+G	amount
Lotus root, cooked	🙂	Free of triggers.		🙂
Maitake mushrooms, raw	¾ 🥄	Tbsp. (15g); 11g in total.		🙂
Morel mushrooms, raw	¾ 🥄	Tbsp. (15g); 11g in total.		🙂
Mung bean sprouts, cooked from fresh	☹️	Avoid consumption!!		☹️
Mung beans, cooked from dried	½ 🥣	Portion (90g); 45g in total.	¾ 🥣	
Mushrooms, batter dipped or breaded	¼ 🥣	Portion (70g); 18g in total.	2½ 🥣	
Okra, raw	2 🥣	Portion (85g); 170g in total.	2 🥣	
Onion, white, yellow or red, raw	1 🥄	Tbsp. (15g); 15g in total.	1 🥄	
Oyster mushrooms, raw	¼ 🥣	Portion (85g); 21g in total.		🙂
Parsnip, cooked	🙂	Free of triggers.		🙂
Pickled beets	3 🥣	Portion (30g); 90g in total.	3 🥣	
Portabella mushrooms, cooked from fresh	½ 🥄	Tbsp. (15g); 8g in total.	12¼ 🥄	
Purslane, raw	58¾ 🥣	Portion (85g); 4,994g in total.		🙂
Radicchio, raw	¾ 🥣	Portion (85g); 64g in total.	¾ 🥣	
Radish, raw	1 🥣	Portion (85g); 85g in total.		🙂
Rutabaga, raw or blanched, marinated in oil mixture	🙂	Free of triggers.		🙂

Vegetables	FRUCTOSE		Standard amount
Lotus root, cooked		☺	Free of fructose.
Maitake mushrooms, raw	B ×½	☺+	Free of fructose. Per Portion (15g) you eat with it, add B-no × F-limit.
Morel mushrooms, raw		☺	Free of fructose.
Mung bean sprouts, cooked from fresh		☺	Free of fructose.
Mung beans, cooked from dried	½	🍽	Portion (90g); 45g in total.
Mushrooms, batter dipped or breaded		☺	Free of fructose.
Okra, raw	2¼	🍽	Portion (85g); 191g in total.
Onion, white, yellow or red, raw		☺	Free of fructose.
Oyster mushrooms, raw	B ×1¾	☺+	Free of fructose. Per Portion (85g) you eat with it, add B-no × F-limit.
Parsnip, cooked	B ×¼	☺+	Free of fructose. Per Portion (85g) you eat with it, add B-no × F-limit.
Pickled beets		☺	Free of fructose.
Portabella mushrooms, cooked from fresh	B ×½	☺+	Free of fructose. Per Portion (15g) you eat with it, add B-no × F-limit.
Purslane, raw	58¾	🍽	Portion (85g); 4,994g in total.
Radicchio, raw	2¼	🍽	Portion (85g); 191g in total.
Radish, raw	B ×½	☺+	Free of fructose. Per Portion (85g) you eat with it, add B-no × F-limit.
Rutabaga, raw or blanched, marinated in oil mixture	B ×1	☺+	Free of fructose. Per Portion (85g) you eat with it, add B-no × F-limit.

Vegetables	SORBITOL Stand.		SORBITOL Low sensitivity amount
Lotus root, cooked	🙂 Free		🙂 Free of sorbitol.
Maitake mushrooms, raw	☹ Avoid	¾ 🥄	Tbsp. (15g); 11g in total.
Morel mushrooms, raw	☹ Avoid	¾ 🥄	Tbsp. (15g); 11g in total.
Mung bean sprouts, cooked from fresh	☹ Avoid	16¾ 🍲	Portion (85g); 1,424g in total.
Mung beans, cooked from dried	🙂 Free		🙂 Free of sorbitol.
Mushrooms, batter dipped or breaded	☹ Avoid	¼ 🍲	Portion (70g); 18g in total.
Okra, raw	🙂 Free		🙂 Free of sorbitol.
Onion, white, yellow or red, raw	☹ Avoid	6 🥄	Tbsp. (15g); 90g in total.
Oyster mushrooms, raw	☹ Avoid	¼ 🍲	Portion (85g); 21g in total.
Parsnip, cooked	🙂 Free		🙂 Free of sorbitol.
Pickled beets	☹ Avoid	15 🍲	Portion (30g); 450g in total.
Portabella mushrooms, cooked from fresh	☹ Avoid	½ 🥄	Tbsp. (15g); 8g in total.
Purslane, raw	🙂 Free		🙂 Free of sorbitol.
Radicchio, raw	🙂 Free		🙂 Free of sorbitol.
Radish, raw	☹ Avoid	1 🍲	Portion (85g); 85g in total.
Rutabaga, raw or blanched, marinated in oil mixture	🙂 Free		🙂 Free of sorbitol.

Vegetables	LACTOSE	Standard amount	
Sauerkraut	🙂	Free of lactose.	
Scallop squash	🙂	Free of lactose.	
Shallot, raw	🙂	Free of lactose.	
Shiitake mushrooms, cooked	🙂	Free of lactose.	
Snow peas (edible pea pods), cooked from fresh	🙂	Free of lactose.	
Sour pickles	🙂	Free of lactose.	
Soybean sprouts, raw	🙂	Free of lactose.	
Soybeans, cooked from dried	🙂	Free of lactose.	
Spaghetti squash	🙂	Free of lactose.	
Spinach, cooked from fresh	🙂	Free of lactose.	
Split pea sprouts, cooked	🙂	Free of lactose.	
Straw mushrooms, canned, drained	🙂	Free of lactose.	
Summer squash, cooked from fresh	🙂	Free of lactose.	
Sun-dried tomatoes, oil pack, drained	🙂	Free of lactose.	
Sweet potato, boiled	🙂	Free of lactose.	
Tempeh	🙂	Free of lactose.	

Vegetables	IBS Standard amount			F+G amount	
Sauerkraut	¾	🥄	Tbsp. (15g); 11g in total.	7	🥄
Scallop squash	4	🍽	Portion (85g); 340g in total.		😊
Shallot, raw	¼	🥄	Tbsp. (15g); 4g in total.	¼	🥄
Shiitake mushrooms, cooked	½	🥄	Tbsp. (15g); 8g in total.		😊
Snow peas (edible pea pods), cooked from fresh	¾	🍽	Portion (85g); 64g in total.	¾	🍽
Sour pickles	1	🍽	Portion (30g); 30g in total.	1	🍽
Soybean sprouts, raw	½	🍽	Portion (85g); 43g in total.	3¾	🍽
Soybeans, cooked from dried	3	🥄	Tbsp. (15g); 45g in total.	3	🥄
Spaghetti squash	😊		Free of triggers.		😊
Spinach, cooked from fresh	4	🍽	Portion (85g); 340g in total.	4	🍽
Split pea sprouts, cooked	1¼	🥄	Tbsp. (15g); 19g in total.	1¼	🥄
Straw mushrooms, canned, drained	¼	🍽	Portion (85g); 21g in total.		😊
Summer squash, cooked from fresh	2	🍽	Portion (85g); 170g in total.	2	🍽
Sun-dried tomatoes, oil pack, drained	½	🥄	Tbsp. (15g); 8g in total.	9¼	🥄
Sweet potato, boiled	😊		Free of triggers.		😊
Tempeh	½	🍽	Portion (85g); 43g in total.	½	🍽

Vegetables	FRUCTOSE		Standard amount
Sauerkraut		☺	Free of fructose.
Scallop squash	4	🥘	Portion (85g); 340g in total.
Shallot, raw		☺	Free of fructose.
Shiitake mushrooms, cooked	B ×1	☺+	Free of fructose. Per Portion (15g) you eat with it, add B-no × F-limit.
Snow peas (edible pea pods), cooked from fresh	B ×3½	☺+	Free of fructose. Per Portion (85g) you eat with it, add B-no × F-limit.
Sour pickles	B ×¼	☺+	Free of fructose. Per Portion (30g) you eat with it, add B-no × F-limit.
Soybean sprouts, raw		☺	Free of fructose.
Soybeans, cooked from dried	5½	🥄	Tbsp. (15g); 83g in total.
Spaghetti squash	B ×¼	☺+	Free of fructose. Per Portion (85g) you eat with it, add B-no × F-limit.
Spinach, cooked from fresh		☺	Free of fructose.
Split pea sprouts, cooked		☺	Free of fructose.
Straw mushrooms, canned, drained		☺	Free of fructose.
Summer squash, cooked from fresh	2¼	🥘	Portion (85g); 191g in total.
Sun-dried tomatoes, oil pack, drained	½	🥄	Tbsp. (15g); 8g in total.
Sweet potato, boiled		☺	Free of fructose.
Tempeh	3¼	🥘	Portion (85g); 276g in total.

Vegetables	SORBITOL Stand.		SORBITOL Low sensitivity amount
Sauerkraut	🙁 Avoid	¾ 🥄	Tbsp. (15g); 11g in total.
Scallop squash	🙂 Free	🙂	Free of sorbitol.
Shallot, raw	🙂 Free	🙂	Free of sorbitol.
Shiitake mushrooms, cooked	🙁 Avoid	½ 🥄	Tbsp. (15g); 8g in total.
Snow peas (edible pea pods), cooked from fresh	🙂 Free	🙂	Free of sorbitol.
Sour pickles	🙁 Avoid	4¼ 🍲	Portion (30g); 128g in total.
Soybean sprouts, raw	🙁 Avoid	½ 🍲	Portion (85g); 43g in total.
Soybeans, cooked from dried	🙁 Avoid	3 🥄	Tbsp. (15g); 45g in total.
Spaghetti squash	🙂 Free	🙂	Free of sorbitol.
Spinach, cooked from fresh	🙁 Avoid	13 🍲	Portion (85g); 1,105g in total.
Split pea sprouts, cooked	🙂 Free	🙂	Free of sorbitol.
Straw mushrooms, canned, drained	🙁 Avoid	¼ 🍲	Portion (85g); 21g in total.
Summer squash, cooked from fresh	🙂 Free	🙂	Free of sorbitol.
Sun-dried tomatoes, oil pack, drained	🙁 Avoid	¾ 🥄	Tbsp. (15g); 11g in total.
Sweet potato, boiled	🙂 Free	🙂	Free of sorbitol.
Tempeh	🙁 Avoid	½ 🍲	Portion (85g); 43g in total.

Vegetables	LACTOSE	Standard amount	
Tomato, cooked from fresh	🙂	Free of lactose.	
Turnip, cooked	🙂	Free of lactose.	
Wax beans (yellow beans), canned, drained	🙂	Free of lactose.	
Winter melon (waxgourd or chinese preserving melon)	🙂	Free of lactose.	
Winter type (dark green or orange) squash, cooked	🙂	Free of lactose.	
Yams, sweet potato type, boiled	🙂	Free of lactose.	
Yellow bell pepper, raw	🙂	Free of lactose.	
Yellow tomato, raw	🙂	Free of lactose.	

Vegetables	IBS	Standard amount	F+G	amount
Tomato, cooked from fresh	¾	Portion (85g); 64g in total.	6½	
Turnip, cooked	2½	Portion (85g); 213g in total.	☺	
Wax beans (yellow beans), canned, drained	¼	Portion (85g); 21g in total.	¼	
Winter melon (waxgourd or chinese preserving melon)	☺	Free of triggers.	☺	
Winter type (dark green or orange) squash, cooked	1¾	Portion (130g); 228g in total.	☺	
Yams, sweet potato type, boiled	☺	Free of triggers.	☺	
Yellow bell pepper, raw	½	Portion (85g); 43g in total.	☺	
Yellow tomato, raw	1	Portion (85g); 85g in total.	6½	

Vegetables	FRUCTOSE		Standard amount
Tomato, cooked from fresh	2¼		Portion (85g); 191g in total.
Turnip, cooked	B ×½		Free of fructose. Per Portion (85g) you eat with it, add B-no × F-limit.
Wax beans (yellow beans), canned, drained			Free of fructose.
Winter melon (waxgourd or chinese preserving melon)			Free of fructose.
Winter type (dark green or orange) squash, cooked	1¾		Portion (130g); 228g in total.
Yams, sweet potato type, boiled			Free of fructose.
Yellow bell pepper, raw	½		Portion (85g); 43g in total.
Yellow tomato, raw	2½		Portion (85g); 213g in total.

Vegetables	SORBITOL Stand.		SORBITOL Low sensitivity amount
Tomato, cooked from fresh	😞 Avoid	¾	Portion (85g); 64g in total.
Turnip, cooked	😞 Avoid	2½	Portion (85g); 213g in total.
Wax beans (yellow beans), canned, drained	😊 Free		Free of sorbitol.
Winter melon (waxgourd or chinese preserving melon)	😊 Free		Free of sorbitol.
Winter type (dark green or orange) squash, cooked	😊 Free		Free of sorbitol.
Yams, sweet potato type, boiled	😊 Free		Free of sorbitol.
Yellow bell pepper, raw	😊 Free		Free of sorbitol.
Yellow tomato, raw	😞 Avoid	1	Portion (85g); 85g in total.

3.8 Ice cream

Ice cream	LACTOSE		Standard amount	
Ben & Jerry's® Ice Cream, Brownie Batter	¼		Portion (110g); 28g in total.	+¼
Ben & Jerry's® Ice Cream, Chocolate Chip Cookie Dough	½		Portion (104g); 52g in total.	+¼
Ben & Jerry's® Ice Cream, Chubby Hubby®	½		Portion (107g); 54g in total.	+½
Ben & Jerry's® Ice Cream, Chunky Monkey®	¼		Portion (107g); 27g in total.	+¼
Ben & Jerry's® Ice Cream, Half Baked	¼		Portion (108g); 27g in total.	+¼
Ben & Jerry's® Ice Cream, Karamel Sutra®	½		Portion (106g); 53g in total.	+¼
Ben & Jerry's® Ice Cream, New York Super Fudge Chunk®	½		Portion (106g); 53g in total.	+½
Ben & Jerry's® Ice Cream, One Sweet Whirled	½		Portion (106g); 53g in total.	+¼
Ben & Jerry's® Ice Cream, Peanut Butter Cup	½		Portion (115g); 58g in total.	+¼
Ben & Jerry's® Ice Cream, Phish Food®	¼		Portion (104g); 26g in total.	+¼
Ben & Jerry's® Ice Cream, Vanilla For A Change	½		Portion (103g); 52g in total.	+¼
Breyers® Ice Cream, Natural Vanilla, Lactose Free	4		Portion (65g); 260g in total.	+3¼
Dreyer's® Grand Ice Cream, Chocolate	1		Portion (65g); 65g in total.	+1
Dreyer's® No Sugar Added Ice Cream, Triple Chocolate	11½		Tsp. (5g); 58g in total.	+9½

Ice cream	IBS	Standard amount	F+G	amount
Ben & Jerry's® Ice Cream, Brownie Batter	¼	Portion (110g); 28g in total.	1¼	
Ben & Jerry's® Ice Cream, Chocolate Chip Cookie Dough	½	Portion (104g); 52g in total.	3¼	
Ben & Jerry's® Ice Cream, Chubby Hubby®	½	Portion (107g); 54g in total.	3½	
Ben & Jerry's® Ice Cream, Chunky Monkey®	¼	Portion (107g); 27g in total.	2½	
Ben & Jerry's® Ice Cream, Half Baked	¼	Portion (108g); 27g in total.	2¼	
Ben & Jerry's® Ice Cream, Karamel Sutra®	½	Portion (106g); 53g in total.	3	
Ben & Jerry's® Ice Cream, New York Super Fudge Chunk®	½	Portion (106g); 53g in total.	3½	
Ben & Jerry's® Ice Cream, One Sweet Whirled	½	Portion (106g); 53g in total.	3	
Ben & Jerry's® Ice Cream, Peanut Butter Cup	½	Portion (115g); 58g in total.	3¼	
Ben & Jerry's® Ice Cream, Phish Food®	¼	Portion (104g); 26g in total.	2¼	
Ben & Jerry's® Ice Cream, Vanilla For A Change	½	Portion (103g); 52g in total.	3¼	
Breyers® Ice Cream, Natural Vanilla, Lactose Free	4	Portion (65g); 260g in total.	23¼	
Dreyer's® Grand Ice Cream, Chocolate	1	Portion (65g); 65g in total.	2¾	
Dreyer's® No Sugar Added Ice Cream, Triple Chocolate	☹	Avoid consumption!	32¾	

Ice cream	FRUCTOSE	Standard amount
Ben & Jerry's® Ice Cream, Brownie Batter	B ×3 ☺+	Free of fructose. Per Portion (110g) you eat with it, add B-no × F-limit.
Ben & Jerry's® Ice Cream, Chocolate Chip Cookie Dough	B ×4¾ ☺+	Free of fructose. Per Portion (104g) you eat with it, add B-no × F-limit.
Ben & Jerry's® Ice Cream, Chubby Hubby®	B ×5 ☺+	Free of fructose. Per Portion (107g) you eat with it, add B-no × F-limit.
Ben & Jerry's® Ice Cream, Chunky Monkey®	B ×2¾ ☺+	Free of fructose. Per Portion (107g) you eat with it, add B-no × F-limit.
Ben & Jerry's® Ice Cream, Half Baked	B ×2¼ ☺+	Free of fructose. Per Portion (108g) you eat with it, add B-no × F-limit.
Ben & Jerry's® Ice Cream, Karamel Sutra®	B ×4¾ ☺+	Free of fructose. Per Portion (106g) you eat with it, add B-no × F-limit.
Ben & Jerry's® Ice Cream, New York Super Fudge Chunk®	58¾ 🍽	Portion (106g); 6,228g in total.
Ben & Jerry's® Ice Cream, One Sweet Whirled	B ×4¾ ☺+	Free of fructose. Per Portion (106g) you eat with it, add B-no × F-limit.
Ben & Jerry's® Ice Cream, Peanut Butter Cup	B ×5¼ ☺+	Free of fructose. Per Portion (115g) you eat with it, add B-no × F-limit.
Ben & Jerry's® Ice Cream, Phish Food®	B ×2¼ ☺+	Free of fructose. Per Portion (104g) you eat with it, add B-no × F-limit.
Ben & Jerry's® Ice Cream, Vanilla For A Change	B ×4½ ☺+	Free of fructose. Per Portion (103g) you eat with it, add B-no × F-limit.
Breyers® Ice Cream, Natural Vanilla, Lactose Free	B ×4¾ ☺+	Free of fructose. Per Portion (65g) you eat with it, add B-no × F-limit.
Dreyer's® Grand Ice Cream, Chocolate	B ×¾ ☺+	Free of fructose. Per Portion (65g) you eat with it, add B-no × F-limit.
Dreyer's® No Sugar Added Ice Cream, Triple Chocolate	☺	Free of fructose.

Ice cream	SORBITOL Stand.	SORBITOL Low sensitivity amount
Ben & Jerry's® Ice Cream, Brownie Batter	☺ Nearly free	☺ Nearly free of sorbitol
Ben & Jerry's® Ice Cream, Chocolate Chip Cookie Dough	☺ Free	☺ Free of sorbitol.
Ben & Jerry's® Ice Cream, Chubby Hubby®	☺ Free	☺ Free of sorbitol.
Ben & Jerry's® Ice Cream, Chunky Monkey®	☺ Nearly free	☺ Nearly free of sorbitol
Ben & Jerry's® Ice Cream, Half Baked	☺ Free	☺ Free of sorbitol.
Ben & Jerry's® Ice Cream, Karamel Sutra®	☺ Free	☺ Free of sorbitol.
Ben & Jerry's® Ice Cream, New York Super Fudge Chunk®	☺ Nearly free	☺ Nearly free of sorbitol
Ben & Jerry's® Ice Cream, One Sweet Whirled	☺ Free	☺ Free of sorbitol.
Ben & Jerry's® Ice Cream, Peanut Butter Cup	☺ Free	☺ Free of sorbitol.
Ben & Jerry's® Ice Cream, Phish Food®	☺ Free	☺ Free of sorbitol.
Ben & Jerry's® Ice Cream, Vanilla For A Change	☺ Free	☺ Free of sorbitol.
Breyers® Ice Cream, Natural Vanilla, Lactose Free	☺ Free	☺ Free of sorbitol.
Dreyer's® Grand Ice Cream, Chocolate	☺ Nearly free	☺ Nearly free of sorbitol
Dreyer's® No Sugar Added Ice Cream, Triple Chocolate	☹ Avoid	☹ Avoid consumption!

Ice cream	LACTOSE	Standard amount	
Drumstick® (sundae cone)	1	Piece (96g); 96g in total.	+¾
Frozen fruit juice Bar	☺	Free of lactose.	
Haagen-Dazs® Desserts Extraordinaire Ice Cream, Creme Brulee	½	Portion (107g); 54g in total.	+¼
Haagen-Dazs® Frozen Yogurt, chocolate or coffee flavors	½	Portion (106g); 53g in total.	+½
Haagen-Dazs® Frozen Yogurt, vanilla or other flavors	½	Portion (106g); 53g in total.	+½
Haagen-Dazs® Ice Cream, Bailey's Irish Cream	½	Portion (102g); 51g in total.	+¼
Haagen-Dazs® Ice Cream, Black Walnut	½	Portion (106g); 53g in total.	+½
Haagen-Dazs® Ice Cream, Butter Pecan	½	Portion (106g); 53g in total.	+½
Haagen-Dazs® Ice Cream, Cherry Vanilla	½	Portion (101g); 51g in total.	+½
Haagen-Dazs® Ice Cream, Chocolate	¼	Portion (106g); 27g in total.	+¼
Haagen-Dazs® Ice Cream, Coffee	¼	Portion (106g); 27g in total.	+¼
Haagen-Dazs® Ice Cream, Cookies & Cream	½	Portion (102g); 51g in total.	+¼
Haagen-Dazs® Ice Cream, Mango	¼	Portion (106g); 27g in total.	+¼
Haagen-Dazs® Ice Cream, Pistachio	½	Portion (106g); 53g in total.	+½
Haagen-Dazs® Ice Cream, Rocky Road	¼	Portion (104g); 26g in total.	+¼

Ice cream	IBS	Standard amount	F+G amount
Drumstick® (sundae cone)	1	Piece (96g); 96g in total.	6¼
Frozen fruit juice Bar	4½	Piece (77g); 347g in total.	
Haagen-Dazs® Desserts Extraordinaire Ice Cream, Creme Brulee	½	Portion (107g); 54g in total.	3
Haagen-Dazs® Frozen Yogurt, chocolate or coffee flavors	½	Portion (106g); 53g in total.	1¾
Haagen-Dazs® Frozen Yogurt, vanilla or other flavors	½	Portion (106g); 53g in total.	3½
Haagen-Dazs® Ice Cream, Bailey's Irish Cream	½	Portion (102g); 51g in total.	1½
Haagen-Dazs® Ice Cream, Black Walnut	½	Portion (106g); 53g in total.	1½
Haagen-Dazs® Ice Cream, Butter Pecan	½	Portion (106g); 53g in total.	2¼
Haagen-Dazs® Ice Cream, Cherry Vanilla	½	Portion (101g); 51g in total.	3¼
Haagen-Dazs® Ice Cream, Chocolate	¼	Portion (106g); 27g in total.	1¼
Haagen-Dazs® Ice Cream, Coffee	¼	Portion (106g); 27g in total.	2½
Haagen-Dazs® Ice Cream, Cookies & Cream	½	Portion (102g); 51g in total.	3¼
Haagen-Dazs® Ice Cream, Mango	¼	Portion (106g); 27g in total.	2¼
Haagen-Dazs® Ice Cream, Pistachio	½	Portion (106g); 53g in total.	½
Haagen-Dazs® Ice Cream, Rocky Road	¼	Portion (104g); 26g in total.	2½

Ice cream	FRUCTOSE		Standard amount
Drumstick® (sundae cone)	B ×2¼	☺ +	Free of fructose. Per Piece (96g) you eat with it, add B-no × F-limit.
Frozen fruit juice Bar	B ×1¼	☺ +	Free of fructose. Per Piece (77g) you eat with it, add B-no × F-limit.
Haagen-Dazs® Desserts Extraordinaire Ice Cream, Creme Brulee	B ×4¾	☺ +	Free of fructose. Per Portion (107g) you eat with it, add B-no × F-limit.
Haagen-Dazs® Frozen Yogurt, chocolate or coffee flavors	B ×¾	☺ +	Free of fructose. Per Portion (106g) you eat with it, add B-no × F-limit.
Haagen-Dazs® Frozen Yogurt, vanilla or other flavors	B ×3	☺ +	Free of fructose. Per Portion (106g) you eat with it, add B-no × F-limit.
Haagen-Dazs® Ice Cream, Bailey's Irish Cream	B ×2¾	☺ +	Free of fructose. Per Portion (102g) you eat with it, add B-no × F-limit.
Haagen-Dazs® Ice Cream, Black Walnut	B ×4¾	☺ +	Free of fructose. Per Portion (106g) you eat with it, add B-no × F-limit.
Haagen-Dazs® Ice Cream, Butter Pecan	B ×4¾	☺ +	Free of fructose. Per Portion (106g) you eat with it, add B-no × F-limit.
Haagen-Dazs® Ice Cream, Cherry Vanilla	B ×4½	☺ +	Free of fructose. Per Portion (101g) you eat with it, add B-no × F-limit.
Haagen-Dazs® Ice Cream, Chocolate	B ×2¾	☺ +	Free of fructose. Per Portion (106g) you eat with it, add B-no × F-limit.
Haagen-Dazs® Ice Cream, Coffee	B ×2¾	☺ +	Free of fructose. Per Portion (106g) you eat with it, add B-no × F-limit.
Haagen-Dazs® Ice Cream, Cookies & Cream	B ×4½	☺ +	Free of fructose. Per Portion (102g) you eat with it, add B-no × F-limit.
Haagen-Dazs® Ice Cream, Mango	B ×2¼	☺ +	Free of fructose. Per Portion (106g) you eat with it, add B-no × F-limit.
Haagen-Dazs® Ice Cream, Pistachio	B ×4¾	☺ +	Free of fructose. Per Portion (106g) you eat with it, add B-no × F-limit.
Haagen-Dazs® Ice Cream, Rocky Road	B ×2¾	☺ +	Free of fructose. Per Portion (104g) you eat with it, add B-no × F-limit.

Ice cream	SORBITOL Stand.	SORBITOL Low sensitivity amount
Drumstick® (sundae cone)	☺ Nearly free	☺ Nearly free of sorbitol
Frozen fruit juice Bar	☹ Avoid	4½ 🍰 Piece (77g); 347g in total.
Haagen-Dazs® Desserts Extraordinaire Ice Cream, Creme Brulee	☺ Free	☺ Free of sorbitol.
Haagen-Dazs® Frozen Yogurt, chocolate or coffee flavors	☺ Nearly free	☺ Nearly free of sorbitol
Haagen-Dazs® Frozen Yogurt, vanilla or other flavors	☺ Free	☺ Free of sorbitol.
Haagen-Dazs® Ice Cream, Bailey's Irish Cream	☺ Nearly free	☺ Nearly free of sorbitol
Haagen-Dazs® Ice Cream, Black Walnut	☺ Free	☺ Free of sorbitol.
Haagen-Dazs® Ice Cream, Butter Pecan	☺ Free	☺ Free of sorbitol.
Haagen-Dazs® Ice Cream, Cherry Vanilla	☺ Free	☺ Free of sorbitol.
Haagen-Dazs® Ice Cream, Chocolate	☺ Nearly free	☺ Nearly free of sorbitol
Haagen-Dazs® Ice Cream, Coffee	☺ Nearly free	☺ Nearly free of sorbitol
Haagen-Dazs® Ice Cream, Cookies & Cream	☺ Free	☺ Free of sorbitol.
Haagen-Dazs® Ice Cream, Mango	☺ Free	☺ Free of sorbitol.
Haagen-Dazs® Ice Cream, Pistachio	☺ Free	☺ Free of sorbitol.
Haagen-Dazs® Ice Cream, Rocky Road	☺ Nearly free	☺ Nearly free of sorbitol

Ice cream	LACTOSE		Standard amount	
Haagen-Dazs® Ice Cream, Strawberry	½		Portion (106g); 53g in total.	+¼
Haagen-Dazs® Ice Cream, Vanilla Chocolate Chip	½		Portion (106g); 53g in total.	+½
Ice cream sandwich	1¼		Piece (72g); 90g in total.	+1
Ice cream, light, no sugar added, with aspartame, vanilla or other flavors (include chocolate chip)	9¾		Tsp. (5g); 49g in total.	+8
Popsicle			Free of lactose.	
Popsicle, sugar free			Free of lactose.	
Sorbet, chocolate			Nearly free of lactose	
Sorbet, coconut	18¾		Portion (106g); 1,988g in total.	+15½
Sorbet, fruit			Free of lactose.	

Ice cream	IBS	Standard amount	F+G	amount
Haagen-Dazs® Ice Cream, Rocky Road	¼	Portion (104g); 26g in total.	2½	
Haagen-Dazs® Ice Cream, Strawberry	½	Portion (106g); 53g in total.	3	
Haagen-Dazs® Ice Cream, Vanilla Chocolate Chip	½	Portion (106g); 53g in total.	3½	
Ice cream sandwich	1¼	Piece (72g); 90g in total.	6¼	
Ice cream, light, no sugar added, with aspartame, vanilla or other flavors (include chocolate chip)	¼	Tsp. (5g); 1g in total.	54¾	
Popsicle	☺	Free of triggers.	☺	
Popsicle, sugar free	☺	Free of triggers.	☺	
Sorbet, chocolate	3	Portion (105g); 315g in total.	3	
Sorbet, coconut	3¼	Portion (106g); 345g in total.	3¼	
Sorbet, fruit	☺	Free of triggers.	☺	

Ice cream	FRUCTOSE		Standard amount
Haagen-Dazs® Ice Cream, Strawberry	B ×4¾	☺ +	Free of fructose. Per Portion (106g) you eat with it, add B-no × F-limit.
Haagen-Dazs® Ice Cream, Vanilla Chocolate Chip	B ×4¾	☺ +	Free of fructose. Per Portion (106g) you eat with it, add B-no × F-limit.
Ice cream sandwich	B ×1½	☺ +	Free of fructose. Per Piece (72g) you eat with it, add B-no × F-limit.
Ice cream, light, no sugar added, with aspartame, vanilla or other flavors (include chocolate chip)		☺	Free of fructose.
Popsicle	B ×1¼	☺ +	Free of fructose. Per Piece (52g) you eat with it, add B-no × F-limit.
Popsicle, sugar free		☺	Free of fructose.
Sorbet, chocolate	B ×3¼	☺ +	Free of fructose. Per Portion (105g) you eat with it, add B-no × F-limit.
Sorbet, coconut	B ×5	☺ +	Free of fructose. Per Portion (106g) you eat with it, add B-no × F-limit.
Sorbet, fruit	B ×5½	☺ +	Free of fructose. Per Portion (106g) you eat with it, add B-no × F-limit.

Ice cream	SORBITOL Stand.		SORBITOL Low sensitivity amount
Haagen-Dazs® Ice Cream, Rocky Road	☺	Nearly free	☺ Nearly free of sorbitol
Haagen-Dazs® Ice Cream, Strawberry	☺	Free	☺ Free of sorbitol.
Haagen-Dazs® Ice Cream, Vanilla Chocolate Chip	☺	Free	☺ Free of sorbitol.
Ice cream sandwich	☺	Free	☺ Free of sorbitol.
Ice cream, light, no sugar added, with aspartame, vanilla or other flavors (include chocolate chip)	☹	Avoid	¼ 🥄 Tsp. (5g); 1g in total.
Popsicle	☺	Free	☺ Free of sorbitol.
Popsicle, sugar free	☺	Free	☺ Free of sorbitol.
Sorbet, chocolate	☺	Free	☺ Free of sorbitol.
Sorbet, coconut	☺	Free	☺ Free of sorbitol.
Sorbet, fruit	☺	Free	☺ Free of sorbitol.

3.9 Ingredients

Ingredients	LACTOSE	Standard amount	
Baking powder	☺	Free of lactose.	
Barley flour	☺	Free of lactose.	
Lemon peel	☺	Free of lactose.	
Orange peel	☺	Free of lactose.	
Rye flour, in recipes not containing yeast	☺	Free of lactose.	
Semolina flour	☺	Free of lactose.	
Spelt flour	☺	Free of lactose.	
Streusel topping, crumb	68¼	Portion (19.56g); 1,335g in total.	+57
Wheat bran, unprocessed	☺	Free of lactose.	
White all-purpose flour, unenriched	☺	Free of lactose.	
White whole wheat flour	☺	Free of lactose.	

Ingredients	IBS	Standard amount	F+G	amount
Baking powder	☺	Free of triggers.		☺
Barley flour	6¼ 🥣	Portion (30g); 188g in total.	6¼	🥣
Lemon peel	☺	Free of triggers.		☺
Orange peel	3¼ 🥄	Tbsp. (15g); 49g in total.		☺
Rye flour, in recipes not containing yeast	1¼ 🥣	Portion (30g); 38g in total.	1¼	🥣
Semolina flour	1¼ 🥣	Portion (30g); 38g in total.	1¼	🥣
Spelt flour	☺	Free of triggers.		☺
Streusel topping, crumb	2¾ 🥣	Portion (19, 56g); 54g in total.	2¾	🥣
Wheat bran, unprocessed	½ 🥄	Tbsp. (15g); 8g in total.	½	🥄
White all-purpose flour, un-enriched	1¼ 🥣	Portion (30g); 38g in total.	1¼	🥣
White whole wheat flour	1¼ 🥣	Portion (30g); 38g in total.	1¼	🥣

Ingredients	FRUCTOSE		Standard amount
Baking powder		☺	Free of fructose.
Barley flour		☺	Free of fructose.
Lemon peel		☺	Free of fructose.
Orange peel	3¼	🥄	Tbsp. (15g); 49g in total.
Rye flour, in recipes not containing yeast	27¾		Portion (30g); 833g in total.
Semolina flour		☺	Free of fructose.
Spelt flour	B ×¼	☺+	Free of fructose. Per Portion (30g) you eat with it, add B-no × F-limit.
Streusel topping, crumb		☺	Free of fructose.
Wheat bran, unprocessed		☺	Free of fructose.
White all-purpose flour, un-enriched		☺	Free of fructose.
White whole wheat flour	33¼		Portion (30g); 998g in total.

Ingredients	SORBITOL Stand.		SORBITOL Low sensitivity amount	
Baking powder	😊	Free	😊	Free of sorbitol.
Barley flour	😊	Free	😊	Free of sorbitol.
Lemon peel	😊	Free	😊	Free of sorbitol.
Orange peel	😊	Free	😊	Free of sorbitol.
Rye flour, in recipes not containing yeast	😊	Free	😊	Free of sorbitol.
Semolina flour	😊	Free	😊	Free of sorbitol.
Spelt flour	😊	Free	😊	Free of sorbitol.
Streusel topping, crumb	😊	Free	😊	Free of sorbitol.
Wheat bran, unprocessed	😊	Free	😊	Free of sorbitol.
White all-purpose flour, un-enriched	😊	Free	😊	Free of sorbitol.
White whole wheat flour	😊	Free	😊	Free of sorbitol.

Glossary

Abbreviation	Meaning
EFSA	European Food Safety Authority.
FDA	Food and Drug Administration.
Fructans	Quickly fermentable carbohydrates that are contained in grain products for example. Included in this group are inulin, kestose and nystose.
Fructose	Oligosaccharide that is primarily contained in fruit.
Galactans	Quickly fermentable carbohydrates that are contained in beans, cabbage, lentils and peas for example (raffinose and stachyose).
Hereditary fructose intolerance	This disease is rare. If you are affected, fructose has a poisonous effect on you. Only a specialist can find out if you are affected and you have to check it before doing a test for fructose intolerance, as it could otherwise be lethal.
Irritable bowel	Definition of this book: an irritable bowel is one that reacts much more intensely to indigestions than it is commonly the case. The presence of trigger cubes in the intestine triggers the symptoms.
Lactose	Oligosaccharide that is primarily contained in dairy products.
Meal	One of three main meals of a given day. The first meal happens at about 7 am the second one at about 1 pm and the third one at about 7 pm. Hence, between each meal there has to be a gap of about six hours in order to avoid overloading your enzyme workers. The tolerable portion sizes refer to this definition of a meal.
NCC	Nutrition Coordination Center of the University of Minnesota.

Abbreviation	Meaning
Sensitivity level	Aside from the standard level, you can use multipliers to determine portion sizes in case you are less sensitive. In the LAXIBA app, we have calculated the tolerable amounts for you. Before increasing your portion sizes to fit another level, you should do a level test to check, if you can tolerate the higher load. There are four levels, see Chapter 3.1.3.
Sorbitol	Sugar alcohol that also limits the tolerance of fructose. Besides, see "sugar-alcohols".
Standard	Portion sizes in this column are based on the usual sensitivity in case of an intolerance towards the respective trigger, i.e. as long as you consume less than the stated maximum amount for this level, you are likely to be untroubled by symptoms from it. It only applies in case of intolerance or certain test - phases. Note that if you consume the maximum portion size for a food at a meal, you cannot eat any other foods that contain the cube at that meal. To combine two foods that contain a certain cube you have to reduce the stated portion sizes accordingly, e.g. by dividing both by two.
Sugar-alcohols	These are contained in some fruit, like apples. Moreover, they are part of many diabetic, dietary and light products as well as chewing gums and mints. They are not contained in stevia. Part of the group of sugar-alcohols besides sorbitol are erythritol, inositol, isomalt, lactitol, maltitol, mannitol, pinitol and xylitol.
Trigger(cube)s	Carbohydrates that fermented in the intestine. To this group belong oligosaccharides (fructose, fructans and galactans, lactose) and sugar-alcohols (like sorbitol).

4

ADVANCED PROCEDURES

4.1 Level test

	Level test tasks	✔
1	You filled out the symptom test sheet for the status quo check.	✔
2	You asked your doctor to refer you to a specialist to do a breath test (if available).	✔
3	You performed the three-week introductory diet and found an improvement to your symptoms at the efficiency check (otherwise please proceed according to Chapter 4.4). If no breath test was available, you performed the substitute test.	✔
4	Now you convince a partner to help you with your tests. Alternatively, you book a personal trainer at *https://laxiba.com/trainer.* The partner will mix your test liquids and interpret your symptom test sheets. You can count on their confidentiality, credibility and availability.	
5	You finished all of the tests, during which your testing partner adhered to the instructions on page 456, and you acted according to the fitting flowchart on pp. 468.	
6	Finish: You talked your result over with your testing partner and entered your new tolerance level into the table on page 136.	

Did your breath or substitute test demonstrate the presence of one or more cube (referring to the example at the beginning of the book) intolerances? Then you should find out whether you can stomach more than the standard amount. Each human differs in the amount he or she can stomach of each trigger. Even in healthy humans the tolerated amount of fructose, for example, fluctuates between 5g and 50g. Moreover, the amount consumed at once for the breath or substitute test is higher than what you would consume in a typical meal. Hence, if your enzyme-workers were able to cope with that amount—you were spared from symptoms after consuming the test does—you can be proud of them, and you can give them a positive interim report: They have mastered all tasks for that trigger with flying colors.

If your crew has ached at the dose, at that point all we know is that the extreme test amount has been too much for them. What it does not mean is that the standard portion sizes used in this book are the highest load your enzyme workers can take. Where is your personal threshold up to which you will not have symptoms? To determine it, you use the level test described in the following. With it, you challenge your enzyme worker gradually and check your sensitivity. With each step, you increase the consumption amount of the tested trigger up to the point at which your enzyme workers ask for a pay raise. The flowcharts from page 468 on depict the procedure. The first three charts only apply if you just have one intolerance. The last one is larger as it is for combined intolerances.

For the level test, you ideally have a test partner preparing the test liquids for you and checking the results. If you have one, only let your partner read the instructions on the pages 452 onward. To increase the reliability, you test each level twice. Otherwise, chance could cause something else to trigger your symptom. Should you consider the matter too private and rather not have someone else included, follow the instructions for self-testers you find on those pages.

Start your test week three days before the test day, as symptoms may occur as many as three days after you consume the trigger containing foods, and you want to start the check uninfluenced from "old" symptoms. On the days before the test, eat according to your current levels. Your current levels are those that you tolerated during the test and retest of the combination test described below. Initially, these are the standard portion sizes in the tables, see page 136. After you have finished the first level test for all tested triggers, whether you perform a combination test and what it looks like depends on your results. It only makes sense if you have a combined intolerance and tolerate at least two triggers at your first level test. For the combination test, you take in the respective triggers together at the higher tolerance level.

How to run a test week

Day 1–3 before the test day	On the test day	Day 1–3 after
Your cube consumption should undercut your current levels by as narrow a margin as possible, but do not force yourself to eat more of anything than you want. Regulate only those levels that your partner confirms to be un-influenced on the test day, as symptoms can occur with three days' delay. If you do not feel as well on the test morning as you did at the end of the introductory diet, reschedule the test until you do.	Fill out the symptom test sheet on the test day and its three subsequent days.	
	At breakfast, lunch and dinner consume only as much of the tested trigger(s) as is part of the test dose and no more. For all other triggers, the current levels hold as described on the left.	Now go back to the levels you were lastly able to tolerate to check an aftereffect. Hence, if you test level 2 of a trigger go back down to level 1 for it and if you test level 3 go down to level 2.

Acceleration option: Perform the tests right after one another. Three days after the last test day, begin the next test day and thus save the three days described in the column on the left.

You do not have to fill out the symptom test sheet during the days leading up to the test (page 53). Instead, you can use the efficiency check sheet as your reference, but from the day of the test to the third day after it, document your symptoms (unless you determine an intolerance earlier).

Before starting, your partner needs to know which ones you want to test. Therefore, your partner needs to see the filled out table on page 481. With that information, the tests can be adapted appropriately. During multiple tests, always ask what your tolerance level after the test is to be able to keep your current restrictions correctly. If you tested and tolerated multiple triggers on one level, a combined test on that level follows.

Your testing partner prepares all test doses except for the fructans (F) and galactans (G). See the level table for F and G below to get a sense of the test quantities. For the test, eat the listed amounts of the following foods at the meals (M) breakfast, lunch and dinner. For the first test, these are the amounts:

Level, amount/Meal	Portion size	Amount per day
Level 1 F: 0.5g, G: 0.5 g	26g peas and 38g couscous	78g peas and 114g couscous
Level 2 F: 1g, G: 1g	53g peas and 77g couscous	159g peas and 231g couscous
Level 3 F: 1.5g, G: 1.5 g	79g peas and 115g couscous	237g peas and 345g couscous

By consuming the listed amounts, you double the consumed amount at Level 1. In the following days, continue eating according to the standard amounts as you find them in the tables (level 0). Then repeat the test at level 1 to cover the result. Tell your testing partner whether your symptoms worsened at the test dose and give her or him the filled out test sheet. Afterward, proceed likewise with the next cube in order of precedence. When you have finished this with all triggers that you want to check, you can perform a combined test of those trigger cube s you were able to stomach at Level 1, do a single level test at a higher level or consider the level tests finished.

When your testing partner confirms you have an intolerance, the level test for that cube is over. Enter the highest tolerated level that cube in the table in Chapter 3.1.3. You might find that you can stomach two triggers separately while keeping the levels for the other one but not both combined. In case that is so, remark that as well and eat accordingly. You can find the precise procedure in the flowcharts in Section 4.2. A level test of table sugar is unnecessary; you will get the tolerated amount by just multiplying the level amount of tolerated fructose by 10 (see Chapter 3.1.3).

For procedural reasons, wait until after you have repeated the test before trying to interpret the results. Please hand your partner remaining sugars and measurement instruments from the substitute test (if taken).

How to handle symptoms

After noting discomforts that were so severe that you told your test collaborate you malabsorbed the load, drink water (up to three liters per day are usually healthy) and take a walk to reduce your symptoms.

Note down the triggers to be tested:

	Fructose	Lactose	Sorbitol	Fruc/Galactans
To be tested? **(Yes/No)**		Begin with TL 2 ☐ TL 1 ☐		
In which sequence **(1, 2, …)**				
My calculated K.O. threshold grade is:				

Choose the triggers for which you want to determine your level. You test fructans and galactans together. For lactose, some keep half the standard amounts at the introductory diet and then test level 1, because they consider themselves more sensible than other with lactose intolerance—mark that in case. If you want to use the mathematical Option B, presented at the end of this Chapter or are using our downloadable tool, also enter your K.O.-grade from the efficiency check or give your partner the filled out excel sheets. Important: disregard triggers that you can stomach—you can consume products containing them just as you did before. Background: if your estimated symptom grade (lid value) after a level test is lower or equal to the estimate K.O. grade, you have tolerated the test load and thereby the level and otherwise you have not.

 ## Summary

As part of the strategy, you first performed the introductory diet to find out, if the diet did reduce your symptoms after all. If it had an effect and you determined your triggers with the breath or substitute test, you can go on to determine your individual sensitivity to avoid unnecessary restrictions.

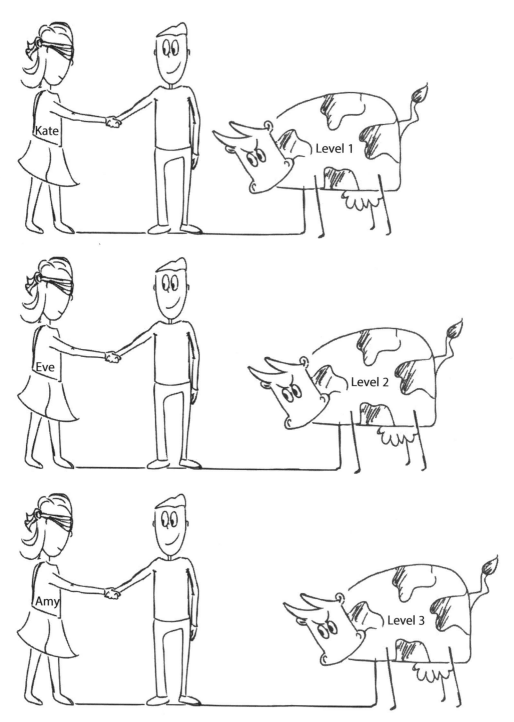

Everyone's sensitivity level is different.

STOP: The following pages are for only your testing partner to read, as they contain information regarding procedural safety—unless you want to do the test alone! Your partner's instructions will depend on your reactions; if you know how your partner is assessing you, you may alter your behavior and distort the results. Continue reading on page 468 to learn about the procedure underlying your partner's tolerance statements. Before and after the three pages for your testing partner are four empty pages. Thus, you can flick back from the end of the book to arrive at page 468 without reading them.

The **instructions** for your testing **partner** follow on page **456**. As the **reader** of the book, you should leave them **unread**, to **produce** a **more accurate** test **result**. Hence, open a new page that is farther **ahead** and then **flick back** to page **468**.

The **instructions** for your testing **partner** follow on page **456**. As the **reader** of the book, you should leave them **unread**, to **produce** a **more accurate** test **result**. Hence, open a new page that is much farther **ahead** and then **flick back** to page **468**.

The **instructions** for your testing **partner** follow on page **456**. As the **reader** of the book, you should leave them **unread**, to **produce** a **more accurate** test **result**. Hence, open a new page that is much farther **ahead** and then **flick back** to page **468**.

The **instructions** for your testing **partner** follow on page **456**. As the **reader** of the book, you should leave them **unread**, to **produce** a **more accurate** test **result**. Hence, open a new page that is much farther **ahead** and then **flick back** to page **468**.

Your friend needs your help! Instructions for testing partners:

You are not the testing partner but the aggrieved party? In case, I caught you! However, of course you also find instructions how to conduct the test yourself. If have a testing partner these lines are not for you, would you please finally move on to page 468!

Now we are in private. Your friend cannot stomach one or more common food ingredients and now wants to find out about the personal tolerance limit. Unfortunately, a placebo effect is quite common in this test. Your role in this test is critical for avoiding a false result. You are going to do two rounds for each ingredient, each test taking about a week. On one of the two days, you are going to hand out a placebo mix instead of the real one. Your friend does not know about the placebo. Just say that the double test is required to get valid results, as you also have to keep track of certain behaviors she or he might exhibit. IMPORTANT: Keep quiet about the placebo until **all** tests are done (use the fitting flowchart pp. 468) and you have talked the results over. Waiting until the end of that final discussion is important, as your friend may want to test another level as well. Between two test days are three monitoring days and three regeneration days. Here is what you need: a beaker, a letter scale, and three 0.5 L bottles. Also, instruct your friend to stop taking another bottle if the symptoms after drinking one are already indicating that the load was too much. Determine the ingredients to you have to do the test for on page 453 and for each of the following triggers, prepare:

> **Note in case you have to do the test without a testing partner:** Prepare the required test bottles on the eve before the test. Make the real and the placebo mix in an equal looking 1-liter-bottle with a non-transparent plastic label (the foil around the bottle on which the brand name shows up). If you use milk, make sure it is still usable for at least two weeks. Now use a pen and write placebo on a colored memo, fold it twice to form a smaller square and put it behind the label of the bottle with the placebo mix. On another note in the same color, you write real mix and put it behind the label of the other bottle. Then you put sticky tape around the tags. Then put both bottles into a non-transparent box that is longer, wider and higher than the bottles. Close it and then turn it around ten times. Thus, you have successfully outwitted yourself: put the bottles in the fridge! On the next morning, you take out one of the bottles, mark it with 1 and drink one third of the mixture in the morning, one third at lunchtime and the rest of the evening (you use one bottle with the daily amount instead of three here, according to the first column of the following tables).

If you find yourself trying to spy at the memo, give yourself a slap on the finger. After the three days following it, where you observed your symptoms, you repeat the test with the other bottle. Again, no fiddling with the label! You have to wait with that until the three observance days of the second bottle are over, too. Now check, how you stomached the placebo versus the real mix.

If your friend has not given you the substances for the test solution, you can order them online or from a pharmacy. You can also ask your pharmacist to weigh the amounts you need. From test to test, increase the level amounts according to the tables on the following pages. Begin with the level 1 (2 for lactose) amounts of the highest ranked ingredient on page 453. Before repeating the test, note whether you first handed out the real or placebo mix and the result. Ideally, you should ask for the symptom test sheet and write down L for reaL and A for plAcebo as well as the result. Then, keep all of the info sheets for the final discussion of all tests. If your friend has given you the K-grade, you can calculate the tolerance (see row L on page 475). If the L-grade is greater than or equal to K, this indicates an intolerance. There are three possible cases after each double test:

Case 1: Neither the placebo nor the real mix causes the symptoms to worsen, i.e., your friend can stomach the amounts of the ingredient, and you can test the next level. Tell her/him that.

Case 2: Only the real mix causes the symptoms to worsen, i.e., your friend is intolerant for the amount. The test series for this ingredient is over, and you can tell your friend.

Case 3: The placebo mix causes symptoms to worsen. Regardless of whether or not the real mix causes symptoms to worsen, as well, repeat the test with the same amount, starting with the placebo mix, but tell her that you reduced the amount to half of the dose. If your friend still reports an intolerance, abort the test and tell her/him that s/he has an intolerance for the amount, and the old levels remain current.

After the test and retest of the first level of the ingredient with rank number 1, test the next one in order (if applicable) also at the first level. After finishing all single tests for the stated ingredients at the first level, continue according to the level test flowchart on pp. 468. On the eve of one of the two test days, hand out three bottles with the real mix, and on the other one, three bottles with the placebo. At breakfast, lunch and dinner your friend drinks one bottle. Find the mixtures for each level in the following explanations and tables:

In the **left column** find the respective **level** and the **total amount** of substances per day, as it is easier to mix the **daily amount in one load** and **then divide** it among the **three bottles**. In the two columns on the right, find the amounts per bottle for the real/placebo substance.

Lactose-intolerance level-test: Required: 1 L reduced-fat milk, 1 L lactose-free cow milk, and vanilla extract. To hide taste differences between the regular, and the lactose-free milk, please add a little bit of vanilla extract (**v.**) to both.

Level and lactose amount as well as milk **sum/day**	Real (R) 3 × bottle with	Placebo (P) 3 × bottle with
Level 1 (3g/meal) per day 180 mL milk and ½ tsp. of **v.**	4 tbsp. (60 mL) milk 1 drop of **v.**	4 tbsp. lactose-free milk 1 drop of **v.**
Level 2 (6g/meal) per day 360 mL milk and ¾ tsp. of **v.**	120 mL milk (100) 2 drops of **v.**	120 mL lactose-free milk 2 drops of **v.**
Level 3 (9g/meal) per day 540 mL milk and 1 tsp. of **v.**	180 mL milk 3 drops of **v.**	180 mL lactose-free milk 3 drops of **v.**

Fructose-intolerance level-test: Required: fructose and table sugar. Mix the following amounts with 200 mL water and add a little bit of vanilla extract (**v.**). Important: you should not dilute the contents:

Level, real/placebo mix **per day**+600 mL water	Real (R) 3 × 200 mL water bottle with	Placebo (P) 3 × 200 mL water bottle with
Level 1, 3 R/3.5 P, 1 tsp. **v.**	1g fructose 3 drops of **v.**	1.17g sugar 3 drops of **v.**
Level 2, 6 R/7 P, 1 tsp. **v.**	2g fructose 3 drops of **v.**	2.34g sugar 3 drops of **v.**
Level 3, 9 R/10.5 P, 1 tsp. **v.**	3g fructose 3 drops of **v.**	3.51g sugar 3 drops of **v.**

Sorbitol-intolerance level-test: Required: 10g of sorbitol and table sugar. Mix the amounts with 200 mL of water and add a little bit of vanilla extract (**v.**). Important: you should not dilute the contents:

Level, real/placebo mix per day+600 mL water	Real (R) 3 × 200 mL water bottle with	Placebo (P) 3 × 200 mL water bottle with
Level 1, 0.3 R/0.2 P, 1 tsp. **v.**	0.1g sorbitol 3 drops of **v.**	0.06g sugar 3 drops of **v.**
Level 2, 1.2 R/0.7 P, 1 tsp. **v.**	0.4g sorbitol 3 drops of **v.**	0.24g sugar 3 drops of **v.**
Level 3, 3 R/1.26 P, 1 tsp. **v.**	0.7g sorbitol 3 drops of **v.**	0.42g sugar 3 drops of **v.**

Combination tests: For the lactose/fructose, lactose/sorbitol and lactose/ sorbitol/fructose combination tests, use the cow milk and lactose freed cow milk together with vanilla extract according to the level amounts for lactose. For the fructose/sorbitol combination test alone, use 200 mL of water. You put all ingredients that you test into the liquids. For each one, use the level amounts according to the single tables for the ingredients. After a tolerated combination test, the new combined tolerance levels hold for all further test days. Continue with another round of single tests for those triggers that your friend stomached well. This time, tell your friend that the new combined tolerance levels hold, and apply the Level 2 amounts for each test.

Thank you very much for your support! Even if you have to overcome scruples to knowingly trick your friend… You do not? Well then, enjoy the white lie for good reason!

The **instructions** for your testing **partner** begin on page **456**. As the **reader** of the book, you should leave them **unread**, to **produce** a **more accurate** test **result**. The book resumes on page 468.

The **instructions** for your testing **partner** begin on page **456**. As the **reader** of the book, you should leave them **unread**, to **produce** a **more accurate** test **result**. The book resumes on page 468.

The **instructions** for your testing **partner** begin on page **456**. As the **reader** of the book, you should leave them **unread**, to **produce** a **more accurate** test **result**. The book resumes on page 468.

The **instructions** for your testing **partner** begin on page **456**. As the **reader** of the book, you should leave them **unread**, to **produce** a **more accurate** test **result**.

4.2   Symptom-based test process

The following flow charts show you the next step, depending on your reaction to the test load. Remember, if you have symptoms after taking the first of three test loads on a test day, abort the test—as this shows that the tested sensitivity level is too high, and there is no point in tantalizing yourself.

You start the test with the first field of the flow chart that is relevant to you. The next step always depends on your test result. If you did not stomach a load, the test is over, and you should stick to the level below, which you did tolerate—at the beginning this is the standard amount in the tables in Chapter 3.

The flow charts

All statements assume that you want to perform the level test to the highest level. However, maybe, it is enough to you to know if you tolerate the next level, in the case just stop after the first test. If you do tolerate more than the standard level, note your level next to the multipliers, see Chapter 3.1.3. You will also be able to select your level when using our mobile phone application. Attention: During the combined level tests, you must not pass any level amount that holds for one of your triggers that you do not check at the time as this may otherwise distort the result. If it does happen, you have to repeat the check.

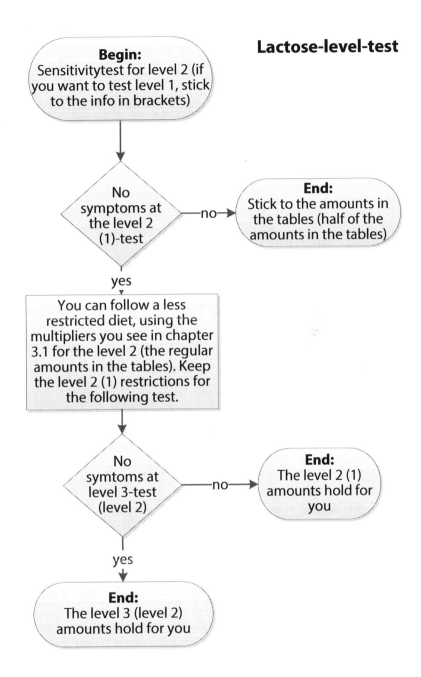

Lactose-level-test

Begin:
Sensitivitytest for level 2 (if you want to test level 1, stick to the info in brackets)

No symptoms at the level 2 (1)-test

—no→ **End:** Stick to the amounts in the tables (half of the amounts in the tables)

yes

You can follow a less restricted diet, using the multipliers you see in chapter 3.1 for the level 2 (the regular amounts in the tables). Keep the level 2 (1) restrictions for the following test.

No symtoms at level 3-test (level 2)

—no→ **End:** The level 2 (1) amounts hold for you

yes

End: The level 3 (level 2) amounts hold for you

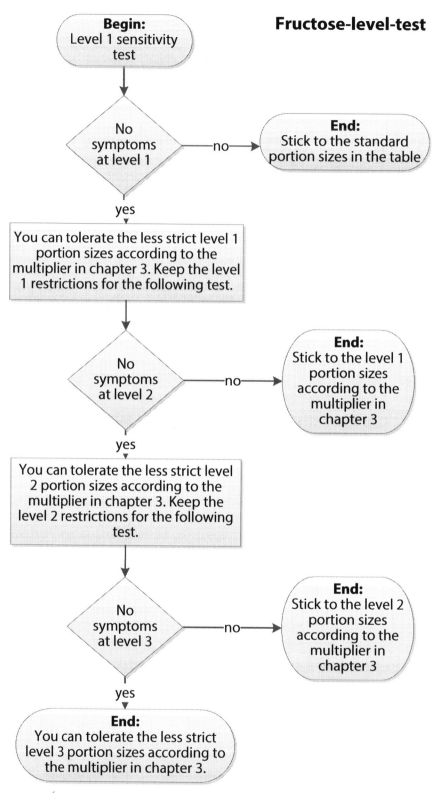

Fructose-level-test

Begin: Level 1 sensitivity test

No symptoms at level 1 —no→ **End:** Stick to the standard portion sizes in the table

yes

You can tolerate the less strict level 1 portion sizes according to the multiplier in chapter 3. Keep the level 1 restrictions for the following test.

No symptoms at level 2 —no→ **End:** Stick to the level 1 portion sizes according to the multiplier in chapter 3

yes

You can tolerate the less strict level 2 portion sizes according to the multiplier in chapter 3. Keep the level 2 restrictions for the following test.

No symptoms at level 3 —no→ **End:** Stick to the level 2 portion sizes according to the multiplier in chapter 3

yes

End: You can tolerate the less strict level 3 portion sizes according to the multiplier in chapter 3.

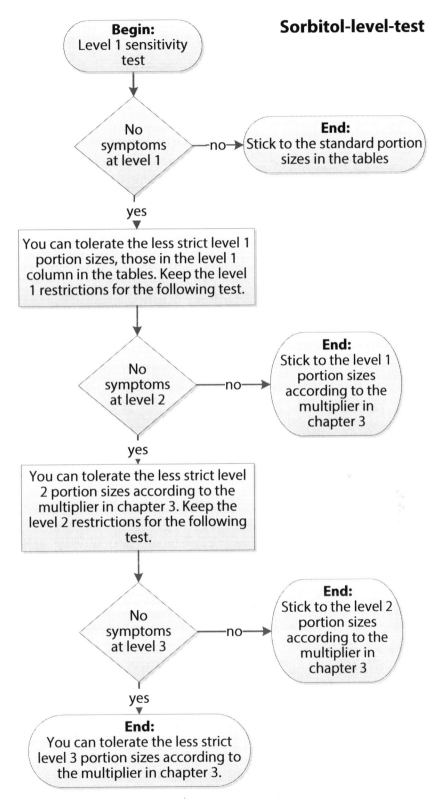

Sorbitol-level-test

Begin: Level 1 sensitivity test

No symptoms at level 1 —no→ **End:** Stick to the standard portion sizes in the tables

yes

You can tolerate the less strict level 1 portion sizes, those in the level 1 column in the tables. Keep the level 1 restrictions for the following test.

No symptoms at level 2 —no→ **End:** Stick to the level 1 portion sizes according to the multiplier in chapter 3

yes

You can tolerate the less strict level 2 portion sizes according to the multiplier in chapter 3. Keep the level 2 restrictions for the following test.

No symptoms at level 3 —no→ **End:** Stick to the level 2 portion sizes according to the multiplier in chapter 3

yes

End: You can tolerate the less strict level 3 portion sizes according to the multiplier in chapter 3.

Flowchart in case of combined intolerances

If you have more than one intolerance, it makes sense to make a combined test. What is its use? Whether you have symptoms depends on the combined amount of trigger cubes passing your enzyme workers to arrive at your large intestine. Let us assume; you tolerated various triggers at the first level—if you consume the maximum portion sizes for that level at the same time you may still suffer from symptoms due to the higher total load of triggers passing the enzyme workers. Hence, with the combination test you see if you can cope with the maximum amount.

An example with fictive triggers

To help you remain impartial, the triggers names refer to actual building materials: granite, wood, and sandstone. You test the trigger "granite" (you ranked as first; see page 453), "sandstone" (ranked second) and "wood" (ranked third). If, according to your testing partner, you could not tolerate "granite" during the first test at level 1, then continue consuming the standard amounts in the tables in Chapter 3 for it. If you were able to tolerate "sandstone" at level 1, however, you could consider this your new level for this trigger if consumed on its own (not in combination with other triggers). You find the factor with which you can multiply the amounts in the tables for your new level in Chapter 3.1.3. Let us say, moreover, that you were able to stomach "wood" at the first level. So next, perform a combined test of "sandstone" and "wood," as you were able to stomach these triggers independently in the single tests. Now, you will consume a mix of the two trigger cubes in your test dilution bottles. While taking this test, eat according to the level 0 portions for "granite." If you can stomach that test load, enter level 1 of "sandstone" and "wood" together with level 0 of "granite," as a new combined level in the table in Chapter 3.1.3.

Afterward, do another round of single level tests. Begin with the level 2 test for "sandstone." The test-dilution-bottle then contains the level 2 amount for "sandstone" and the level 1 amount for "wood." On the test days, keep "granite" at level 0. On the three days, that follow; eat according to the level 1 portion sizes of "sandstone" and "wood." Let us say you tolerate the level 2 amount of "sandstone" well but not that of wood. Now, you would enter level 2 for "sandstone" for the combined level 1 for "wood". Moreover, you could test the level 3 for "sandstone." At this test, again add the level 1 amount of "wood". If you can stomach it, note down level 3 for "sandstone" with level 1 for "wood".

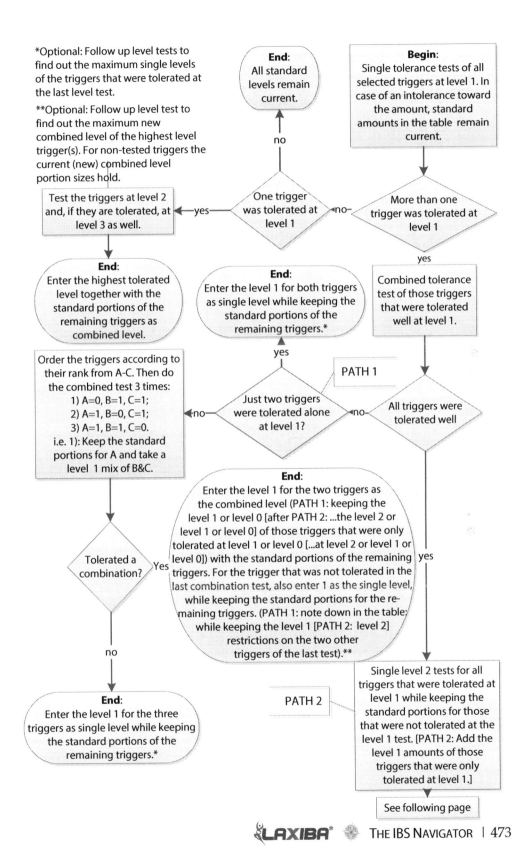

*Optional: Follow up level tests to find out the maximum single levels of the triggers that were tolerated at the last level test.

**Optional: Follow up level test to find out the maximum new combined level of the highest level trigger(s). For non-tested triggers the current (new) combined level portion sizes hold.

Begin: Single tolerance tests of all selected triggers at level 1. In case of an intolerance toward the amount, standard amounts in the table remain current.

End: All standard levels remain current.

More than one trigger was tolerated at level 1

One trigger was tolerated at level 1

Test the triggers at level 2 and, if they are tolerated, at level 3 as well.

End: Enter the highest tolerated level together with the standard portions of the remaining triggers as combined level.

End: Enter the level 1 for both triggers as single level while keeping the standard portions of the remaining triggers.*

Combined tolerance test of those triggers that were tolerated well at level 1.

PATH 1

Order the triggers according to their rank from A-C. Then do the combined test 3 times:
1) A=0, B=1, C=1;
2) A=1, B=0, C=1;
3) A=1, B=1, C=0.
i.e. 1): Keep the standard portions for A and take a level 1 mix of B&C.

Just two triggers were tolerated alone at level 1?

All triggers were tolerated well

End: Enter the level 1 for the two triggers as the combined level (PATH 1: keeping the level 1 or level 0 [after PATH 2: ...the level 2 or level 1 or level 0] of those triggers that were only tolerated at level 1 or level 0 [...at level 2 or level 1 or level 0]) with the standard portions of the remaining triggers. For the trigger that was not tolerated in the last combination test, also enter 1 as the single level, while keeping the standard portions for the re-maining triggers. (PATH 1: note down in the table: while keeping the level 1 [PATH 2: level 2] restrictions on the two other triggers of the last test).**

Tolerated a combination?

End: Enter the level 1 for the three triggers as single level while keeping the standard portions of the remaining triggers.*

PATH 2

Single level 2 tests for all triggers that were tolerated at level 1 while keeping the standard portions for those that were not tolerated at the level 1 test. [PATH 2: Add the level 1 amounts of those triggers that were only tolerated at level 1.]

See following page

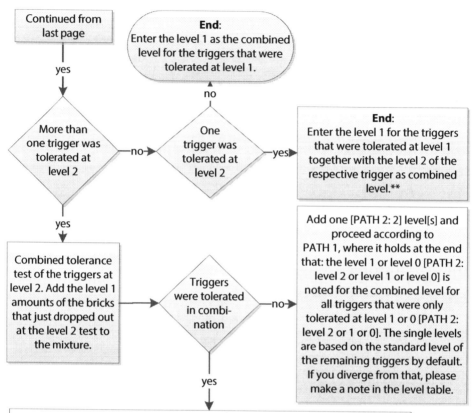

Proceed according to PATH 2, and depending on the field, add a level or follow the instructions in the squared brackets. Or, if you arrive at this field for the second time, note the highest tolerated levels of the triggers as the combined levels. The single levels are regularly based on the standard level of the remaining trigger. If you diverge from that, please make a note in the level table.

4.3 Test result calculation table

You have two calculation options: option **A** is slightly simpler than option **B**. Real cracks immediately start with **B**. **B** saves time at any further check, and you get a statement on your tolerance. [5]

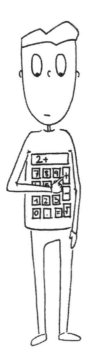

---

[5] From a statistical point of view the survey is slim and the result vague.

4.3.1　The efficiency check calculation table

You use the following table and enter the total intensity of bloating of the respective day into the row **A**. Into the first four cells of that row, you enter the results of the **efficiency check days**, i.e. the last days of your introductory diet. Into the remaining four fields of that row, you enter the values of the **status-quo-days** (the four days before starting your introductory diet, hence, before reducing your trigger consumption).

Calculation option A: Determine $A1$ = total stool grade at the first day of your efficiency check, i.e. your grade in the morning (you calculate your stool grade by multiplying your stool value by the number of defecations you had in the morning) plus the grade at lunchtime plus the grade at the evening. Likewise, you proceed with all other **A**-numbers. Afterward, you determine the **B**-numbers: $B1 = A1$ plus the bloating grade at the first efficiency-check-day plus the pain grade on that day. You calculate $B2$ likewise with the grades for day 2 and so on. Next, you calculate $C2$ and afterward $D2$, which is the average of the status-quo-check-days. To interpret the result, you compare $D2$ with the highest day-grade of the efficiency-check-days, the highest grade of the group $B1$ to $B4$. When checking the success of the introductory diet, it holds that the greater $D2$ lies above the maximum grade of the group the more likely it is that the introductory diet was successful in lowering your symptoms.

Calculation Option B: You calculate $A1$ to $A8$ as well as $B1$ to $B8$ according to the calculation option **A**. Afterward, you estimate $C1$ and $D1$, as well as $C2$ and $D2$ and proceed with the steps described in the table up to K. To interpret the result you compare the $D2$-value with the K-value, i.e. the K. O.[6] threshold grade. At the introductory diet, it holds that: If $D2$ is bigger or equal to the K-grade; this indicates that the diet successfully lowered your symptoms.

If the diet fails, however, try sensitivity level zero if you are lactose intolerant and otherwise a fructans and galactans diet or check alternative triggers, see page 482.

---

[6] K = if L tops this K.-O.-threshold, the level test amount is too much for your enzyme workers.

	Efficiency check day-				Status-quo-check-day before introductory diet			
	1:	2:	3:	4:	1:	2:	3:	4:
A	A1	A3	A3	A4	A5	A6	A7	A8

Enter the total stool grade for each day into the A-cells

	1:	2:	3:	4:	1:	2:	3:	4:
B	B1	B2	B3	B4	B5	B6	B7	B8

B5 = stool- + bloating- + pain grade on status-quo-check-day 1

C	C1	C1 = B1 + B2 + B3 + B4 Sum of cells B1 to B4	C2
		C2 = B5 + B6 + B7 + B8 Sum of cells B5 to B8	
D	D1	D1 = C1 ÷ 4 Divide your result in cell C1 by 4	D2
		D2 = C2 ÷ 4 Divide your result in cell C2 by 4	

E	E1	E2	E3	E4	E1 = B1 - D1, E2 = B2 - D1 etc. To calculate E1, subtract D1 from B1. Negative results are possible.
F	F1	F2	F3	F4	F1 = E1 x E1, F2 = E2 x E2 etc. To calculate F1, multiply E1 by itself. As minus times minus is plus, all results are positive.

G	G	G = F1 + F2 + F3 + F4 Add your results of the cells F1 to F4
H	H	H = G ÷ 4 Divide G by 4
I	I	I = Take the root of H Take the root of your result in H. On your calculator the root symbol looks like this: $\sqrt{\ }$.
J	J	J = I x 2 Multiply I by 2
K	K	K = J + D1 Add the result of cell J to the one in cell D1. The K-grade is the K. O. threshold grade as the success of the introductory diet depends on it. The diet lowered your symptoms if D2 is bigger than K (D2 > K). In addition, you can assess the success of the sensitivity level test with it. You tolerated the tested level if L is not bigger than K (L ≤ K). Please transfer the K-grade to the level test table.

1. Efficiency check calculation with page 55-56 values

	Efficiency-check-day-				Status-quo-check-day before introductory diet				
	1:	**2:**	**3:**	**4:**	**1:**		**2:**	**3:**	**4:**
A	A1	A3	A3	A4	A5		A6	A7	A8
	3	2	3	2		16	14	12	14

Enter the total stool grade for each day into the A-cells

B	B1	B2	B3	B4	B5		B6	B7	B8
	9	8	11	8		30	30	31	28

B5 = stool- + bloating- + pain grade on status-quo-check-day 1

C	C1	C1 = B1 + B2 + B3 + B4 Sum of cells B1 to B4	C2
	36	C2 = B5 + B6 + B7 + B8 Sum of cells B5 to B8	119
D	D1	D1 = C1 ÷ 4 Divide your result in cell C1 by 4	D2
	9	D2 = C2 ÷ 4 Divide your result in cell C2 by 4	29.75

E	E1	E2	E3	E4	E1 = B1 - D1, E2 = B2 - D1 etc.
					To calculate E1, subtract D1 from B1. Negative
	0	-1	2	-1	results are possible.
F	F1	F2	F3	F4	F1 = E1 x E1, F2 = E2 x E2 etc.
					To calculate F1, multiply E1 by itself. As minus
	0	1	4	1	times minus is plus, all results are positive.

G	G	G = F1 + F2 + F3 + F4
	6	Add your results of the cells F1 to F4
H	H	H = G ÷ 4
	1.5	Divide G by 4
I	I	I = Take the root of H Take the root of your result in H. On your
	1.22	calculator the root symbol looks like this: √.
J	J	J = I x 2
	2.45	Multiply I by 2
K	K	K = J + D1
		Add the result of cell J to the one in cell D1. The K-grade is called
	11.45	K. O. threshold grade as the success of the introductory diet (D2 >
		K) and the sensitivity level test (L ≤ K) depend on it.

Calculation method A

D2 is 29.75 and thus way larger than the highest day grade, 11, (B3) of the group B1 to B4, which indicates the success of the introductory diet.

Calculation method B

D2 = 29.75 is bigger than K = 11.45, and that shows the success of the diet. Had D2 been smaller or equal to K, try a fructans and galactans diet or a lactose diet at sensitivity level 0 or a check for alternative triggers (see Chapter 4.4).

4.3.2   The level test calculation table

Use the following table and enter the grades of the level test days. You only need to estimate the grades from the level test sheet (enter them into B5 to B8. If you used math option B, just enter the K value, and you are ready to determine your result. If you use math option A, you have to calculate D1. Having done the introductory diet is, of course, necessary.

Calculation option A: *A1* = stool grade at the first efficiency-check-day, i.e. grade in the morning (multiply the stool value in the morning by the number of defecations you had in the morning) plus stool grade at lunchtime plus stool grade at the evening. Enter your total stool grade into the cell with the *A1* in italic. Likewise, you proceed with all other **A**-Numbers. Afterward, estimate the **B-grades**: *B1* = *A1* plus total bloating grade plus total pain grade on the test day. You calculate *B2* with the grades for the first day after the test day and so on. Next, you determine *C1* and afterward *D1*, i.e. the average of the efficiency-check days. To interpret the result, compare *D1* with the highest day grade of the level test days, *B5* to *B8*. When checking the success of the diet, it holds that the much greater the largest day grade is compared to *D1*, the rather you did not tolerate the load of the tested sensitivity level. If that is the case, stick to the portion sizes of a lower sensitivity level.

Calculation option B: If you calculated *K* at the efficiency check—you should have as doing a level test before checking the efficiency of the diet makes no sense—just copy it to this table. Aside from it, all you need is to estimate *B1* to *B8* according to calculation option **A** and determine *L*. For the assessment, you compare the *L*-, i.e. the level grade with the *K*-grade, the K.-O.-threshold grade. It holds: if *L* is bigger than *K*, this means that the amount consumed during the test has triggered symptoms. Therefore, you should stick to the portion sizes of the sensitivity level below at which your symptoms improved. If *L* is lower than *K*, you tolerated the level amount and can have the less restricted diet according to that level. What is more, you can check an even higher sensitivity level if you want.

	Efficiency-check-day-				Level-test	day after test day-		
	1:	**2:**	**3:**	**4:**	**Test day**	**1:**	**2:**	**3:**
A	A1	A3	A3	A4	A5	A6	A7	A8

Enter the total stool grade for each day into the A-cells

B	B1	B2	B3	B4	B5	B6	B7	B8

B5 = stool- + bloating- + pain grade on status-quo-check-day 1

C	C1	$C1 = B1 + B2 + B3 + B4$ Sum of the cells B1 to B4
D	D1	$D1 = C1 \div 4$ Divide your results in cell C1 by 4
K	K	Please copy the K grade you estimated at the end of the introductory diet to this field. If you have not yet calculated it, do it now as described in the efficiency-check-calculation-table.
L	L	L = is the biggest grade of the group: B5, B6, B7, B8. This group contains the results of the level test day (B5) and the three days following it (B6 to B8). With the L-grade, you evaluate the current Level test. Assessment:

L > K, if L is bigger than K, it means that the tested load for that level caused you symptoms and that you, therefore, should adjust your diet to a lower sensitivity level.

L ≤ K, if L is lower or equal to K, it means that you tolerated the load of that level per meal.

1. Level test calculation with the page 55-56 values

	Efficiency-check-day-				Level-test	day after test day-		
	1:	**2:**	**3:**	**4:**	**Test day**	**1:**	**2:**	**3:**
A	A1	A3	A3	A4	A5	A6	A7	A8
	3	2	3	2	16	14	12	14
	Enter the total stool grade for each day into the A-cells							
B	B1	B2	B3	B4	B5	B6	B7	B8
	9	8	11	8	30	30	31	28
	B5 = stool- + bloating- + pain grade on status-quo-check-day 1							
C	C1	C1 = B1 + B2 + B3 + B4 Sum of the cells B1 to B4						
	36							
D	D1	D1 = C1 ÷ 4 Divide your results in cell C1 by 4						
	9							
K	K	*Please copy the K grade you estimated at the end of the introductory diet to this field. If you have not yet calculated it, do it now as described in the efficiency-check-calculation-table.*						
	11.45							
L	L	L = is the biggest grade of the group: B5, B6, B7, B8. This group contains the results of the level test day (B5) and the three days following it (B6 to B8). With the L-grade, you evaluate the current Level test. Assessment:						
		L > K, if L is bigger than K, it means that the tested load for that level caused you symptoms and that you, therefore, should adjust your diet to a lower sensitivity level.						
	31	L ≤ K, if L is lower or equal to K, it means that you tolerated the load of that level per meal.						

Calculation method A

The highest total grade of a day of the group B5 to B8, B7 = 31 is way above D1 = 9, which indicates that you did not tolerate the level amount. If the highest grade of the group B5 to B8 had been smaller or equal to 9, you would have tolerated the sensitivity level amount and could have taken a less restricted diet according to the amounts of that level. Moreover, you could have tested the next level for people that are even less sensitive.

Calculation method B

As L = 31 is bigger than K = 11.45, you have not tolerated the level load of that trigger. Had L been smaller or equal to 11.45, you would have endured the level amount and could have followed the less strict diet for that level. Moreover, you could have tested the next higher tolerance level.

4.4 Alternative strategies

General causes of abdominal discomfort

The following foods show up as triggers most often in an analysis of nutrition diaries. On a subjective scale from **1 (seldom) to 5 (very often)**:

5 wheat, milk, coffee, eggs and potatoes
4 nuts
2 rye, barley, corn 2, oats 2, banana 2, onions 2, peas 2.

One can explain the malabsorptions for all of these foods except for coffee, corn, eggs, nuts, and potatoes by malabsorptions of one of our core triggers fructose, lactose, fructans, and galactans or sorbitol based on the scientific analysis checked by the author. The author was unable to find studies that analyzed the fructans and galactanscontent of eggs, coffee, and nuts.

Alternative diet strategy

Sometimes a product such as coffee causes discomfort or acts as a trigger for reasons other than the carbohydrates (triggers) that are the focus of this book. There may be a relation between your symptoms and your coffee consumption? Alternatively, you have an assumption concerning a food or an ingredient like aspartame, carrageenan, chicory root, guar gum, inulin, potassium benzoate, maltodextrin, modified starch (often included in drugs) or xanthan. In these cases, I recommend you take an alternative introductory diet. What you need for that is a filled out status-quo-ckeck-symptom test sheet. Note down your symptoms in the following four days if you have not done so, yet.
Then, you abstain from coffee, corn, eggs, nuts, and potatoes, as well as up to two to four other products or ingredients that you suspect might be causing you trouble. Before starting the diet take note of the greatest amount, you are likely to consume of the affected foods at breakfast, lunch and dinner in gram or pieces. You need that sheet later to find out which of the foods if any, caused your symptoms. Hence, keep that sheet well. Then at the end of the three test weeks, use the symptom test sheet again to determine the efficiency of the diet by comparing it with your former status quo sheet. If you want, you can also employ the mentioned calculation methods, using the final sheet from your alternative diet as your efficiency check sheet. Even if I repeat myself, before starting the diet, discuss potential personal risks with your doctor.

If the diet successfully relieved your symptoms (D2 is larger than K), you now move on with it testing each of the foods or ingredients you abstained from alone with three days in between. To do that, first, look at the notes you made regarding your usual portion sizes of the foods included in the test. If you avoid ingredients, you use products you usually eat and that contain it. Choose one of the foods or ingredients, and on test day, eat the amounts that are typical for you at the times you usually eat them. Let us say you start with coffee. So on the test day, you drink it as you usually did before the diet. On the three following days, you avoid it just like the other foods you are testing and note down your symptoms, as you did on the test day. If then if your symptoms have worsened, then coffee triggers them. If you are using math Option B (see page 475), you estimated your L-grade for coffee and found it to be greater than the K grade. During the test weeks, continue to avoid the foods you still have to test and those for which the test showed an intolerance. If you had no symptoms during the test, it indicates that you can safely consume the given food as you did before the alternative introductory diet.

If you malabsorbed a food or an ingredient, you have two options: either you can completely avoid the food, or you can determine a tolerable portion size by performing a level test. For the level test, you divide your usual portion by four. Starting three days before the test, refrain from all symptom-inducing foods you found. On the test day, eat the to-be-tested portion size at the times you normally have your three main meals. Start with one-fourth of your regular portion size. If your symptoms do not worsen, you use the level test calculation method and determine L, repeat the test on the fourth day after your test day with half of your typical portion size. If you can stomach this amount, repeat the test with three-fourths of your regular portion. If you were not able to stomach one-fourth of your average portion size, you could choose to avoid the food or ingredient or test it further at a reduced test portion size. If symptoms arose at half your usual portion size, then consider your tolerable amount to be one-fourth of a full portion for you; if they arose at three-fourths, your tolerable amount is a half-portion. If you could not narrow your symptoms down to a critical food or ingredient, return to your usual diet. Probably, the foods and ingredients you tested are not triggering your symptoms. You could check other foods afterward. If this did not help either, low dosage antidepressants, like loperamide in the case of bloating and diarrhea, constitute one possible remaining alternative for addressing your symptoms. Moreover, other causes like a histamine intolerance or multiple chemical sensitivity (MCS) are possible. Consult your doctor to discuss these options further.

Sources

Ali, M., Rellos, P., & Cox, T. M. (1998). Heriditary fruktose intolerance. *Journal of Medical Genetics*, 35(5), 353-365.

American Cancer Society (2015). *Colorectal cancer and early detection*. Retrieved from: www.cancer.org/acs/groups/cis/documents/webcontent/003170-pdf.pdf.

Ananthakrishnan, A. N., Higuchi, L. M., Huang, E. S., Khalili, H., Richter, J. M., Fuchs, C. S., & Chan, A. T. (2012). Aspirin, nonsteroidal anti-inflammatory drug use, and risk for Crohn disease and ulcerative colitis: a cohort study. *Annals of Internal Medicine*, 156(5), 350-359.

Barrett, J. S., Gearry, R. B., Muir, J. G., Irving, P. M., Rose, R., Rosella, O., ... & Gibson, P. R. (2010). Dietary poorly absorbed, short-chain carbohydrates increase delivery of water and fermentable substrates to the proximal colon. *Alimentary Pharmacology & Therapeutics*, 31(8), 874-882.

Balasubramanya, N. N., Sarwar, & Narayanan, K. M. (1993). Effect of stage of lactation on oligosaccharides level in milk. *Indian Journal of Dairy & Biosciences*, 4, 58-60.

Belitz, H.-D., Grosch, W., & Schieberle, P. (2008). *Lehrbuch der Lebensmittelchemie* (6th ed.). Berlin Heidelberg: Springer.

Berekoven, L., Eckert, W., Ellenrieder, P. (2009). Marktforschung: *Methodische Grundlagen und praktische Anwendung* (12th ed.). Wiesbaden: Gabler.

Bernstein, C. N., Fried, M., Krabshuis, J. H., Cohen, H., Eliakim, R., Fedail, S., ... & Watermeyer, G. (2010). World Gastroenterology Organization Practice Guidelines for the diagnosis and management of IBD in 2010. *Inflammatory Bowel Diseases*, 16(1), 112-124.

Biesiekierski, J. R., Rosella, O., Rose, R., Liels, K., Barrett, J. S., Shepherd, S. J., ... & Muir, J. G. (2011). Quantification of fructans, galacto-oligosacharides and other short-chain carbohydrates in processed grains and cereals. *Journal of Human Nutrition and Dietetics*, 24(2), 154-176.

Binnendijk, K. H., & Rijkers, G. T. (2013). What is a health benefit? An evaluation of EFSA opinions on health benefits with reference to probiotics. *Beneficial Microbes*, 4(3), 223-230.

Blumenthal, M. (1998). *The Complete German Commission E Monographs; Therapeutic Guide to Herbal Medicine*. Boston, MA: Integrative Medicine Communications.

Boehm, G., & Stahl, B. (2007). Oligosaccharides from milk. *The Journal of Nutrition*, 137(3), 847S-849S.

Bowden, P. (2011). *Telling It Like It Is*. Paul Bowden.

Briançon, S., Boini, S., Bertrais, S., Guillemin, F., Galan, P., & Hercberg, S. (2011). Long-term antioxidant supplementation has no effect on health-related quality of life: The randomized, double-blind, placebo-controlled, primary prevention SU.VI.MAX trial. *International Journal of Epidemiology*, 40(6), 1605-1616.

Campbell, J. M., Fahey, G. C., & Wolf, B. W. (1997). Selected indigestible oligosaccharides affect large bowel mass, cecal and fecal short-chain fatty acids, pH and microflora in rats. *The Journal of Nutrition*, 127(1), 130-136.

Chi, W. J., Chang, Y. K., & Hong, S. K. (2012). Agar degradation by microorganisms and agar-degrading enzymes. *Applied Microbiology and Biotechnology*, 94(4), 917-930.

Choi, Y. K; Johlin Jr., F. C.; Summers, R.W., Jackson, M., & Rao, S. S. C. (2003). Fruktose intolerance: an under-recognized problem. *The American Journal of Gastroenterology*, 98(6) 2003, S. 1348-1353.

CIAA (n. d.). *CIAA agreed reference values for GDAs* [Table]. Retrieved from http://gda.fooddrinkeurope.eu/asp2/gdas_portions_rationale.asp?doc_id=127.

Connor, W. E. (2000). Importance of n− 3 fatty acids in health and disease. *The American Journal of Clinical nutrition*, 71(1), 171S-175S.

Coraggio, L. (1990). *Deleterious Effects of Intermittent Interruptions on the Task Performance of Knowledge Workers: A Laboratory Investigation* (Doctoral Dissertation). Retrieved from http://arizona.openrepository.com.

Corazza, G. R., Strocchi, A., Rossi, R., Sirola, D., & Fasbarrini, G. (1988). Sorbitol malabsorption in normal volunteers and in patients with celiac disease. *Gut*, 29(1), 44-48.

Cummings, J. H. (1981). Short chain fatty acids in the human colon. *Gut*, 22(9), 763-779.

Cummings, J. H., & Macfarlane, G. T. (1997). Role of intestinal bacteria in nutrient metabolism. *Journal of Parental and Enteral Nutrition*, 21(6), 357-365.

DGE (2013). Vollwertig essen und trinken nach den 10 Regeln der DGE. 9th Edition, Bonn.

Donker, G. A., Foets, M., & Spreeuwenberg, P. (1999). Patients with irritable bowel syndrome: health status and use of healthcare services. *British Journal of General Practice*, 49(447), 787-792.

Drossman, D. A., Li, Z., Andruzzi, E., Temple, R. D., Talley, N. J., Thompson, W. G. ...Corazziari, E. et al. (1993). US householder survey of functional gastrointestinal disorders: prevalence, sociodemography, and health impact. *Digestive Diseases and Sciences*, 38(9), 1569-1580.

Dukas, L., Willett, W. C., & Giovannucci, E. L. (2003). Association between physical activity, fiber intake, and other lifestyle variables and constipation in a study of women. *The American Journal of Gastroenterology*, 98(8), 1790-1796.

EFSA (2007). Opinion of the scientific panel on dietetic products, nutrition and allergies on a request from the commission related to a notification from epa on lactitol pursuant to article 6, paragraph 11 of directive 2000/13/ec- for permanent exemption from labeling. *The EFSA Journal*, 5(10), 565-570.

EFSA (2012a). Scientific opinion on dietary reference values for protein. *The EFSA Journal*, 10(2), 2557-2622.

EFSA (2012b). Scientific opinion on the substantiation of health claims related to lactobacillus casei dg cncm i-1572 and decreasing potentially pathogenic gastro-intestinal microorganisms (id 2949, 3061, further assessment) pursuant to article 13(1) of regulation (ec) no 1924/2006. *The EFSA Journal*, 10(6), 2723-2637.

EFSA (2012c). Scientific opinion on the tolerable upper intake level of eicosapentaenoic acid (epa), docosahexaenoic acid (dha) and docosapentaenoic acid (dpa). *The EFSA Journal*, 10(7), 2815-2862.

EFSA (2013). scientific opinion on the substantiation of a health claim related to bimuno® gos and reducing gastro-intestinal discomfort pursuant to article 13(5) of regulation (ec) no 1924/2006. *The EFSA Journal*, 11(6), 3259-3268.

Eisenführ, F., Weber, M., & Langer, T. (2010): *Rational Decision Making*, Heidelberg, Berlin: Springer.

Erdman, K., Tunnicliffe, J., Lun, V. M., & Reimer, R. A. (2013). Eating patterns and composition of meals and snacks in elite canadian athletes. *International Journal Of Sport Nutrition & Exercise Metabolism*, 23(3), 210-219.

Evans, J. M., McMahon, A. D., Murray, F. E., McDevitt, D. G., & MacDonald, T. M. (1997). Non-steroidal anti-inflammatory drugs are associated with emergency admission to hospital for colitis due to inflammatory bowel disease. *Gut*, 40(5), 619-622.

Falony, G., Verschaeren, A. De Bruycker, F., De Preter, V., Verbecke, F. L., & De Vuyst L. (2009b). In vitro kinetics of prebiotic inulin-type fructan fermentation by butyrate-producing colon bacteria: implementation of online gas chromatography for quantitative analysis of carbon dioxide and hydrogen gas production. *Applied Environmental Microbiology*, 75(18), 5884-5892.

FAO (2008). Fats and fatty acids in human nutrition. *FAO Food and Nutrition Paper*, 91, 9-20.

Farquhar, P. H., & Keller, L. R. (1989). Preference intensity measurement. *Annals of Operations Research*, 19(1), 205-217.

Farshchi, H. R., Taylor, M. A., & Macdonald, I. A. (2004). Regular meal frequency creates more appropriate insulin sensitivity and lipid profiles compared with irregular meal frequency in healthy lean women. *European Journal of Clinical Nutrition*, 58(7), 1071-1077.

Fasano, A., & Catassi, C. (2001). Current approaches to diagnosis and treatment of celiac disease: an evolving spectrum. *Gastroenterology*, 120(3), 636-651.

Fass, R., Fullerton, S., Naliboff, B., Hirsh, T., & Mayer, E. A. (1998). Sexual dysfunction in patients with irritable bowel syndrom and non-ulcer dyspepsia. *Digestion*, 59(1), 79-85.

Fernández-Bañares, F., Esteve-Pardo, M., de Leon, R., Humbert, P., Cabré, E., Llovet, J. M., & Gassull, M. A. (1993). Sugar malabsorption in functional bowel disease: clinical implications. *American Journal of Gastroenterology*, 88(12), 2044-2050.

Fox, K. (2013). N. t.. In Wells, V., Wyness, L., & Coe, S. (Eds.). The British Nutrition Foundation's 45th anniversary conference: behaviour change in relation to healthier lifestyles. *Nutrition Bulletin*, 38(1), 100-107.

Gaby, A. R. (2005). Adverse effects of dietary fruktose. *Alternative medicine review*, 10(4).

Gay-Crosier, F., Schreiber, G., & Hauser, C. (2000). Anaphylaxis from inulin in vegetables and processed food. *The New England Journal of Medicine*, 342(18), 1372.

German, J., Freeman, S., Lebrilla, C., & Mills, D. (2008). Human milk oligosaccharides: evolution, structures and bioselectivity as substrates for intestinal bacteria, *Nestlé Nutrition Workshop, Pediatric Program*, 62, 205-222.

Gibson, P. R., Newnham, E., Barrett, J. S., Shepherd, S. J., & Muir, J. G. (2007). Review article: Fruktose malabsorption and the bigger picture. *Alimentary Pharmacology & Therapeutics*, 25(4), 349-363.

Gibson, P. R., & Shepherd, S. J. (2010). Evidence-based dietary management of functional gastrointestinal symptoms: the fodmap approach. *Journal of Gastroenterology and Hepatology*, 25(2), 252-258.

Gilbert, P. (2013). N. t.. In Wells, V., Wyness, L., & Coe, S. (Eds.). The British Nutrition Foundation's 45th anniversary conference: behaviour change in relation to healthier lifestyles. *Nutrition Bulletin*, 38(1), 100-107.

Goldstein, R., Braverman, D., & Stankiewicz, H. (2000). Carbohydrate malabsorption and the effect of dietary restriction on symptoms of irritable bowel syndrome and functional bowel complaints. *Israel Medical Association Journal*, 2(8), 583-587.

Gralnek, I. M., Hays, R. D., Kilbourne, A., Naliboff, B., & Mayer, E. A. (2000). The impact of irritable bowel syndrome on health-related quality of life. *Gastroenterology*, 119(3), 654-660.

Hahn, B. A., Kirchdoerfer, L. J., Fullerton, S., & Mayer, S. (1997). Patient perceived severity of irritable bowel syndrome in relation to symptoms, health resource utilization and quality of life. *Alimentary Pharmacology and Therapeutics*, 11(3), 553-559.

Hallert, C., Grant, C., Grehn, S., Grännö, C., Hultén, S., Midhagen, G., ... & Valdimarsson, T. (2002). Evidence of poor vitamin status in coeliac patients on a gluten-free diet for 10 years. *Alimentary Pharmacology & Therapeutics*, 16(7), 1333-1339.

Hanauer, S. B. (2006). Inflammatory bowel disease: epidemiology, pathogenesis, and therapeutic opportunities. *Inflammatory Bowel Diseases*, 12(5), S3-S9.

Hawthorne, B., Lambert, S., Scott, D., & Scott, B. (1991). Food intolerance and the irritable bowel syndrome. *Journal of Human Nutrition and Dietetics*, 4(1), 19–23.

Hawking, S. (n. d.). *Publications*. Retrieved from http://hawking.org.uk/publications.html.

Hillson, M. (2013). N. t.. In Wells, V., Wyness, L., & Coe, S. (Eds.). The British Nutrition Foundation's 45th anniversary conference: behaviour change in relation to healthier lifestyles. *Nutrition Bulletin*, 38(1), 100-107.

Hoekstra, J. H., van Kempen, A. A. M. W., & Kneepkens, C. M. F. (1993). Apple juice malabsorption: fruktose or sorbitol?. *Journal of Pediatric Gastroenterology and Nutrition*, 16(1), 39-42.

Huether, G. (Lecturer) (2014*). Interview mit Prof. Dr. Gerald Hüther zu Angst & Berufung*. Retrieved from http://www.coach-your-self.tv/Startseite/TV/InterviewmitProfDrH%c3%BCtherzuAngstBerufung/tabid/1341/Default.aspx

Hyams, J. S. (1983). Sorbitol intolerance: an unappreciated cause of functional gastrointestinal complaints. *Gastroenterology*, 84(1)1, 30-33.

Hyams, J. S., Etienne, N. L., Leichtner, A. M., & Theuer, R. C. (1988). Carbohydrate malabsorption following fruit juice ingestion in young children. *Pediatrics*, 82(1), 64-68.

Itzkowitz, S. H. & Daniel, H. (2005). Concensus Coference: colorectal cancer screening and surveillance in inflammatory bowel disease. *Inflammatory Bowel Disease*, 11(3).

Jameson, S. (2000). Coeliac disease, insulin-like growth factor, bone mineral density, and zinc. *Scandinavian Journal of Gastroenterology*, 35(8), 894-896.

Jemal, A., Siegel, R., Ward, E., Murray, T., Xu, J. Smigal, C., & Thun, M. J. (2006). Cancer statistics, 2006. *CA: A Cancer Journal for Clinicians*, 56(2), 106-130.

Jensen, R. G., Blanc, B., & Patton, S. (1995). Particulate constituents in human and bovine milks. In Jensen, R. G. (Ed.), *Handbook of Milk Composition* (pp. 51-62). San Diego: Academic Press.

Kennedy, E. (2004). Dietary diversity, diet quality, and body weight regulation. *Nutrition Reviews*, 62(s2), S78-S81.

Kneepkens, C. M. F., Vonk, R. J., & Fernandes, J. (1984). Incomplete intestinal absorption of fruktose. *Archives of Disease in Childhood*, 59(8), 735-738.

Kneepkens, C. M. F., Jakobs, C., & Douwes, A. C. (1989): Apple juice, fruktose, and chronic nonspecific diarrhoea. *Pediatrics*, 148(6), 571-573.

Knudsen, B. K., & Hessov, I. (1995). Recovery of inulin from Jerusalem artichoke (Helianthus tuberosus L.) in the small intestine of man. *British Journal of Nutrition*, 74(01), 101-113.

Komericki, P., Akkilic-Materna, M., Strimitzer, T., Weyermair, K., Hammer, H. F., & Aberer, W. (2012). Oral xylose isomerase decreases breath hydrogen excretion and improves gastrointestinal symptoms in fruktose malabsorption – a double-blind, placebo-controlled study. *Alimentary Pharmacology & Therapeutics*, 36(10), 980-987.

Kornbluth, A., & Sachar, D. B. (2004). Ulcerative colitis practice guidelines in adults (update): American College of Gastroenterology, Practice Parameters Committee. *The American Journal of Gastroenterology*, 99(7), 1371-1385.

Kuhn, R., & Gauhe, A. (1965). Bestimmung der bindungsstelle von sialinsäureresten in oligosacchariden mit hilfe von perjodat. *Chemische Berichte*, 98(2), 395-314.

Kupper, C. (2005). Dietary guidelines and implementation for celiac disease. *Gastroenterology*, 128(4), 121-127.

Kushi, L. H., Doyle, C., McCullough, M., Rock, C. L., Demark-Wahnefried, W. Bandera, E. V., ... & Gansler, T. (2012). American cancer society guidelines on nutrition and physical activity for cancer prevention. *CA: A Cancer Journal for Clinicians*, 62(1), 30-67.

Ladas, S. D., Grammenos, I., Tassios, P. S., & Raptis, S. A. (2000). Coincidental malabsorption of laktose, fruktose, and sorbitol ingested at low doses is not Common in normal adults. *Digestive Diseases and Sciences*, 45(12), 2357-2362.

Langkilde, A. M., Andersson, H., Schweizer, T. F., & Würsch, P. (1994). Digestion and absorption of sorbitol, maltitol and isomalt from the small bowel. A study in ileostomy subjects. *European Journal of Clinical Nutrition*, 48(11), 768-775.

Latulippe, M. E., & Skoog, S. M. (2011). Fruktose malabsorption and intolerance: effects of fruktose with and without simultaneous glucose ingestion. *critical Reviews in Food Science and Nutrition*, 51(7), 583-592.

Le, A. S., & Mulderrig, K. B. (2001). *Sorbitol and Mannitol*. Nabors, O'B. (Ed.). New York, NY: Marcel Dekker.

Ledochowski, M., Sperner-Unterweger, B., Widner, B., & Fuchs, D. (1998a). Fruktose malabsorption is associated with early signs of mentral depression. *European Journal of Medical Research*, 3(6), 295-298.

Ledochowski, M., Sperner-Unterweger, B., & Fuchs, D. (1998b). Laktose malabsorption is associated with early signs of mental depression in females – a preliminary report. *Digestive Diseases and Sciences*, 43(11), 2513-2517.

Ledochowski, M., Überall, F., Propst, T., & Fuchs, D. (1999). Fruktose malabsorption is associated with lower plasma folic acid concentrations in middle-aged subjects. *Clinical Chemistry*, 45(11), 2013-2014.

Ledochowski, M., Widner, B., Bair, H., Probst, T., & Fuchs, D. (2000a). Fruktose-and sorbitol-reduced diet improves mood and gastrointestinal disturbances in fruktose malabsorbers. *Scandinavian Journal of Gastroenterology*, 35(10), 1048-1052.

Ledochowski, M., Widner, B., Sperner-Unterweger, B., Probst, T., Vogel, W., & Fuchs, D. (2000b). Carbohydrate malabsobtion syndromes and early signs of mental depression in females. *Digestive Diseases and Sciences*, 45(12), 1255-1259. [Anm. d. Verf.: Die Studie ist für Männer nicht aussagekräftig, da die Stichprobengröße zu klein ist.]

Leinoel (n. d.). *Leinöl(Leinsamen)*. Retrieved from http://www.vitalstoff-journal.de/vitalstoff-lexikon/l/leinoel-leinsamen.

Lewis, S. J., & Heaton, K. W. (1997). Stool form scale as a useful guide to intestinal transit time. *Scandinavian Journal of Gastroenterology*, 32(9), 920-924.

Lifschitz, C. H. (2000). Carbohydrate absorption from fruit juices in infants. *Pediatrics*, 105(1), e4.

Lombardi, D. A., Jin, K., Courtney, T. K., Arlinghaus, A., Folkard, S., Liang, Y., & Perry, M. J. (2014). The effects of rest breaks, work shift start time, and sleep on the onset of severe injury among workers in the People's Republic of China. *Scandinavian Journal of Work, Environment & Health*, 40(2), 146-155.

Lomer, M. C. E., Parkes, G. C., & Sanderson, J. D. (2008). Review article: Laktose intolerance in clinical practice – myths and realities. *Alimentary Pharmacology & Therapeutics*, 27(2), 93-103.

Longstreth, G. F., Thompson, W. G., chey, W. D., Houghton, L. A., Mearin, F., & Spiller, R. C. (2006). Functional bowel disorders. *Gastroenterology*, 130(5), 1480-1491.

Maintz, L., & Novak, N. (2007). Histamine and histamine intolerance. *The American Journal of Clinical Nutrition*, 85(5), 1185-1196.

Makras, L., Van Acker, G., & De Vuyst, L. (2005). Lactobacillus paracasei subsp. paracasei 8700: 2 degrades inulin-type fructans exhibiting different degrees of polymerization. *Applied and Environmental Microbiology*, 71(11), 6531-6537.

Mccoubrey, H., Parkes, G. C., Sanderson, J. D., & Lomer, M. C. E. (2008). Nutritional intakes in irritable bowel syndrome. *Journal of Human Nutrition and Dietetics*, 21(4), 396-397.

McKenzie, Y. A., Alder, A., Anderson, W. Goddard, L, Gulia, P., Jankovich, E. …Lomer, M. C. E. (2012). British dietic association evidence-based guidelines for the dietary management of irritable bowel syndrome in adults. *Journal of Human Nutrition and Dietics*, 25(3), 260-274.

Meyrand, M., Dallas, D. C., caillat, H., Bouvier, F., Martin, P., & Barile, D. (2013). Comparison of milk oligosaccharides between goats with and without the genetic ability to synthesize αs1-casein. *Small Ruminant Research*, 113(2), 411-420.

Michel, G., Nyval-Collen, P., Barbeyron, T., czjzek, M., & Helbert, W. (2006). Bioconversion of red seaweed galactans: a focus on bacterial agarases and Carrageenases. *Applied Microbiology and Biotechnology*, 71(1), 23-33.

Michie, S. (2013). N. t.. In Wells, V., Wyness, L., & Coe, S. (Eds.). The British Nutrition Foundation's 45th anniversary conference: Behaviour change in relation to healthier lifestyles. *Nutrition Bulletin*, 38(1), 100-107.

Mishkin, D., Sablauskas, L., Yalovsky, M., & Mishkin, S. (1997). Fruktose and sorbitol malabsorption in ambulatory patients with functional dyspepsia: comparison with laktose maldigestion/malabsorption. *Digestive Diseases and Sciences*, 42(12), 2591-2598.

Molodecky N. A., Soon, I. S., Rabi, D. M., et al. (2012). Increasing incidence and precalence of the inflammatory bowel diseases with time, based on systematic review. *Gastroenterology*, 142(1), 46-54.

Monash University (2014). *The Monash University Low Foodmap Diet* [Software]. Available from http://www.med.monash.edu/cecs/gastro/fodmap/education.html

Montalto, M., Curigliano, V., Santoro, L., Vastola, M., Cammarota, G., Manna, R., ... & Gasbarrini, G. (2006). Management and treatment of laktose malabsorption. *World Journal of Gastroenterology*, 12(2), 187.

Molis, C., Flourié, B., Ouarne, F., Gailing, M. F., Lartigue, S., Guibert, A., Bornet, F., & Galmiche, F. P. (1996). Digestion, excretion, and energy value of fructooligosaccharides in healthy humans. *The American Society for Clinical Nutrition*, 64(3), 324-328.

Mosby's Medical Dictionary (8th ed.). St. Louis, MO: Mosby.

Moshfegh, A. J., James, E. F., Goldman, J. P., & Ahuja, J. L. C. (1999). Presence of inulin and oligofruktose in the diets of Americans. *The Journal of Nutrition*, 129(7), 1407S-1411S.

Mount Sinai (n. d.). *Fiber Chart*. Retrieved from https://www.wehealny.org/healthinfo/dietaryfiber/fibercontentchart.html.

Mozaffarian, D., & Wu, J. H. (2011). Omega-3 fatty acids and cardiovascular disease effects on risk factors, molecular pathways, and clinical events. *Journal of the American College of Cardiology*, 58(20), 2047-2067.

Muir, J. G., Shepherd, S. J., Rosella, O., Rose, R., Barrett, J. S., & Gibson, P. R. (2007). Fructan and free fruktose content of common Australian vegetables and fruit. *Journal of Agricultural and Food Chemistry*, 55(16), 6619-6627.

Muir, J. G., Rose, R., Rosella, O., Liels, K., Barrett, J. S., Shepherd, S. J., & Gibson, P. R. (2009). Measurement of short-chain carbohydrates in common Australian vegetables and fruits by high-performance liquid chromatography (HPLC). *Journal of Agricultural and Food Chemistry*, 57(2), 554-565.

Nanda, R., James, R., Smith, H., Dudley, C. R. K., & Jewell, D. P. (1989). Food intolerance and the irritable bowel syndrome. *Gut*, 30(8), 1099-1104.

National Digestive Diseases Information Clearinghouse (2014). Crohn's disease. *NIH Publication*, 14-3410.

National Digestive Diseases Information Clearinghouse (2014). Diverticular disease. *NIH Publication*, 13-1163.

National Digestive Diseases Information Clearinghouse (2014). Ulcerative colitis. *NIH Publication*, 14-1597.

Necas, J., Bartosikova, L. (2013). Carageenan: a review. *Veterinarni Medicina*, 58(4), 187-205.

Nelis, G. F., Vermeeren, M. A., & Jansen, W. (1990). Role of fruktose-sorbitol malabsorbtion in the irritable bowel syndrome. *Gastroenterology*, 99(4), 1016-1020.

Newburg, D. S. & Neubauer, S. H. (1995). Carbohydrates in milks: analysis, quantities, and significance. In Jensen, R. G. (Ed.), *Handbook of Milk Composition* (pp. 273-349). San Diego: Academic Press.

NICNAS (2008). Multiple chemical sensitivity: identifying key research needs. *Scientific Review Report.*

Nucera, G., Gabrielli, M., Lupascu, A., Lauritano, E. C., Santoliquido, A., cremonini, F., ...Gasbarrini, A. (2005). Abnormal breath tests to laktose, fruktose and sorbitol in irritable bowel syndrome may be explained by small intestinal bacterial overgrowth. *Alimentary Pharmacology & Therapeutics*, 21(11), 1391-1395.

O'Connell, J. B., Maggard, M. A., & Ko, C. Y. (2004). Colon cancer survival rates with the new American Joint Committee on Cancer sixth edition staging. *Journal of the National Cancer Institute*, 96(19), 1420-1425.

O'Connell, S., & Walsh, G. (2006). Physicochemical characteristics of commercial lactases relevant to their application in the alleviation of laktose intolerance. *Applied Biochemistry and Biotechnology*, 134(2), 179-191.

Ong, D., Mitchell, S., Barrett, J., Shepherd, S., Irving, P., Biesiekierski, J., & ... Muir, J. (2010). Manipulation of dietary short chain carbohydrates alters the pattern of gas production and genesis of symptoms in irritable bowel syndrome. *Journal of Gastroenterology & Hepatology*, 25(8), 1366-1373.

Park, Y. K., & Yetley, E. A. (1993). Intakes and food sources of fruktose in the United States. *The American Journal of Clinical Nutrition*, 58(5), 737S-747S.

Parker, T. J., Naylor, S. J., Riordan, A. M., & Hunter, J. O. (1995). Management of patients with food intolerance in irritable bowel syndrome. The development and use of an exclusion diet. *Journal of Human Nutrition and Dietetics*, 8(3), 159-166.

Peery, A. F., Barrett, P. R. Park, D., et al. (2012). A high-fiber diet does not protect against asymptomatic diverticulosis. *Gastroenterology*, 142(2), 266-272.

Petitpierre, M., Gumowski, P., & Girard, J. P. (1985). Irritable bowel syndrome and hypersensitivity to food. *Annals of Allergy, Asthma & Immunology*, 54(6), 538-540.

Quigley, E., Fried, M., Gwee, K. A., Olano, C., Guarner, F., Khalif, I., ... & Le Mair, A. W. (2009). Irritable bowel syndrome: a global perspective. *WGO Practice Guideline.*

Quigley, E., M., M., Hunt, R. H., Emmanuel, A., & Hungin, A. P. S. (2013). *Irritable bowel syndrome (ibs): what is it, what causes it and can i do anything about it?* Retrieved from http://client.blueskybroadcastcom/WGO/ index.html.

Raithel, M., Weidenhiller, M., Hagel, A.-F.-K., Hetterich, U., Neurath, M. F., & Konturek, P. C. (2013). The malabsorption of commonly occurring mono and disaccharides: levels of investigation and differential diagnoses. *Dtsch Arztebl Int*, 110(46), 775-782.

Rex, D. K., Johnson, D. A., Anderson, J. C., Schoenfeld, P. S., Burke, C. A., & Inadomi, J. M. (2009). American College of Gastroenterology guidelines for colorectal cancer screening 2008. *The American Journal of Gastroenterology*, 104(3), 739-750.

Riby, J. E., Fujisawa, T., & Kretchmer, N. (1993). Fruktose absorption. *The American Journal of Clinical Nutrition*, 58(5), 748S-753S.

Ross, A. C., Manson, J. E., Abrams, S. A., Aloia, J. F., Brannon, P. M., Clinton, S. K., ... & Shapses, S. A. (2011). The 2011 report on dietary reference intakes for calcium and vitamin D from the Institute of Medicine: what clinicians need to know. *Journal of Clinical Endocrinology & Metabolism*, 96(1), 53-58.

Rubio-Tapia, A., Hill, I. D., Kelly, C. P., Calderwood, A. H., & Murray, J. A. (2013). ACG clinical guidelines: diagnosis and management of celiac disease.*The American Journal of Gastroenterology*, 108(5), 656-676.

Rumessen, J. J., & Gudmand-Høyer, E. (1986). Absorption capacity of fruktose in healthy adults. comparison with sucrose and its constituent monosaccharides. *Gut*, 27(10), 1161-1168.

Rumessen, J. J., & Gudmand-Høyer, E. (1987). Malabsoption of fruktose-sorbitol mixtures. Interactions causing abdominal distress. *Scandinavian Journal of Gastroenterology*, 22(4), 431-436.

Rumessen, J. J. (1992). Fruktose and related food carbohydrates. sources, intake, absorbtion, and clinical implications. *Scandinavian Journal of Gastroenterology*, 27(10), 819-828.

Ruppin, H., Bar-Meir, S., Soergel, K. H., Wood, C. M., & Schmitt Jr, M. G. (1980). Absorption of short-chain fatty acids by the colon. *Gastroenterology*, 78(6), 1500-1507.

Rycroft, C. E., Jones, M. R., Gibson, G. R., & Rastall, R. A. (2001). A comparative in vitro evaluation of the fermentation properties of prebiotic oligosaccharides. *Journal of Applied Microbiology*, 91(5), 878-887.

Scientific Community on Food (2000*). Opinion of the Scientific Committee on Food on the tolerable upper intake level of folate.* Retrieved from: www.ec.europa.eu/food/fc/sc/scf/out80e_en.pdf

Shepherd, S. J., & Gibson, P. R. (2006). Fruktose malabsorption and symptoms of irritable bowel syndrome: guidelines for effective dietary management. *Journal of the American Dietetic Association*, 106(10), 1631-1639.

Shepherd, S. J., Parker, F. C., Muir, J. G., & Gibson, P. R. (2008). Dietary triggers of abdominal symptoms in patients with irritable bowel syndrome: randomized placebo-controlled evidence. *Clinical Gastroenterology and Hepatology*, 6(7), 765-771.

Silk, D. B. A., Davis, A., Vulevic, J., Tzortzis, G., & Gibson, G. R. (2009). Clinical trial: the effects of a trans-galactooligosaccharide prebiotic on faecal microbiota and symptoms in irritable bowel syndrome. *Alimentary Pharmacology & Therapeutics*, 29(5), 508-518.

Simopoulos, A. P. (1999). Essential fatty acids in health and chronic disease. *The American Journal of Clinical Nutrition*, 70(3), 560s-569s.

Speier, C., Vessey, I., & Valacich, J. S. (2003). The effects of interruptions, task complexity, and information presentation on computer-supported decision-making performance. *Decision Sciences*, 34(4), 771-797.

Stefanini, G. F., Saggioro, A., Alvisi, V., Angelini, G., capurso, L., Di, L. G., ...Melzi, G. (1995). Oral cromolyn sodium in comparison with elimination diet in the irritable bowel syndrome, diarrheic type. multicenter study of 428 patients. *Scandinavian Journal of Gastroenterology*, 30(6), 535–541.

Stockwell, M. (n. d.). *Awards/Events*. Retrieved from www.melissastock well.com/Melissa_Stockwell/Awards.html.

Stubbs, J. (2013). N. t.. In Wells, V., Wyness, L., & Coe, S. (Eds.). The British Nutrition Foundation's 45th anniversary conference: behaviour change in relation to healthier lifestyles. *Nutrition Bulletin*, 38(1), 100-107.

Suarez, F. L., Savaiano, D. A., & Levitt, M. D. (1995). A comparison of symptoms after the consumption of milk or lactose-hydrolyzed milk by people with self-reported severe lactose intolerance. *New England Journal of Medicine*, 333(1), 1-4.

Suarez, F. L., Springfield, J., Furne, J. K., Lohrmann, T. T., Kerr, P. S., & Levitt, M. D. (1999). Gas production in humans ingesting a soybean flour derived from beans naturally low in oligosaccharides. *The American Journal of Clinical Nutrition*, 69(1), 135-139.

Sundhedsstyrelsen og Fødevareministeriet (2009). *Cøliaki og mad uden Gluten* (4th ed.). København: Sundhedsstyrelsen.

Tarpila, S., Tarpila, A., Grohn, P., Silvennoinen, T., & Lindberg, L. (2004). Efficacy of ground flaxseed on constipation in patients with irritable bowel syndrome. *Current Topics in Nutraceutical Research*, 2(2), 119–125.

Test (2008). Schneller, schöner, stärker. *test – Journal Gesundheit*, 43(02), 88-92.

Teuri, U., Vapaatalo, H., & Korpela, R. (1999). Fructooligosaccharides and lactulose cause more symptoms in laktose maldigesters and subjects with pseudohypolactasia than in control laktose digesters. *The American Journal of Clinical Nutrition*, 69(5), 973-979.

Thompson, Kyle (2006). *Bristol Stool Chart* [Graphical illustration]. Retrieved from http://commons.wikimedia.org/wiki/File:Bristol_Stool_chart.png

Nanda, R., Shu, L. H., & Thomas, J. R. (2012). A fodmap diet update: craze or credible. *Practical Gastroenterology*, 10(12), 37-46.

Toschke, A. M., Thorsteinsdottir, K. H., & von Kries, R. (2009). Meal frequency, breakfast consumption and childhood obesity. *International Journal of Pediatric Obesity*, 4(4), 242-248.

Tou, J. C., Chen, J., & Thompson, L. U. (1998). Flaxseed and its lignan precursor, secoisolariciresinol diglycoside, affect pregnancy outcome and reproductive development in rats. *The Journal of Nutrition*, 128(11), 1861-1868.

Truswell, A. S., Seach, J. M., & Thorburn, A. W. (1988). Incomplete absorption of pure fruktose in healthy subjects and the facilitating effect of glucose. *The American Journal of Clinical Nutrition*, 48(6), 1424-1430.

U. S. Department of Agriculture and U. S. Department of Health and Human Services (2010). *Dietary Guidelines for Americans* (7th ed.). Washington, Dc: U. S. Government Printing Office.

U. S. Department of Agriculture, Agricultural Research Service (2013). *USDA National Nutrient Database for Standard Reference*, Release 26. Retrieved from: http://www.ars.usda.gov/ba/bhnrc /ndl.

van Loo, J., Coussement, P., De Leenheer, L., Hoebregs, H., & Smits, G. (1995). On the presence of inulin and oligofruktose as natural ingredients in the western diet. *Critical Reviews in Food Science and Nutrition*, 35(6), 525–552.

Varea, V., de Carpi, J. M., Puig, C., Alda, J. A., camacho, E., Ormazabal, A., ... & Gómez, L. (2005). Malabsorption of carbohydrates and depression in Children and adolescents. *Journal of Pediatric Gastroenterology and Nutrition*, 40(5), 561-565.

Verhoef, P., Stampfer, M. J., Buring, J. F., Gaziano, J. M., Allen, R. H., Stabler, S. P., ... & Willett, W. C. (1996). Homocysteine metabolism and risk of myocardial infarction: relation with vitamins B6, B12, and folate. *American Journal of Epidemiology*, 143(9), 845-859.

Vernia, P., Ricciardi, M. R., Frandina, C., Bilotta, T., & Frieri, G. (1995). laktose malabsorption and irritable bowel syndrome. Effect of a long-term laktose-free diet. *The Italian Journal of Gastroenterology*, 27(3), 117-121.

Vesa, T. H., Korpela, R. A., & Sahi, T. (1996). Tolerance to small amounts of laktose in laktose maldigesters. *The AmericanJournal of Clinical Nutrition*, 64(2), 197-20.

Virtanen, S. M., Räsänen, L., Mäenpää, J., & Åkerblom, H. K. (1987). Dietary survey of Finnish adolescent diabetics and non-diabetic controls. *Acta Paediatrica*, 76(5), 801-808.

Vos, M. B., Kimmons, J. E., Gillespie, C., Welsh, J., & Blanck, H. M. (2008). Dietary fruktose consumption among US children and adults: the third National Health and Nutrition Examination Survey. *The Medscape Journal of Medicine*, 10(7), 160.

Watson, B. D. (2008). Public health and carrageenan regulation : a review and analysis. *Journal of Applied Phycology*, 20(5), 505-513.

Webb, F. S., & Whitney, E. N. (2008). *Nutrition: Concepts and Controversies* (11th ed.). Belmont, CA: Thomson/ Wadsworth.

Wedlake, L., Slack, N., Andreyev, H. J. N., & Whelan, K. (2014). Fiber in the treatment and maintenance of inflammatory bowel disease: a systematic review of randomized controlled trials. *Inflammatory bowel diseases*, 20(3), 576-586.

Welch, C. E., Allen, A. W., & Donaldons, G. A. (1953). An appraisal of resection of the colon for diverticulitis of the sigmoid. *Annals of Surgery*, 138(3), 332-343.

Wells, N. E. J., Hahn, B. A., & Whorwell, P. J. (1997). Clinical economics review: irritable bowel syndrome. *Allimentary Pharmacology and Therapeutics*, 11, 1019-1030.

—

Sources regarding the prevalence of IBS:
USA
Longstreth, G. F., & Wolde-Tsadik, G. (1993). Irritable bowel-type symptoms in hmo examinees. *Digestive Diseases and Sciences*, 38(9), 1581-1589.

Talley, N. J., Zinsmeister, A. R., van Dyke, C., & Melton, L. J. (1991). Epidemiology of colonic symptoms and the irritable bowel syndrome. *Gastroenterology*, 101(4), 927-934.

O'Keefe, E. A., Talley, N. J., Zinsmeister, A. R., & Jacobsen, S. J. (1995). Bowel disorders impair functional status and quality of life in the elerdly: a population-based study. *Journal of Gastroenterology*, 50A, M184-M189.

Great Britain
Jones, R., & Lydeard, S. (1992). Irritable bowel syndrom in the general population. *British Medical Journal*, 304(6819), 87-90.

Japan and the Netherlands

Schlemper, R. J., van der Werf, S. D. J., Vandenbroucke, J. P., Blemond, I., & Lamers, C. B. H. W. (1993). Peptic ulcer, non-ulcer dysepsia and irritable bowel syndrom in the Netherlands and Japan. *Scandinavian Journal of Gastroenterology*, 28(200), 33-41.

Nigeria

Olubuykle, I. O., Olawuyl, F., & Fasanmade, A. A. (1995). A study of irritable bowel syndrom diagnosed by manning Criteria in an African population. *Digestive Diseases and Sciences*, 40(5), 983-985.

—

Wilder-Smith, C. H., Materna, A., Wermelinger, C., & Schuler, J. (2013). Fruktose and laktose intolerance and malabsorption testing: the relationship with symptoms in functional gastrointestinal disorders. *Alimentary Pharmacology and Therapeutics*, 37(11), 1074-1083.

Winterfeldt, D. von, & Edwards, W. (1986). *Decision Analysis and Behavioral Research*. Cambridge: Cambridge University Press.

Wittstock, A. (1949). *Marc Aurel – Selbstbetrachtungen*. Stuttgart: Reclam.

Zohar, D. (1999). When things go wrong: The effect of daily work hassles on effort, exertion and negative mood. *Journal of Occupational and Organizational Psychology*, 72(3), 265-283.

Food Index

Basmati rice, cooked in unsalted water 340

BBQ roasted jalapeno sauce 348

Beef bacon (kosher) 326

Beef steak, chuck, visible fat eaten 326

Beef with noodles soup, condensed 306

Beer 146

Beer, low alcohol 146

Beer, low carb 146

Beer, non alcoholic 146

Beets, raw 402

Ben & Jerry's® Ice Cream, Brownie Batter 430

Ben & Jerry's® Ice Cream, Chocolate Chip Cookie Dough 430

Ben & Jerry's® Ice Cream, Chubby Hubby® 430

Ben & Jerry's® Ice Cream, Chunky Monkey® 430

Ben & Jerry's® Ice Cream, Half Baked 430

Ben & Jerry's® Ice Cream, Karamel Sutra® 430

Ben & Jerry's® Ice Cream, New York Super Fudge Chunk® 430

Ben & Jerry's® Ice Cream, One Sweet Whirled 430

Ben & Jerry's® Ice Cream, Peanut Butter Cup 430

Ben & Jerry's® Ice Cream, Phish Food® 430

Ben & Jerry's® Ice Cream, Vanilla For A Change 430

Biscotti, chocolate, nuts 266

BK Big Fish® 348

BK Fresh Apple Slices 348

Black beans, cooked from dried 402

Black cherry juice 182

Black currant juice 182

Black olives 402

Black Russian 146

Blackberries, fresh 384

Blackberry juice 182

Bloody Mary 146

BLT Salad® with TenderCrisp chicken (no dressing or croutons) 348

Blue cheese 222

Blueberries, fresh 384

Bockwurst 326

Bok choy, raw 402

Bologna, beef ring 222

Bologna, combination of meats, light (reduced fat) 222

Boston Market® 1/4 white rotisserie chicken, with skin 326

Boston Market® macaroni and cheese 306

Boston Market® roasted turkey breast 326

Boston Market® sweet corn 340

Bourbon 146

Boysenberries, fresh 384

Brandy 146

Bratwurst 326

Bratwurst, beef 326

Bratwurst, light (reduced fat) 326

Bratwurst, made with beer 326

Bratwurst, made with beer, cheese-filled 326

Bratwurst, turkey 326

Braunschweiger 326

Brazil nuts, unsalted 254

Breath mint, regular 286

Breath mint, sugar free 286

Breyers® Ice Cream, Natural Vanilla, Lactose Free 430

Breyers® Light! Boosts Immunity Yogurt, all flavors 236

Breyers® No Sugar Added Ice Cream, Vanilla 236

Breyers® YoCrunch Light Nonfat Yogurt, with granola 236

Brie cheese 222
Broccoli flower (green cauliflower), cooked 402
Broccoli, raw 402
Brown mushrooms (Italian or Crimini, raw 402
Brown sugar 286
Brownie, chocolate, fat free 266
Brussels sprouts, cooked from fresh 402
Bulgur, home cooked 340
Burgundy wine, red 150
Burgundy wine, white 150
Butter cracker 266
Butter, light, salted 222
Butter, unsalted 222
Buttermels® (Switzer's®) 286
Butternut squash soup 306

C
Cabbage, green, cooked 406
Cabbage, red, cooked 406
Cabbage, savoy, raw 406

Cabot® Non Fat Yogurt, plain 236
Cabot® Non Fat Yogurt, vanilla 236
Caesar Salad (no dressing or croutons) 348
Caesar salad dressing 356
Cafe au lait, without flavored syrup 168
Cafe latte, flavored syrup 168
Cafe latte, without flavored syrup 168
Calzone, cheese 306
Camembert cheese 222
Camomile tea 168
Campari® 150
Candy necklace 286
Canfield's® Root Beer 192
Canfield's® Root Beer, diet 192
Cantaloupe, fresh 384
Cape Cod 150
Cappuccino, canned 168
Cappuccino, decaf, with flavored syrup 168

Cappuccino, decaf, without flavored syrup 168
Capri Sun®, all flavors 182
Carambola (starfruit), fresh 384
Caramel or sugar coated popcorn, store bought 254
Carrot cake, glazed, homemade 266
Carrot juice 182
Carrots, cooked from fresh 406
Carrots, raw 406
Cascadian Farm® Organic Gran. Bar, Dark Chocolate Cranberry 210
Cashews, raw 254
Casserole (hot dish), with tomato 337
Casserole (hot dish), rice with beef, tomato base, vegetables other than dark green, cheese or gravy 306
Cauliflower, cooked from frozen 406
Caviar 326

Celeriac (celery root), cooked from fresh 406
Celery, cooked 406
Chai tea 168
Chalupas Supreme® with beef, beans, cheese 376
Champagne punch 150
Champagne, white 150
Chard, raw or blanched, marinated in oil 406
Chardonnay 150
Chayote squash, cooked 406
Cheddar cheese 368
Cheddar cheese, natural 222
Cheerios® Snack Mix, all 210
Cheese cracker 254
Cheese gnocchi 340
Cheese sauce, store bought 222
Cheeseburger 348
Cheesecake, plain or flavored, homemade 266
Cherry Coke® 192

Cherry pie, bottom crust only 266
Chestnuts, boiled, steamed 406
Chestnuts, roasted 254
Chewing gum 286
Chewing gum, sugar free 286
Chia seeds 254
Chicken and dumplings soup, condensed 306
Chicken breast, spicy crispy 356
Chicken cake or patty 337
Chicken fricassee with gravy, American style 326
Chicken Littles with sauce 356
Chicken noodle soup with vegetables, can 306
Chicken with cheese sauce, vegetables other than dark green 337
Chicken wonton soup, prepared from condensed can 306

Chicory coffee 168
Chicory coffee powder, unprepared 406
Chicory greens, raw 406
Chili with beans, beef, canned 306
Chipotle southwest salad dressing 368
Chips Ahoy!® Chewy Gooey Caramel Cookies (Nabisco®) 266
Chobani® Nonfat Greek Yogurt, Black Cherry 236
Chobani® Nonfat Greek Yogurt, Lemon 236
Chobani® Nonfat Greek Yogurt, Peach 236
Chobani® Nonfat Greek Yogurt, Raspberry 236
Chobani® Nonfat Greek Yogurt, Strawberry 236
Chocolate cake, glazed, store 266
Chocolate Chex® (General Mills®) 210
Chocolate chip cookie 368

Chocolate chip cookies, store bought 270
Chocolate chunk cookie 368
Chocolate cookies, iced, store bought 270
Chocolate pudding, store bought 236
Chocolate pudding, store bought, no sugar 236
Chocolate sandwich cookies, double filling 270
Chocolate sandwich cookies, sugar free 270
Chocolate truffles 286
Chop suey, chicken 310
Chop suey, tofu, no noodles 310
Cinnamon crispas 270
Cinnamon toast crunch® (General Mills®) 210
Cinnamon Toasters® (Malt-O-Meal®) 210
Clams, with mushroom, onions, & bread 326

Classic Fruit Chocolates (Liberty Orchards®) 286
Clementine, fresh 384
Clif Bar®, Chocolate Chip 138
Clif Bar®, Crunchy Peanut Butter 138
Clif Bar®, Oatmeal Raisin Walnut 138
Club soda 150
Cocoa Krispies® (Kellogg's®) 210
Cocoa Puffs® (General Mills®) 210
Coconut Bars, nuts 286
Coconut cream (liquid from grated meat) 254
Coconut milk, fresh (liquid from grated meat, water added) 254
Coconut, dried, shredded or flaked, unsweetened 254
Coconut, fresh 254
Coffee substitute, prepared 168

Coffee, prepared from flavored mix, no sugar 168
Cognac 150
Cointreau® 150
Coke Zero® 192
Coke® 192
Coke® with Lime 192
Colby Jack cheese 222
Cole slaw 356
Coleslaw, with apples and raisins, mayo dressing 406
Coleslaw, with pineapple, mayo dressing 406
Collards, raw 406
Corn Chex® (General Mills®) 210
Corn Flakes (Kellogg's®) 210
Cornbread, from mix 340
Cornbread, homemade 340
Cottage cheese, 1% fat, lactose reduced 222
Cottage cheese, uncreamed dry curd 236
Couscous, cooked 340

Cracked wheat bread, with raisins 204
Cranberries, dried (Craisins®) 388
Cranberries, fresh 388
Cranberry juice cocktail, with apple juice 182
Cranberry juice cocktail, with blueberry juice 182
Cream cheese spread 226
Cream cheese, whipped, flavored 226
Cream cheese, whipped, plain 226
Cream of asparagus soup, condensed can 310
Cream of broccoli soup, condensed 310
Cream of celery soup, homemade 310
Cream of chicken soup, condensed 310
Cream of mushroom soup, from condensed can 310

Cream of potato soup mix, dry 310
Cream of spinach soup mix, dry 310
Creamed chicken 337
Creamy buffalo sauce 356
Creme de Cocoa 150
Creme de menthe 150
Crepe, plain 270
Crispy Chicken Caesar Salad 356
Crispy Twister without sauce 356
Crispy Twister® with sauce 356
Croissant, chocolate 270
Croissant, fruit 270
Crunchy Nut Roasted Nut & Honey (Kellogg's®) 210
Cucumber, raw, with peel 410

Cucumber, raw, without peel 410
Curacao 150
Currants, fresh, black 388
Currants, fresh, red and white 388

D

Daiquiri 150
Dairy Queen® Foot Long Hot Dog 310
Dandelion tea 172
Danish pastry, frosted, with cheese filling 270
Dannon® Activia® Light Yogurt, vanilla 240
Dannon® Activia® Yogurt, plain 240
Dannon® Greek Yogurt Honey 240
Dannon® Greek Yogurt, Plain 240
Dannon® la Crème Yogurt, fruit flavors 240
Dare Breaktime Ginger Cookies 270
Dare® Lemon Crème Cookies 270
Dark chocolate Bar 50% 286
Dark chocolate Bar 60%-69% cacao 290
Dark chocolate Bar 70%-85% cacao 290

Dark chocolate Bar, sugar free 290

Dark Fruit Chocolates (Liberty Orchards®) 290

Dark Fruit Chocolates, Sugar Free (Liberty Orchards®) 290

Dates 388

Demitasse 172

Diet 7 UP® 192

Diet Coke® 192

Diet Dr. Pepper® 192

Diet Pepsi®, fountain 192

Doritos® Tortilla Chips, Nacho Cheese 254

Doughnut, glazed, coconut topping 270

Doughnut, glazed, plain 270

Doughnut, sugared 270

Dove® Promises, Milk Chocolate 172

Dreyer's® Grand Ice Cream, Chocolate 430

Dreyer's® No Sugar Added Ice Cream, Triple Chocolate 430

Drumstick® (sundae cone) 434

E

Earl Grey, strong 172

Edam cheese 226

EGG® bread roll 270

Eggnog, regular 150

Eggplant, cooked 410

Elderberries, fresh 388

Electrolyte drink 138

Elephant ear (crispy) 270

Endive, curly, raw 410

English muffin bread 204

English muffin, whole wheat, with raisins 274

Enoki mushrooms, raw 410

Espresso, raw 172

Essentials Oat Bran cereal (Quaker®) 210

Evaporated milk, diluted, 2% fat (reduced fat) 240

Evaporated milk, skim (fat free) 172

Evaporated milk, whole 240

Extra Crispy Tenders 356

F

Falafel 340

Familia Swiss Muesli® 210

Fanta Zero®, fruit flavors 192

Fanta® Red 192

Fanta®, fruit flavors 192

Fennel bulb 410

Fennel tea 172

Feta cheese 240

Feta cheese, fat free 240

Fettuccini Alfredo®, no meat, carrots or dark green veggies 310

Fettuccini Alfredo®, no meat, vegetables except dark green 310

Fettuccini noodles 340

Fiber One Original® (General Mills®) 214

Fiber One® Nutty Clusters & Almonds (General Mills®) 214

Fifty 50® Sugar Free Butterscotch Hard Candy 290

Figs, dried, cooked, sweetened 388

Figs, fresh 388

Filberts, raw 254

Fish croquette 337

Fish or seafood with cream or white sauce 337

Fish sticks, patties / nuggets, breaded, 330

Fish with breading 330

Flax seeds, not fortified 254

Fleischmann's® Butter Margarine, tub, whipped 226

Focaccia bread 204

Fondue sauce 240

Frappuccino® 172

Frappuccino®, bottled or canned 172

Frappuccino®, bottled light 172

French Burnt Peanuts 290

French fries 348

French or Vienna roll 204

French toast 274

Froot Loops® (Kellogg's®) 214

Frosted Flakes®
(Kellogg's®) 214
Frosted Flakes®
Reduced Sugar
(Kellogg's®) 214
Frosted Mini-
Wheats Big Bite®
(Kellogg's®) 214
Frozen custard,
chocolate or cof-
fee flavors 274
Frozen fruit juice
Bar 434
Fruit drink or
punch 182
Fruit punch, alco-
holic 150
Fruit sauce, jelly-
based 310

G
Garbanzo beans
canned 340
Garlic, fresh 410
Gatorade®, all fla-
vors 138
Gelatin, jello 290
German choco-
late cake, glazed,
homemade 274
German style po-
tato salad, with
bacon and vine-
gar dressing 310
GG® Scandina-
vian Bran Crisp-
bread 204

Gibson 154
Gin 154
Ginger ale 192
Ginger root, raw
410
Ginko nuts, dried
258
Girl Scout® Lem-
onades 274
Girl Scout® Pea-
nut Butter Patties
274
Girl Scout® Sa-
moas® 274
Girl Scout® Short-
bread® 274
Girl Scout® Thin
Mints 274
Glaceau® Vita-
minwater 138
Gluten free bread
204
GO Veggie!™
Rice Slices 240
Goat cheese, hard
226
GoLEAN® Crisp!
Cereal, Cinna-
mon Crumble
(Kashi®) 214
GoLEAN®
Crunch! Cereal,
Honey Almond
Flax (Kashi®) 214
Gooseberries,
fresh 388
Gorgonzola
cheese 226

Gorton's® Bat-
tered Fish Fillets
330
Gorton's® Pop-
corn Shrimp,
Original 330
Gouda cheese 226
Goulash, with
beef, noodles, to-
mato base 330
Grand Marnier®
154
Grapefruit juice,
white 182
Grapefruit, fresh,
pink or red 388
Grapes, fresh 388
Grasshopper 154
Greek yogurt,
plain, nonfat, 240
Green beans
(string beans),
cooked 410
Green bell pep-
pers 410
Green olives 410
Green pea soup
310
Green peas, raw
340
Green tea, strong
172
Green tomato,
raw 410
Grits (polenta)
410
Guava (guayaba),
fresh, 388

Gum drops 290
Gum drops,
sugar free 290
Gummi bears 290
Gummi bears,
sugar free 290
Gummi dino-
saurs 290
Gummi dino-
saurs, no sugar
290
Gummi worms
290
Gummi worms,
sugar free 294

H
Haagen-Dazs®
Creme Brulee 434
Haagen-Dazs®
Frozen Yogurt,
chocolate or cof-
fee flavors 434
Haagen-Dazs®
Frozen Yogurt,
vanilla or other
flavors 434
Haagen-Dazs® Ice
Cream, Bailey's
Irish Cream 434
Haagen-Dazs® Ice
Cream, Black
Walnut 434
Haagen-Dazs® Ice
Cream, Butter Pe-
can 434

Haagen-Dazs® Cherry Vanilla 434

Haagen-Dazs® Ice Cream, Chocolate 434

Haagen-Dazs® Ice Cream, Coffee 434

Haagen-Dazs® Ice Cream, Cookies & Cream 434

Haagen-Dazs® Ice Cream, Mango 434

Haagen-Dazs® Ice Cream, Pistachio 434

Haagen-Dazs® Ice Cream, Rocky Road 434

Haagen-Dazs® Ice Cream, Strawberry 438

Haagen-Dazs® Ice Cream, Vanilla Chocolate Chip 438

Half and half 240

Halvah 274

Ham croquette 337

Ham Sandwich with Veggies, no mayo 368

Hamburger 348

Hard candy 294

Hard candy, sugar free 294

Hardee's® Loaded Omelet Biscuit 310

Harvey Wallbanger 154

Health Valley® Multigrain Chewy Granola Bar, Chocolate Chip 214

Herbal tea 172

Herring, pickled 330

Hershey's® Bliss Hot Drink White Chocolate, prepared 172

Hershey's® Caramel Filled Chocolates no sugar 294

Hershey's® Milk Chocolate Bar 294

Hickorynuts 258

High-protein Bar, generic 138

Honey 214

Honey BBQ sauce 356

Honey mustard dressing 368

Honey Nut Chex® (General Mills®) 214

Honey Oat bread 368

Honey Smacks® (Kellogg's®) 214

Honeydew 388

Hot chili peppers, green, cooked 410

Hot chili peppers, red, cooked from fresh 410

Hot chocolate, homemade 172

Hot dog, combination of meats, plain 226

Hot wings 356

House side salad 356

Hubbard squash 414

I

Ice cream sandwich 438

Ice cream, light 438

Instant coffee mix, unprepared 172

Irish coffee with alcohol and whipped cream 172

Italian BMT® Sandwich with Veggies, no mayo 368

J

Jackfruit, fresh 388

Jam 226

Jam no sugar or sweetener 230

Jasmine tea 176

Jelly beans® 294

Jelly beans®, sugar free 294

Jerusalem artichoke raw 414

Jujyfruits® 294

K

Kale, raw 414

Kamikaze 154

Kashi® Chewy Granola Bar, Cherry Dark Chocolate 214

Kashi® Layered Granola Bar, Pumpkin Pecan 294

Kefir 240

Kelp, raw 414

Ken's® Apple Cider Vinaigrette dressing 348

Kern's® Mango-Orange Nectar 182

Kern's® Strawberry Nectar 182

Kidney beans, cooked from dried 414

Kirsch 154

Kit Kat® 294

Kit Kat® White 294

Kiwi fruit, gold 388

Kiwi fruit, green 388

Kohlrabi, cooked 414

Kraft® Cheese Spread, Roka Blue 230

L

Lasagna, home-made, beef 314

Lasagna, home-made, cheese, no vegetables 314

Lasagna, home-made, spinach, no meat 314

Laughing Cow® Mini Babybel®, Cheddar 240

Laughing Cow® Mini Babybel®, Original 244

Lay's® Potato Chips 258

Lay's® Potato Chips, Sour Cream & Onion 258

Lay's® Stax Potato Crisps, Cheddar 258

Lay's® Stax Potato Crisps, Hot 'n Spicy 258

Lebkuchen (German ginger bread) 274

Leeks, leafs 414

Leeks, root 414

Leeks, whole 414

Lemon juice, fresh 186

Lemon peel 442

Lemon, fresh 392

Lentil soup, condensed 314

Lentils, cooked from dried 340

Lettuce, Boston, bibb or butterhead 414

Lettuce, green leaf 414

Lettuce, iceberg 414

Lettuce, red leaf 414

Lettuce, romaine or cos 414

Libby's® Apricot Nectar 186

Libby's® Banana Nectar 186

Libby's® Juicy Juice®, Apple Grape 186

Libby's® Juicy Juice®, Grape 186

Libby's® Pear Nectar 186

Licorice 294

Licuado, mango 244

Light beer 154

Light cream 244

Lima beans, cooked from dried 414

Limburger cheese 230

Lime juice, fresh 186

Lime, fresh 392

Lipton® Iced Tea Mix, sweetened with sugar, prepared 196

Lipton® Instant 100% Tea, unsweetened, prepared 196

Liqueur, coffee flavored 154

Little Debbie® Coffee Cake, Apple Streusel 274

Little Debbie® Fudge Brownies with Walnuts 274

Little Debbie® Nutty Bars 294

Liver pudding 330

Loaf cold cut, spiced 337

Loganberries, fresh 392

Long Island iced tea 154

Long John or bismarck, glazed, cream or custard filled & nuts 274

Lotus root, cooked 418

Lowbush cranberries (lingonberries) 392

Lychees (litchis), fresh 392

Lycium (wolf or goji berries) 392

Lyonnaise (potatoes and onions) 314

M & M® cookie 368

M & M's® Peanut 294

Macadamia nuts, raw 258

Macaroni or pasta salad, with meat, egg, mayo dressing 314

Mai Tai 154

Maitake mushrooms, raw 418

Malt liquor 154

Mamba® Fruit Chews 294

Mamba® Sour Fruit Chews 294

M

Mandarin orange, fresh 392

Mango nectar 186

Mango, fresh 392

Mangosteen, fresh 392

Manhattan 154

Maple syrup, pure 214

Margarine, diet, fat free 230

Margarine, tub, salted, sunflower oil 230

Margarita, frozen 154

Marmalade, sugar free with aspartame 230

Marmalade with saccharin 230

Marmalade, sugar free with sucralose 230

Marshmallow 298

Martini® 154

Mascarpone 230

Mashed potatoes with gravy 356

McDonald's® apple slices 360

McDonald's® Barbecue sauce 360

McDonald's® Big Mac® 360

McDonald's® caramel sundae® 360

McDonald's® Cheeseburger 360

McDonald's® Chicken McNuggets® 360

McDonald's® chocolate chip cookies 360

McDonald's® chocolate milk 360

McDonald's® Crispy Chicken Snack Wrap with ranch sauce 360

McDonald's® Double Cheeseburger 360

McDonald's® Filet-O-Fish® 360

McDonald's® French fries 360

McDonald's® Hamburger 360

McDonald's® hot fudge sundae® 360

McDonald's® hot mustard 360

McDonald's® M & M McFlurry® 364

McDonald's® McCafe shakes, chocolate 364

McDonald's® McCafe shakes, vanilla or other flavors 364

McDonald's® McChicken® 364

McDonald's® McDouble® 364

McDonald's® McRib® 364

McDonald's® Newman's Own® Creamy Caesar dressing 364

McDonald's® Newman's Own® Low Fat Balsamic Vinaigrette salad dressing 364

McDonald's® orange juice 364

McDonald's® Quarter Pounder 364

McDonald's® Sausage & EGG® McMuffin® 364

McDonald's® side salad 364

McDonald's® smoothies, all flavors 364

McDonald's® Southwestern chipotle Barbecue sauce 364

McDonald's® sweet and sour sauce 364

Meat ravioli, with tomato sauce 314

Meatloaf, pork 337

Meatloaf, tuna 337

Melba Toast®, Classic (Old London®) 258

Mentos® 298

Merlot, red 154

Merlot, white 158

Milk chocolate Bar, cereal 298

Milk chocolate Bar, cereal, sugar free 298

Milk chocolate Bar, sugar free 298

Milk Chocolate covered raisins 298

Milk Maid® Caramels (Brach's®) 298

Milk, low lactose Lactaid®, skim (fat free) 244

Milk, lactose reduced Lactaid®, fortified 214

Milk, low lactose Lactaid® 176

Milk, unprepared dry powder, 176

Mineral Water 196

Minestrone soup, condensed 314

Pancake, whole wheat, homemade 278
Pancakes and syrup 352
Panda Express® Orange Chicken 314
Papaya, fresh 392
Parmesan cheese, dry (grated) 244
Parmesan cheese, dry (grated), nonfat 244
Parmesan Oregano bread 368
Parsnip, cooked 418
Passion fruit (maracuya), fresh 392
Passion fruit juice 186
Pasta salad with vegetables, Italian dressing 314
Peach juice 186
Peach pie, bottom crust only 278
Peach, fresh 392
Peanut butter, unsalted 258
Peanuts, dry roasted, salted 258
Pear juice 186
Pear, fresh 396
Pecan praline 298

Pepperidge Farm® Soft Sugar Cookies 282
Pepperidge Farm® Turnover, Apple 282
Pepsi® 196
Pepsi® Max 196
Pepsi® Twist 196
Persimmon, fresh 396
Pho soup (Vietnamese soup) 318
Picante taco sauce 352
Pickled beef 330
Pickled beets 418
Pillsbury® Big White Chunk Macadamia Nut Cookies 282
Pillsbury® Cinnamon Roll with Icing, all flavors 282
Pina colada 158
Pine nuts, pignolias 258
Pineapple juice 186
Pineapple orange drink 186
Pineapple, dried 396
Pineapple, fresh 396
Pistachio nuts, raw 258

Pizza Hut® cheese bread stick 318
Pizza Hut® Pepperoni Lover's pizza, stuffed crust 318
Pizza Hut® Personal Pan, supreme 318
Pizza, homemade or restaurant, cheese, thin crust 318
Plain dumplings for stew, biscuit type 340
Plantains, green, boiled 396
Plum, fresh 396
Polenta 344
Pomegranate juice 186
Pomegranate, fresh (arils-seed/juice sacs) 396
Poore Brothers® Potato Chips, Salt & Cracked Pepper 258
Popcorn, store bought (prepopped), "buttered" 282
Popsicle 438
Popsicle, sugar free 438

Pork cutlet, visible fat eaten 330
Port wine 158
Portabella mushrooms 418
Potato bread 204
Potato chips, salted 258
Potato dumpling (Kartoffelkloesse) 344
Potato gnocchi 344
Potato pancakes 344
Potato salad, with egg, mayo dressing 318
Potato soup with broccoli and cheese 318
Potato sticks 262
Potato, boiled, with skin 344
Potato, boiled, without skin 344
Power Bar® 20g Protein Plus, Chocolate Crisp 138
Power Bar® 20g Protein Plus, Chocolate Peanut Butter 138
Power Bar® 30g Protein Plus, Chocolate Brownie 142

Power Bar® Harvest Energy®, Double Chocolate Crisp 142

Power Bar® Performance Energy® 142

Powerade®, all flavors 142

Pretzels, hard, unsalted, sticks 262

Pringles® Light Fat Free Potato Crisps, Barbecue 262

Pringles® Potato Crisps, Loaded Baked Potato 262

Pringles® Potato Crisps, Original 262

Pringles® Potato Crisps, Salt & Vinegar 262

Pudding mix, other flavors, cooked type 244

Pumpernickel roll 204

Pumpkin or squash seeds 262

Purslane, raw 418

Q

Quince, fresh 396

Quinoa 344

R

Radicchio, raw 418

Radish, raw 418

Raisins, uncooked 396

Rambutan, canned in syrup 396

Ranch Crispy Chicken Wrap 352

Ranch salad dressing 372

Raspberries, fresh, red 396

Raspberry juice 190

Ratatouille 318

Red beans and rice soup mix, dry 318

Red Bull® Energy Drink 200

Red Bull® Energy Drink Sugar Free 200

Rhubarb pie, bottom crust only 282

Rhubarb, fresh 396

Ribs, beef, spare, visible fat eaten 330

Rice bread 204

Rice cake 262

Rice Krispies® (Kellogg's®) 218

Rice milk 244

Rice noodles, fried 344

Rice pudding (arroz con leche), coconut, raisins 244

Rice pudding (arroz con leche), plain 244

Rice pudding (arroz con leche), raisins 244

Ricotta cheese, part skim milk 248

Riesen® 298

Riesling 158

Ritz Cracker (Nabisco®) 262

Roast Beef Sandwich with Veggies, no mayo 372

Rob Roy 158

Rockstar Original® 200

Rockstar Original® Sugar Free 200

Rompope (eggnog with alcohol) 158

Root beer 158

Roquefort cheese 230

Rose hips 396

Rose wine, other types 158

Rum 158

Rum and cola 158

Rusty nail 158

Rutabaga, raw or blanched, marinated in oil mixture 418

Rye bread 204

Rye flour, in recipes not containing yeast 442

Rye roll 204

S

Sake 162

Salami, beer or beerwurst, beef 330

Salmon, red (sockeye), smoked 330

Sambuca 162

Sandwich cookies, vanilla 282

Sangria 162

Santa Claus melon 396

Sapodilla, fresh 396

Sauerbraten 335

Sauerkraut 422

Scallop squash 422

Scallops 335

Schnapps, all flavors 162

Schweppes® Bitter Lemon 200

Scotch and soda 162

Scrambled egg, made with bacon 318

Screwdriver 162

Sea Pak® Seasoned Shrimp, Roasted Garlic 335

Sea Pak® Shrimp Scampi in Parmesan Sauce 335

Seabreeze 162

Semolina flour 442

Sesame chicken 318

Sesame sticks 262

Shake, chocolate 352

Shake, strawberry 352

Shake, vanilla or other 352

Shallot, raw 422

Shiitake mushrooms, cooked 422

Singapore sling 162

Slim-Fast® Easy to Digest, Vanilla, ready-to-drink can 248

Sloe gin 162

Sloe gin fizz 162

Smart Balance® Light with Flax Oil Margarine, tub 230

Smart Balance® Margarine 230

Smarties® 298

Snickers® 298

Snickers®, Almond 298

Snow peas, cooked 422

Sorbet, chocolate 438

Sorbet, coconut 438

Sorbet, fruit 438

Sorghum 218

Souffle, meat 337

Soup base 318

Sour cherries, fresh 396

Sour cream 248

Sour pickles 422

Sourdough bread 204

Soursop (guanabana), fresh 400

Southern Comfort® 162

Soy bread 208

Soy chips 262

Soy Kaas Fat Free, all flavors 234

Soy milk, chocolate, sweetened with sugar, not fortified 176

Soy milk, plain or original, with artificial sweetener, ready 248

Soy milk, vanilla or other flavors, sugar, fat free, ready 248

Soybean sprouts, raw 422

Soybeans, cooked from dried 422

Spaetzle (spatzen) 344

Spaghetti squash 422

Spaghetti, with carbonara sauce 318

Spearmint tea 200

Special K® Blueberry cereal (Kellogg's®) 218

Special K® Cinnamon Pecan cereal (Kellogg's®) 218

Special K® Original cereal (Kellogg's®) 218

Special K® Red Berries cereal (Kellogg's®) 218

Spelt flour 442

Spiced ham loaf, canned 335

Spicy Italian Sandwich with Veggies, no meat 372

Spinach ravioli, with tomato sauce 318

Spinach, cooked from fresh 422

Splenda® 176

Split pea sprouts, cooked 422

Spring roll 318

Sprinkles Cookie Crisp® (General Mills®) 218

Sprite® 200

Sprite® Zero 200

Squash ravioli, with sauce 318

Starbucks® Hot Cocoa Double Chocolate 176

Starbucks® Hot Cocoa Salted Caramel, prepared 176

Starburst®, Original 302

Steak & Cheese Sandwich with Veggies 372

Stewed green peas & sofrito 322

Sticky bun 282

Stonyfield® Oikos Greek Yogurt, Blueberry 248

Stonyfield® Oikos Greek Yogurt, Caramel 248

Stonyfield® Oikos Greek Yogurt, Chocolate 248

Stonyfield® Oikos Greek Yo-gurt, Strawberry 248

Straw mushrooms, canned, drained 422

Strawberries, fresh 400

Strawberry milk, prepared 248

Strawberry pie, bottom crust only 282

Strawberry Shake 380

Streusel topping, crumb 442

Suckers®, sugar free 302

Sugar cookies, iced, store bought 282

Sugar, white granulated 302

Summer squash, cooked 422

Sunbelt Bakery® Granola Bar, Banana Harvest 218

Sunbelt Bakery® Chewy Granola Bar, Blueberry Harvest 218

Sunbelt Bakery® Chewy Granola Bar, Golden Almond 218

Sunbelt Bakery® Granola Bar, Low Fat Oatmeal Raisin 218

Sunbelt Bakery® Chewy Granola Bar, Oats & Honey 218

Sunbelt Bakery® Fudge Dipped Chewy Granola Bar, Coconut 218

Sundaes®, caramel 352

Sundaes®, chocolate fudge 352

Sundaes®, mini M & M® 352

Sundaes®, Oreo® 352

Sundaes®, strawberry 352

Sun-dried tomatoes, oil pack 422

Sunflower seeds, raw 262

Sushi, with fish 322

Sushi, with fish and vegetables in seaweed 322

Sushi, with vegetables 322

Swedish Meatballs 322

Sweet and sour chicken 322

Sweet and sour sauce 356

Sweet cherries, fresh 400

Sweet corn 356

Sweet Onion Chicken Teriyaki Sandwich with Veggies, no mayo 372

Sweet onion salad dressing 372

Sweet potato bread 282

Sweet potato, boiled 422

Sweetened condensed milk 176

Sweetened condensed milk, reduced fat 248

Swiss cheese, natural 234

Swiss cheese 234

Swiss Miss® Hot Cocoa Sensible Sweets Diet, sugar free, prepared 180

Sylvaner 162

T

Taco Bell® 7-Layer Burrito 322

Taco Bell® Beef Enchirito 376

Taco Bell® Caramel Apple Empanada 376

Taco Bell® Cheesy Fiesta Potatos 376

Taco Bell® cheesy gordita crunch 376

Taco Bell® Cinnamon Twists 376

Taco Bell® Combo Burrito 376

Taco Bell® Crunchwrap Supreme 322

Taco Bell® Double Decker Taco Supreme®, beef 376

Taco Bell® Mexican Pizza 322

Taco Bell® Nachos Supreme 322

Taco Bell® Pintos 'n Cheese 376

Taco John's® nachos 262

Taco with beans, cheese 322

Taffy 302

Tap water 200

Tempeh 422

TenderCrisp® Chicken Sandwich 352

Tequila 162

Tequila sunrise 162

Tic Tacs® 302

Tilsit cheese 234
Tiramisu 282
Toast, cinnamon and sugar, whole wheat bread 208
Toast, butter 208
Toblerone® Swiss Dark Chocolate with Honey & Almond Nougat 302
Toblerone® Swiss Milk Chocolate with Honey & Almond Nougat 302
Toblerone® Swiss White Confection with Honey & Almond Nougat 302
Toffee 302
Toffifay® 302
Tofu, raw (not silken), cooked, low fat 248
Tokaji Wine 162
Tomato juice 190
Tomato relish 322
Tomato soup mix, dry 322
Tomato, cooked from fresh 426
Tonic water 200
Tonic water, diet 200
Tootsie Pops® 302

Tortilla 262
Triple Sec 166
Triticale bread 208
Tuna Sandwich with Veggies, no mayo 372
Tuna 335
Turkey Breast & Ham Sandwich with Veggies 372
Turkey Breast Sandwich with Veggies 372
Turnip 426
Twix® 282

V
V-8® 100% A-C-E Vegetable Juice 190
Vanilla Coke® 200
Vegetable soup, condensed 322
Veggie Delite Salad 372
Veggie Delite Sandwich 372
Venison or deer, stewed 335
Veryfine Cranberry Raspberry 190
Vichyssoise 322
Vinegar 372
Vodka 166

W
Waffles, bran 282
Waffles mix 282
Walnuts 262
Watermelon, fresh 400
Wax beans 426
Weetabix® Organic Crispy 218
Wendys' 380
Werther's® Original Caramel Coffee Hard Candies 302
Wheat bran 442
Wheaties® 218
Whipped cream 180
Whipped cream, chocolate 248
Whipped cream, fat free 248
Whiskey 166
Whiskey sour 166
White flour 442
White bean stew with sofrito 322
White bread 208
White chip macadamia nut cookie 372
White chocolate Bar 302
White Russian 166
White tea 180
White whole grain wheat bread 208

White whole wheat flour 442
Whole wheat bread 208
Whopper® with cheese 352
Wild 'n Fruity Gummi Bears (Brach's®) 302
Windmill cookies 282
Wine spritzer 166
Winter melon 426
Winter type squash 426
Wise Onion Flavored Rings 262
Wrap bread 372

Y
Yams, sweet potato type 426
Yellow bell pepper, raw 426
Yellow tomato, raw 426
Yerba® Mate tea 200
Yogurt with aspartame 252
Yogurt wth sucralose 252
Yogurt, fruited, whole milk 252

Z
Zesty onion ring sauce 352
Zsweet® 302

Made in the USA
San Bernardino, CA
04 February 2019